Thyroiditis

Editors

Virginia A. LiVolsi
Associate Professor of Pathology
Yale University School of Medicine
New Haven, Connecticut

and

Paul LoGerfo
Assistant Professor of Surgery
Columbia University College of Physicians & Surgeons
New York, New York

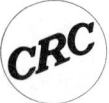

CRC Press, Inc.
Boca Raton, Florida

Library of Congress Cataloging in Publication Data

Main entry under title:

Thyroiditis.

   Bibliography: p.
   Includes index.
   1. Thyroiditis. I. LiVolsi, Virginia A.
II. LoGerfo, Paul. [DNLM: 1. Thyroiditis.
WK 200 T551]
RC657.5.T48T48   616.4'4   81-2642
ISBN 0-8493-5705-5   AACR2

This book represents information obtained from authentic and highly regarded sources. Reprinted material is quoted with permission, and sources are indicated. A wide variety of references are listed. Every reasonable effort has been made to give reliable data and information, but the author and the publisher cannot assume responsibility for the validity of all materials or for the consequences of their use.

All rights reserved. This book, or any parts thereof, may not be reproduced in any form without written consent from the publisher.

Direct all inquiries to CRC Press, Inc., 2000 N.W. 24th Street, Boca Raton, Florida 33431.

© 1981 by CRC Press, Inc.

International Standard Book Number 0-8493-5705-5

Library of Congress Card Number 81-2642
Printed in the United States

PREFACE

The purpose of this monograph is to present the various aspects of a group of non-neoplastic thyroid disorders, generally termed "thyroiditis". Etiologies are reviewed: infectious, autoimmune disorders, drug effects, perineoplastic reactions, and traumatic. In each subgroup of thyroiditis, clinical, diagnostic, pathologic, pathogenetic, and prognostic features are described. The role of newer diagnostic methods, especially needle biopsy and cytology, is discussed. Experimental models of thyroiditis in various species are reviewed with an overview of the contributions made by these models to our understanding of the pathogenetic and immunologic mechanisms operative in human thyroiditis.

THE EDITORS

Virginia A. LiVolsi is an Associate Professor of Pathology, Yale University School of Medicine, New Haven, Connecticut.

Dr. LiVolsi received a B.S. degree in Chemistry in 1965 from the College of Mount Saint Vincent in New York City and an M.D. degree in 1969 from Columbia University College of Physicians and Surgeons in New York. She served an internship, residency and fellowship in Pathology at the Columbia-Presbyterian Medical Center. During her training, which focused on surgical pathology, she developed an interest in thyroid pathology and physiology. This interest has continued in her present position at Yale University where she serves as an attending pathologist at the Yale-New Haven Hospital and Associate Professor of Pathology.

Dr. LiVolsi has published many articles focusing on thyroid histopathology, thyroid tumors, lesions of parafollicular cells, and immunohistochemistry of thyroid lesion.

Paul LoGerfo is an Associate Professor of Surgery at Columbia College of Physicians & Surgeons, Columbia University, New York, N.Y.

Dr. LoGerfo received his B.S. degree in Biology from Rensselaer Polytechnic Institute, Troy, N.Y. in 1961, and his M.D. from Upstate Medical Center, Syracuse, N.Y. in 1967. He served his internship and residency training at Columbia Presbyterian Medical Center in New York City. In addition to his surgical training he spent 1½ years developing a tumor immunology laboratory in the Department of Surgery. Currently, a large share of his surgical practice centers on the treatment of thyroid and parathyroid diseases. He is the recipient of an NIH career development award #5KO4CA00192, and is Assistant Director of the Clinical Research Cancer Center in Presbyterian Hospital.

Dr. LoGerfo has published many papers dealing with tumor immunology, thyroid, and parathyroid disease. In addition, he has published a number of articles dealing with thyroglobulin in benign and malignant thyroid disease.

CONTRIBUTORS

Thomas A. Colacchio, M.D.
Clinical Teaching Fellow in Surgery
College of Physicians and Surgeons
Columbia University
New York, New York

Carey Dolgin, M.D.
Visiting Clinical Fellow in Surgery
College of Physicians and Surgeons
Columbia University
New York, New York

Hannibal Edwards, M.D.
Surgical Resident
Presbyterian Hospital
New York, New York

Virginia A. LiVolsi, M.D.
Assistant Professor of Pathology
Director, Laboratory of Cytology
Yale University School of Medicine
New Haven, Connecticut

Paul LoGerfo, M.D.
Assistant Professor of Surgery
College of Physicians and Surgeons
Columbia University
New York, New York

Alan H. Seplowitz, M.D.
Assistant Professor of Clinical
  Medicine
College of Physicians and Surgeons
Columbia University
New York, New York

ACKNOWLEDGMENTS

The editors realize that many people contribute directly or indirectly to an undertaking of this kind. We wish to thank those individuals who guided us in our clinical understanding of thyroid disorders: Drs. Carl R. Feind, Sidney Werner, Kenneth Sterling; and those who taught us the recognition of many pathologic expressions of thyroiditis: Drs. Raffaele Lattes and Karl H. Perzin.

We are grateful to Ms. Aurelia Chattock for her careful evaluation of cytologic specimens, to Ms. Brooke Wheeler for invaluable research assistance, to Mrs. Maria Silberberg for secretarial assistance, and to Mr. John Braslin for photomicrography. We thank Dr. David Lowell for his allowing us to examine and illustrate interesting and unusual thyroid lesions from his practice, and many endocrinologists and surgeons from both our institutions for case material and cooperation. We appreciate the help of Dr. Gary Pasternak for translating some classic works, Dr. Maria Merino for lending us her photographic expertise, and many of the Yale University Pathology Housestaff for bringing unusual thyroid cases to our attention, particularly Drs. Susan Putnam and Craig Dise.

We thank the contributing authors for their efforts in reviewing many areas of thyroiditis.

Finally we wish to thank our families for their patience, and the editors of CRC Press for their unending assistance.

TABLE OF CONTENTS

Chapter 1
Introduction: History 1
Virginia A. LiVolsi

Chapter 2
Acute Thyroiditis 5
Hannibal Edwards

Chapter 3
Other Infectious Thyroiditides 13
Hannibal Edwards and Virginia A. LiVolsi

Chapter 4
Subacute Thyroiditis 21
Hannibal Edwards and Virginia A. LiVolsi

Chapter 5
Palpation Thyroiditis 43
Virginia A. LiVolsi

Chapter 6
Hashimoto's Thyroiditis 53
Alan Seplowitz

Chapter 7
Chronic Thyroiditis: Pathologic Aspects 65
Virginia A. LiVolsi

Chapter 8
Drug-Associated Thyroiditis 99
Virginia A. LiVolsi

Chapter 9
Radiation-Associated Thyroiditis 109
Virginia A. LiVolsi

Chapter 10
Thyroiditis Associated with Thyroid Tumors 119
Virginia A. LiVolsi

Chapter 11
Riedel's Struma 133
Virginia A. LiVolsi

Chapter 12
Laboratory Diagnostic Methods in Thyroiditis 147
Hannibal Edwards

Chapter 13
Needle Biopsy and Cytology in the Diagnosis of Thyroiditis 163
Virginia A. LiVolsi and Paul LoGerfo

Chapter 14
Surgical Management of Thyroiditis 173
Carey Dolgin and Paul LoGerfo

Chapter 15
Experimental Thyroiditis: A Review 179
Thomas A. Colacchio

Chapter 1

INTRODUCTION; HISTORY

Virginia A. LiVolsi

TABLE OF CONTENTS

I. History 2
    A. Discovery of the Thyroid Gland 2
    B. Classical Descriptions of Thyroiditis 2

II. The Problems in Understanding Thyroiditis 2

III. Outline of Topics Covered 2

IV. Classification of Thyroiditis 3

References 3

I. HISTORY

A. Discovery of the Thyroid Gland

According to Rolleston,[1] Galen initially noted the existence of the thyroid; Vesalius in the sixteenth century described it, and Wharton named it.[1] The discovery of the thyroid gland represented the beginning of a search for an understanding of its function and diseases. The present monograph will review one of the gland's major maladies: thyroiditis.

B. Classical Descriptions of Thyroiditis

Thyroiditis, or strumatitis, stands alone as a disease to which three major eponyms are attached. These include those individuals who described subacute and chronic thyroiditides: de Quervain, Hashimoto, and Riedel. In 1904, and later, in 1935, de Quervain[2,3] described subacute granulomatous thyroiditis and separated it from acute and tuberculous infection involving the thyroid. Hashimoto[4] reported four cases of chronic thyroiditis and separated struma lymphomatosa from other inflammatory conditions affecting the thyroid. This author distinguished the disease he detailed from that disorder described 16 yr earlier by Riedel.[5]

Following these now classical descriptions, the literature showed much confusion and engendered debate since all three thyroiditides were considered interrelated by many authors. Thus, Riedel's struma was believed to represent the end result of either, or both, subacute or Hashimoto's thyroiditis. However, more modern views fail to support such definite interrelationships, and these views will be described further.

II. THE PROBLEMS IN UNDERSTANDING THYROIDITIS

Attempts toward understanding these thyroid disorders have continued to the present day. Modern techniques including tissue culture, electron microscopy, radioimmunoassay, and the armamentaria of immunology, virology, and endocrinology have solved some of the problems in understanding the pathogenesis of thyroiditis. However, many more questions have been raised. Thus, although evidence for a viral etiology for subacute thyroiditis has accumulated from serological, epidemiological, and ultrastructural studies, what specific viruses are implicated? What is the nature of the various autoimmune phenomena and genetics involved in classic Hashimoto's disease? What is the relationship between classic Hashimoto's and chronic, nonspecific lymphoid thyroiditis; do they represent variants or grades of the same disorder or separate entities? How are Hashimoto's thyroiditis and Graves' disease related? Is Reidel's struma a disorder *of*, or merely *involving*, the thyroid gland? These include only a few unanswered questions in this field.

III. OUTLINE OF TOPICS COVERED

This book will examine these issues and others, and it will review what is presently known about the various forms of thyroiditis, methods of diagnosis, differential diagnosis, pathology, clinical correlations, and prognosis. Pathological curiosities which might be confused with significant lesions are reviewed, i.e., palpation thyroiditis. The effects of exogenous agents such as drugs and radiation on the gland are discussed. Where pertinent, immunological data will be described.

A chapter is devoted to an evaluation of the various laboratory and radiologic techniques used in the diagnosis of thyroiditis (Chapter 12). This supplements the discussions of diagnostic methods for the individual forms of thyroiditis included in earlier

Table 1
FORMS OF THYROIDITIS

Acute (including abscess)
  Bacterial
  Fungal
  Parasitic
  Viral
Subacute
  Infectious, ? viral
  Sarcoid associated
  Etiology unknown
Palpation (traumatic thyroiditis)
Chronic lymphocytic
  Hashimoto's disease and variants
  Chronic "nonspecific" thyroiditis
  Focal thyroiditis
Drug-associated
Radiation
Thyroiditis associated with other thyroid disorders
  Neoplasms
  Graves' disease
Riedel's disease

chapters describing each of these entities. In addition, a chapter outlining the techniques and yields of needle biopsy and aspiration cytology of the thyroid is included (Chapter 13). The surgical approach to the thyroid in thyroiditis and the value of surgery in these conditions is discussed in Chapter 14. Finally, the pathogenesis of the major forms of thyroiditis as elucidated by experimental models is discussed (Chapter 15).

IV. CLASSIFICATION OF THYROIDITIS

It seems appropriate to list in this introduction the classification of thyroiditis as used by the present authors. Our system is not new and follows closely in its major headings that of Hazard,[6] Skillern,[7] and Volpe[8] (Table 1). Subsequent chapters will follow this classification scheme.

REFERENCES

1. **Rolleston, H. D.**, *The Endocrine Organs in Health and Disease,* Oxford University Press, London, 1936.
2. **de Quervain, F.**, Die akute, nicht eiterige Thyreoiditis und die Beteiligung der Schilddruse an akuten Intoxikationen und Infektionen uberhaupt, *Mitt. Grenzgeb. Med. Chir.,* 2 (Suppl.), 1, 1904.
3. **de Quervain, F. and Giordanengo, G.**, Die akute und subakute Nichteitrige Thyreoditis, *Mitt. Grenzgeb. Med. Chir.,* 44, 538, 1935.
4. **Hashimoto, H.**, Zur Kenntniss der lymphomatosen Veranderung der Schilddruse (Struma lymphomatosa), *Arch. Klin. Chir.,* 97, 219, 1912.
5. **Riedel, B. M. C. L.**, Die chronische, zur Bildung eisenharter Tumoren fuhrende Entzundung der Schilddruse, *Verhandl. Dtsch. Ges. Chir.,* 25, 101, 1896.
6. **Hazard, J. B.**, Thyroiditis: a review, *Am. J. Clin. Pathol.,* 25, 289, 1955.
7. **Skillern, P. G.**, Thyroiditis, in *The Thyroid Gland,* Vol. 2, Pitts-Rivers, R. and Trotter, W. R., Eds., Butterworths, Inc., Washington, D.C., 1964, 130.
8. **Volpe, R.**, Etiology, pathogenesis and clinical aspects of thyroiditis, II, *Pathol. Annu.,* 13, 399, 1978.

Chapter 2

ACUTE THYROIDITIS

Hannibal Edwards

TABLE OF CONTENTS

I.	Introduction	6
II.	Historical Aspects	6
III.	Incidence	6
IV.	Clinical Features	6
V.	Physical Findings	7
VI.	Laboratory Findings	7
VII.	Pathogenesis	8
VIII.	Etiology	8
IX.	Pathology	8
X.	Diagnosis	9
XI.	Differential Diagnosis	9
XII.	Course	10
XIII.	Treatment	10
XIV.	Prognosis	10
References		11

JOB 5705:::::4 GALLEY 1x ....

I. INTRODUCTION

Although the terminology remains confused and some authors include viral and subacute nonsuppurative thyroiditis under the classification of acute thyroiditis,[1-4] the present author agrees with Volpe[1-3] that "acute thyroiditis" be reserved for those inflammations of the thyroid gland which are produced by infections with bacterial or fungal organisms. These glands show a suppurative or necrotizing granulomatous inflammation.[1,2] Clinically, this condition is usually associated with septic manifestations.

II. HISTORICAL ASPECTS

Historically, acute suppurative thyroiditis was described initially by Bauchet in 1857.[5] Robertson[6] reported an epidemic of suppurative thyroiditis which occurred in St. Etienne in 1864. In these initial reports, it was noted that acute bacterial thyroiditis was uncommon, ranging from 0.1 to 1% of all thyroid diseases.[7-12]

In the modern antibiotic era, acute thyroiditis is considered rare. Concomitantly, morbidity and mortality from this disease have decreased.[1-3] Hazard,[7] who reviewed the condition in 1955, credited Mygind[13] with distinguishing acute thyroiditis occurring in a previously normal gland from "acute strumitis", that is, infection in a nodular goiter.[14] The latter infections tend to suppurate more frequently than the former.

III. INCIDENCE

According to Hazard,[7] the incidence of acute thyroiditis is unknown because some authors have included cases now known to represent subacute thyroiditis. In addition, adequate microbiological documentation is lacking in many cases.[7] Burhans[15] accepted only 200 cases of infectious thyroiditis until 1928; by 1943, Higbee[16] could add only 24 more documented cases. In the more recent literature, acute infectious thyroiditis has been reported in children, in the elderly, in debilitated individuals, or in immunologically impaired patients.

IV. CLINICAL FEATURES

Acute (bacterial) thyroiditis is a rare but often severe illness. Burhans[15] noted that the disease may occur at any age from 18 months to 77 yr. A peak incidence of 20 to 40 yr[6,7,16] was found in the older literature, with 60% of the cases diagnosed before age 50.[15] More recent reports indicate that this disorder tends to affect patients at the two extremes of age: childhood and old age.[1-3,17,18]

In most series, the sex ratio is about equal,[1-4,7] although a female predominance has been noted by some authors.[7,15] Thus, Robertson[6] found a 5:3 female to male ratio in his 96 cases and Burhans[15] reported 47 females and 20 males in his group.

This disorder is seen most often in association with an infection elsewhere in the neck (e.g., pharyngitis, tonsillitis) or with generalized sepsis.[1,3,7,19] On initial presentation, not readily identifiable source of infection may be apparent. A urinary tract infection is often the associated, underlying condition in these patients. Acute thyroiditis may follow major trauma to the neck, allowing a portal of entry for microorganisms.[7,15,20,21]

Most often, patients present a septic picture with malaise, tachycardia, chills, fever, and a painful swollen neck.[1,4] The pain may be referred to the ear, jaw, or skull[1] and it is accentuated by movement of the neck. Although the process may involve the

Table 1
SIGNS OF ACUTE THYROIDITIS[a]

Sign	% Patients showing sign
Fever	90
Tachycardia	90
Neck tenderness	95
Neck swelling	50
Erythema	45
Partial ptosis	<10
Corneal anesthesia	<10
Thyrotoxicosis	rare

[a] Adapted from References 1-4, 7, 15, and 19.

thyroid diffusely, it often remains confined to one lobe. Even in those instances in which diffuse glandular involvement is found, one lobe tends to be affected predominantly.

Acute bacterial thyroiditis usually begins very abruptly. Often, the first symptom is neck (perithyroidal) pain. Burhans[15] found this symptom in 50% of his cases. The pain is lancinating, and radiates to the mandible, occiput, or ear. Robertson[6] describes the characteristic "acute thyroiditis" posture: the head is bowed and the chin is supported by the hand.

Chills and fever initiate the disease in ⅓ of the cases.[15] A discernible prodrome is rarely described. Coughing, which is typically dry and nonproductive, is identified in 15 to 20% of the patients. Rarely, blood-tinged mucus may be expectorated. This indicates that the suppurative process has extended into the trachea[14,19] and must be regarded as a serious symptom.

Hoarseness occurs in 20% of cases; rarely, aphonia will develop. These voice changes have been attributed to venous congestion and compression of the recurrent laryngeal nerves.[15] Dyspnea may be identified in half of the patients. This symptom is produced by edema of the trachea with resulting decrease in airway. Rarely will the dyspnea be severe enough to necessitate tracheostomy.[15] Dysphagia is described in only 3 to 4% of affected individuals initially, although it may develop in up to 20% of the patients during the course of the disease.

V. PHYSICAL FINDINGS

Physical examination discloses fever (38 to 40°C), elevated pulse rate, and neck swelling with tenderness elicited by palpation, swallowing, and movement. The classic signs of acute inflammation are found; thus, the thyroid may feel hot and even fluctuant and the skin over it appears red. Lymphadenopathy and extension of the inflammation to other cervical tissues may be noted.[1-4,7,19] Rarely, partial ptosis with corneal anesthesia may be seen. This has been attributed to sympathetic nerve impairment as a result of neck inflammation.[15] Thyrotoxicosis has been described rarely[1,15] (Table 1).

VI. LABORATORY FINDINGS

Elevations of white blood cell count and sedimentation rate are found commonly. Blood cultures are positive in most cases.[1-4] Thyroid function tests tend to remain normal and the patient is euthyroid unless the gland is almost totally involved.[1-4] Mild changes may be noted: the protein-bound iodine (PBI), T_4, and T_3 may increase slightly, presumably as a result of release of stored hormone.[1,7,19,22] Yet, these increases still remain close to, or within, the normal range. The PBI is invariably elevated to a greater level than T_4 and T_3. In this way, the laboratory values resemble those in subacute thyroiditis. However, in the latter condition, PBI and thyroid hormones are increased beyond the normal range.[1-4,19]

Radioiodine uptake is often normal or low normal.[1-4,19] Scintiscans of the thyroid show decreased uptake in the region of major involvement; this may simulate a cold nodule.[19] Thyroid autoantibodies do not appear during the illness.[1-4,19] The changes in thyroid function in acute bacterial thyroiditis are short-lived. In most cases, they may be so mild that random serum samples will miss the changes.

VII. PATHOGENESIS

Volpe[1] and Hazard[7] have summarized the possible routes of infection to the thyroid:

1. Hematogenous spread from a distant focus of infection
2. Direct invasion from infected cervical tissues, e.g., tonsils, pharynx, or lymph nodes
3. Direct trauma to the thyroid allowing organisms to enter
4. Spread via lymphatics
5. Infection of a thyroglossal duct cyst extending into the gland

Although the thyroid is richly vascularized, the rarity of acute suppurative thyroiditis suggests resistance of the gland to infection. The commonly affected population groups tend to show some degree of immunologic impairment which may account for hematogenous infection in some cases.[1,19] Infection of the normal gland usually produces a diffuse lesion, whereas in nodular goiter, abscess is commonly seen.[23]

Experimentally, Farrant[24] showed that bacterial toxins injected into the thyroid (from staphylococci and streptococci) produced colloid depletion followed by desquamation and degeneration of follicular epithelium; then, vascularity increased and regeneration of follicular cells, at first resembling hyperplasia, ensues. Cole et al.[25] demonstrated that these experimental lesions could be prevented by administering iodine.

VIII. ETIOLOGY

The organisms most commonly involved in acute thyroiditis include gram-positive bacteria, especially *Streptococcus, Staphylococcus,* and *Pneumococcus*.[1,4,7,18,19,26-29] Other bacteria[30] including gram-negative organisms have been reported to cause acute thyroiditis (*Escherichia coli*,[16,22,31] *Salmonella*,[23,32] *Klebsiella*,[17] *Bacteroides*,[18,25,33] *Pseudomonas*,[34] gas forming organisms,[35-37] and mixed infections[18]) but these are rare. (Granulomatous suppuration with organisms such as mycobacteria does occur — see Chapter 3; acute viral thyroiditis is discussed in Chapter 4.)

IX. PATHOLOGY

In previously normal glands, the inflammation appears diffuse; whereas in nodular goiter, more localized lesions are seen.[7] Usually one lobe is affected more severely than the other although the process involves the entire gland.[7] The histopathology of acute thyroiditis is the pathology of suppuration (Figure 1). The major focus shows follicular destruction and polymorphonuclear cell infiltration and colloid depletion is noted. Frequently, microabscess formation is found. Bacteria can be demonstrated in tissue sections.[2,3,7]

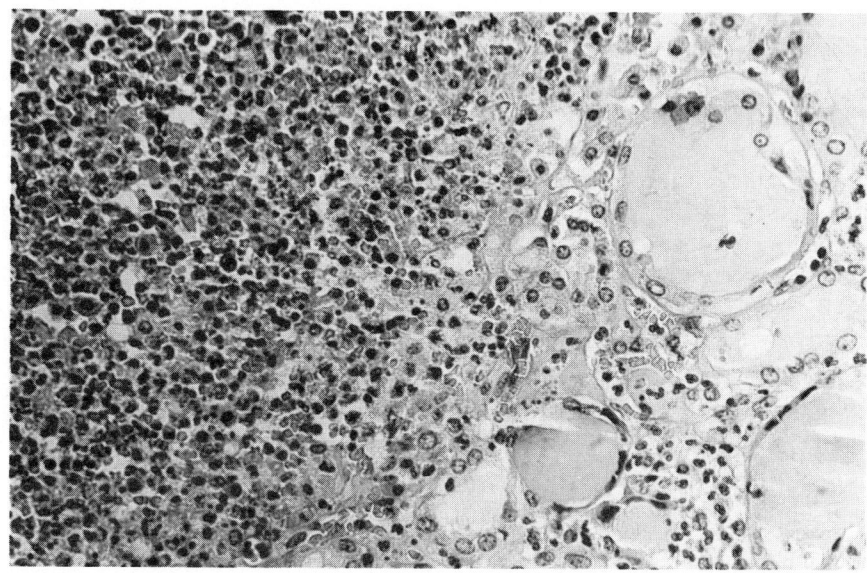

FIGURE 1. Microabscess in thyroid in a case of acute bacterial thyroiditis. Note extension of inflammatory cells into and between normal follicles on right. (Hematoxylin-eosin; magnification × 200.)

X. DIAGNOSIS

In the classical case, the diagnosis is made easily. Volpe stresses that, occasionally, the symptoms develop slowly and misdiagnoses of subacute thyroiditis, hemorrhage into a thyroid cyst, or even carcinoma may be rendered. Usually, follow-up will disclose the correct diagnosis.[1,4]

Ultrasound evaluation of acute thyroiditis has been described rarely and its use remains rudimentary.[22] The value of this technique in diagnosis of acute thyroiditis awaits further study.

Needle aspiration or biopsy of the thyroid may prove valuable in diagnosing acute thyroiditis.[19,38] If pus is obtained, gram stains can be performed and cultures taken. On the basis of the gram-stain results, therapy can be instituted quickly.[39] Adler et al.[39] recommend biopsy and culture studies to establish diagnosis and prompt institution of therapy.

XI. DIFFERENTIAL DIAGNOSIS

Some of the conditions which may mimic acute thyroiditis are: (1) subacute thyroiditis, (2) sudden hemorrhage into the thyroid, or into an adenoma of the thyroid, (3) glossitis and abscess formation at the base of the tongue, and (4) thyroglossal cysts.

Differentiating between acute thyroiditis and the above conditions is not difficult for the most part. Occasionally, a patient with subacute thyroiditis may present a rapidly evolving disease which may mimic acute thyroiditis. However, invariably the patient with subacute thyroiditis shows greater derangement of thyroid function. Solely on clinical grounds it may be impossible to distinguish between the early phase of subacute thyroiditis and acute thyroiditis.[1,3,19] Needle aspiration or biopsy may prove useful in differentiating the two conditions.[19,39] Without therapy, the patient with bacterial thyroiditis becomes more ill, whereas individuals with the subacute form recover.[39]

Hemorrhage into the thyroid gland is characterized by a sudden onset of pain and swelling in the thyroid. The pain begins to subside gradually shortly after its onset. In acute thyroiditis, the pain increases over a period of time. Often, the patient with hemorrhage into the thyroid will present a history of a preexisting mass which might represent a cyst or a neoplasm. This finding is unusual in acute thyroiditis.

While glossitis and abscess formation at the base of the tongue can result in neck tenderness and fever, oral examination will distinguish these conditions from thyroiditis.[1,4] Hemorrhage or infection in thyroglossal cysts can mimic acute thyroiditis. These cysts usually lie cephalad to the thyroid but, since acute thyroiditis may affect the pyramidal lobe, the correct diagnosis may only be made at exploration.[19] When acute bacterial thyroiditis presents a classical picture, the diagnosis is easy. The difficulty arises at the initial stages of the disease when the physical changes may be minimal or confusing. In such cases, one may have to await the further development of symptoms to arrive at the correct diagnosis.

XII. COURSE

The course is progressive and without treatment, and complications may ensue. These include rupture of an abscess, septicemia, and thrombophlebitis of neck veins including the internal jugular vein.[1,4,22,40,41] Mortality was high (25 to 30%) before the availability of antibiotics.[1,4] With appropriate therapy, recovery is expected.[42]

XIII. TREATMENT

Modern therapy is directed toward identification of the offending organism and institution of appropriate antibiotic medication. Penicillin and related compounds, as well as tetracycline, are used most often since the commonly involved gram positive organisms are usually susceptible to them.[1,42,43] If unusual organisms are found to be the causative agents, antibiotic sensitivities should serve as a guide to proper therapy. If an abscess develops, surgical drainage or even lobectomy may be required[1,4,42-46] (see Chapter 14).

XIV. PROGNOSIS

The prognosis of acute bacterial thyroiditis is good if the disease is recognized and treated appropriately. Most forms of acute thyroiditis resolve in 3 to 4 weeks if managed properly.[1-4,7,42-44]

The suppurative form of thyroiditis may be complicated by extension of the infection into cervical soft tissues, mediastinum, esophagus, or trachea.[7] Deaths in the preantibiotic era occurred commonly (25%) in the suppurative type of acute thyroiditis. With modern therapy, the prognosis is excellent and total recovery may be expected in most patients. The lesions rarely recur,[25,47] although chronic infection may result.[1-3] Thyroid function remains normal after recovery. Fibrosis of the gland occurs rarely, but permanent hypothyroidism is most unusual.[1,46]

REFERENCES

1. **Volpe, R.,** Acute suppurative thyroiditis, in *The Thyroid,* Werner, S. C. and Ingbar, S. H., Eds., Harper and Row Inc., New York, 1971, 849.
2. **Volpe, R.,** The pathology of thyroiditis, *Human Pathol.,* 9, 429, 1978.
3. **Volpe, R.,** Etiology, pathogenesis and clinical aspects of thyroiditis, II, *Pathol. Annu.,* 13, 399, 1978.
4. **DeGroot, L. J. and Stanbury, J. B.,** *The Thyroid and Its Diseases,* John Wiley and Sons, New York, 1975, 572.
5. **Bauchet, L. J.,** De la thyroidite (goitre aigu) et die goitre enflamme (goitre chronique enflamme), *Gazz. Hedb. Med. Chir.,* 4, 19, 1857.
6. **Robertson, W. S.,** Acute inflammation of the thyroid gland, *Lancet,* 1, 930, 1911.
7. **Hazard, J. B.,** Thyroiditis: a review, *Am. J. Clin. Pathol.,* 25, 289, 1955.
8. **Cleland, J. B.,** Purulent infiltration in and around the thyroid gland, *Med. J. Aust.,* 1, 790, 1927.
9. **Clute, H. M. and Smith, L. W.,** Acute thyroiditis, *Surg. Gynecol. Obstet.,* 44, 23, 1927.
10. **Henderson, J.,** Abscess of thyroid, *Am. J. Surg.,* 29, 36, 1935.
11. **Lahey, F. H.,** Thyroiditis: its differentiation from malignancy, *Lahey Clin. Found. Bull.,* 3, 194, 1944.
12. **Young, T. O.,** Inflammatory disease of the thyroid gland, *Minn. Med.,* 23, 105, 1940.
13. **Mygind, H.,** Thyroiditis acuta simplex, *Hosp. tid. Tjbenh.,* 2, 1181, 1894.
14. **Brenizer, A. G.,** Suppurative strumitis caused by *Salmonella typhosa, Ann. Surg.,* 133, 247, 1951.
15. **Burhans, E. C.,** Acute thyroiditis, *Surg. Gynecol. Obstet.,* 47, 748, 1928.
16. **Higbee, D.,** Acute thyroiditis in relationship to deep infections of the neck, *Ann. Otol. Rhinol. Laryngol.,* 52, 620, 1943.
17. **Mann, C. H.,** Thyroid abscess in a 3 ½ year old child, *Arch. Otolaryngol.,* 103, 299, 1977.
18. **Bussman, Y. C., Wong, M. C., Bell, M. J., and Santiago, J. V.,** Suppurative thyroiditis with gas formation due to mixed anaerobic infection, *J. Pediatr.,* 90, 321, 1977.
19. **Hurley, J. R.,** Thyroiditis, *Disease-A-Month,* December, 1977.
20. **Bishop, H. M. and Durman, D. C.,** Traumatic rupture of the thyroid gland, *Am. J. Surg.,* 75, 524, 1948.
21. **Stein, O.,** Acute inflammation of the thyroid gland, *Laryngoscope,* 22, 1020, 1912.
22. **Himsworth, R. L. and Kark, A. E.,** Studies on a case of suppurative thyroiditis, *Acta Endocrinol.,* 85, 55, 1977.
23. **Womack, N. A.,** Thyroiditis, *Surgery,* 16, 770, 1944.
24. **Farrant, R.,** Cited by Rundles, F. F., in *Joll's Diseases of the Thyroid Gland,* Heinemann, Ltd., London, 1951, 317.
25. **Cole, W. H., Womack, N. A., and Gray, S. H.,** Cited by Rundles, F. F., in *Joll's Diseases of the Thyroid Gland,* Heinemann, Ltd., London, 1951, 317.
26. **Hagan, A. D., Goffinet, J., and Davis, J. W.,** Acute streptococcal thyroiditis, *JAMA,* 202, 282, 1967.
27. **Abe, K., Taguchi, T., Okuno, A., Matsuura, N., Takebayashi, K., and Sasaki, H.,** Recurrent acute suppurative thyroiditis, *Am. J. Dis. Child.,* 132, 990, 1978.
28. **Altemieir, W. A.,** Acute pyogenic thyroiditis, *Arch. Surg.,* 61, 76, 1950.
29. **Hagan, A. D., Goffinet, J., and Davis, J. W.,** Acute streptococcal thyroiditis, *JAMA,* 202, 282, 1967.
30. **Alsever, R. N., Stiver, H. G., Dinerman, N., Dahl, C. R., and Eickhoff, T. C.,** Hemophilus influenza pericarditis and empyema with thyroiditis in an adult, *JAMA,* 230, 1426, 1974.
31. **Saksouk, F. and Salti, I. S.,** Acute suppurative thyroiditis caused by *Escherichia coli, Br. Med. J.,* 2, 23, 1977.
32. **Van Heerden, J. A. and O'Connell, P.,** Acute suppurative thyroiditis due to *Salmonella enteritides, Va. Med. Mon.,* 98, 556, 1971.
33. **Sharma, R. K. and Rapkin, R. H.,** Acute suppurative thyroiditis caused by *Bacteroides melaninogenicus, JAMA,* 299, 1470, 1974.
34. **Weissel, M., Wolf, A., and Linkesch, W.,** Acute suppurative thyroiditis caused by *Pseudomonas aeruginosa, Br. Med. J.,* 2, 580, 1977.
35. **Warren, C. P. W. and Mason, B. J.,** *Clostridium septicum* infection of the thyroid gland, *Postgrad. Med. J.,* 46, 586, 1970.
36. **Gaajor, A. and El-Baren, F.,** Acute thyroiditis with gas formation, *Laryngol. Otol.,* 89, 323, 1975.
37. **Joffe, N. and Schamroth, L.,** Gas-forming infection of the thyroid gland, *Clin. Radiol.,* 17, 95, 1966.
38. **Kohler, P. O., Floyd, W. L., and Wynn, J.,** Indications for thyroid needle biopsy: suppurative thyroiditis, *South. Med. J.,* 59, 182, 1966.

39. **Adler, M. E., Jordan, G., and Walter, R. M.**, Acute suppurative thyroiditis, *West. J. Med.*, 128, 165, 1978.
40. **Montgomery, G. H.**, Acute thyroiditis progressing to suppuration, *J. Med. Assoc. Ala.*, 30, 497, 1961.
41. **Hawbaker, E. L.**, Thyroid abscess, *Am. Surg.*, 37, 290, 1971.
42. **Volpe, R.**, Treatment of thyroiditis, *Mod. Treatment*, 6, 474, 1969.
43. **Volpe, R.**, Acute and subacute thyroiditis, *Pharmacol. Ther.*, 1, 171, 1976.
44. **Thomas, C. G.**, Acute suppurative thyroiditis: surgical treatment, in *The Thyroid,* Werner, S. C. and Ingbar, S. H., Eds., Harper and Row, New York, 1971, 852.
45. **Kirkland, R. T., Kirkland, J. L., Rosenberg, H. S., Harbert, F. J., Librik, L., and Clayton, G.**, Solitary thyroid nodules in 30 children and report of a child with a thyroid abscess, *Pediatrics*, 51, 85, 1973.
46. **Greenfield, J. and Curtis, G. M.**, Acute suppurative thyroiditis during childhood, *Am. J. Dis. Child.*, 58, 837, 1939.
47. **Szego, P. L. and Levy, R. P.**, Recurrent acute suppurative thyroiditis, *Can. Med. Assoc. J.*, 103, 631, 1970.

Chapter 3

OTHER INFECTIOUS THYROIDITIDES

Hannibal Edwards and Virginia A. LiVolsi

TABLE OF CONTENTS

I.	Introduction	14
II.	Etiology	14
	A. Unusual Organisms Producing Thyroiditis	14
	B. Tuberculosis Thyroidites	14
	C. Fungal Thyroiditis	14
III.	Clinical Features	15
IV.	Laboratory Findings	17
V.	Diagnosis	17
VI.	Differential Diagnosis	18
	A. Clinical	18
	B. Pathological	18
VII.	Course and Prognosis	18
VIII.	Treatment	18
References		19

I. INTRODUCTION

For reasons which are not understood, the thyroid gland appears to resist infection even in the face of overwhelming sepsis.[1] The marked vascularity of the gland would suggest a special susceptibility, but this is not found. As noted in Chapter 2, acute thyroiditis is rare. This chapter will briefly review other even less common infections of the thyroid. In the modern era, when infectious thyroiditis does occur, it arises almost always in patients with abnormal immune systems.

II. Etiology

A. Unusual Organisms Producing Thyroiditis

Rare reports of uncommon organisms producing acute or subacute (smoldering) thyroiditis have appeared. These organisms include *Brucella* sp.,[2] *Treponema* sp.,[3,4] *Actinomyces* sp.,[5] and *Ecchinococcus*.[6]

B. Tuberculous Thyroiditis

Thyroiditis caused by acid-fast organisms and fungi has been reported, but occurs rarely. A wide range of clinical presentations from acute to chronic thyroiditis has been described.

Reports prior to 1950 indicate that many cases of subacute thyroiditis were produced by mycobacterial infection of the gland. Thus, a diagnosis of tuberculous thyroiditis was made if the histology of the gland showed a granulomatous character.[7] Jaffe,[7] however, pointed out that the majority of cases diagnosed as tuberculosis of the thyroid represented subacute thyroiditis, a disease of unknown, possibly viral, etiology (see Chapter 4). This author reviewed 21 cases of tuberculous thyroiditis and found neither caseation nor acid-fast organisms in most of these. Similarly, Klassen and Curtis[8] described 17 cases of tuberculous infection of the thyroid but in only 7 of these, were organisms identified.

Adequately documented tuberculous thyroiditis is indeed very rare.[9] Patients with pulmonary, gastrointestinal, genitourinary, or even miliary tuberculosis rarely show evidence of thyroid involvement.[10]

Early investigators felt that the thyroid gland was immune to tuberculosis. Experimentally, however, injecting tubercle bacilli into the thyroid artery[11] or carotid artery[12] led to infection of the gland although other organs, i.e., testis and spleen, appear more susceptible to the organism.[13] Nevertheless, for reasons which remain unclear, thyroid involvement in patients with tuberculosis rarely occurs.[7,8] Most individuals who have documented tuberculous thyroiditis will also have pulmonary disease. In these subjects, a hematogenous route of infection has been postulated.[8] Atypical mycobacteria can produce thyroiditis on rare occasions.[14,15] The incidence of these infections remains extremely low, however.

C. Fungal Thyroiditis

Candida, Aspergillus, and *Coccidioidomycosis* have been described as producing thyroiditis.[16-18] These infections occur only in the clinical setting of impaired immunologic status. Hence, the patient of Robinson et al.[16] had received immunosuppressive drugs for Goodpasture's syndrome, the individual reported by Halazun et al.[17] suffered from chronic granulomatous disease of childhood, and a patient of Loeb et al.[18] had polyarteritis nodosa. Thus, fungal thyroiditis is associated with fungemia and the organisms reach the thyroid by a hematogenous route.

One of the present authors (VAL) has studied two patients with *Aspergillus* thyroiditis. In both of these individuals, thyroid involvement by the fungus was documented only at autopsy:

Case 1 — this elderly female had a history of poorly differentiated lymphocytic lymphoma treated for several years with various drug regimens. When she died of overwhelming pulmonary infection due to *Aspergillus*, a small white nodule was noted in the thyroid gland. On histologic section, this lesion showed a microabscess containing many fungal forms. The remaining thyroid appeared normal.

Case 2 — a 28-year-old female was admitted complaining of fever and chills of 1 week duration. In 1974, she developed sinusitis and arthalgias. A biopsy of the nasal septum revealed vasculitic changes and granulomas, most consistent with Wegener's granulomatosis. She was started on Imuran and prednisone therapy. Chronic renal failure developed, necessitating hemodialysis.

On admission, chest X-ray disclosed a left upper lobe cavity. Her hematocrit was 21.8 with a hemoglobin of 7.2 and a white count of 3500. The impression at the time of admission was fever and chills, secondary either to Wegener's granulomatosis or superimposed infection. She was treated with gentamycin and Keflin, initially. Vomiting, nausea and abdominal pain developed and elevations of amylase and lipase were found. At exploratory laparotomy, an acutely perforated and gangrenous gallbladder was seen. The pathology of the specimen showed acute and chronic cholecystitis without stones. Cytomegalovirus inclusions were seen in the mucosa. Postoperatively, she was treated with gentamycin, ampicillin, and Cleocin. The peritoneal fluid grew *Serratia* and *Candida*. She was begun on Amphoteracin B. Two weeks postoperatively, Cytoxan was begun but was soon discontinued because of neutropenia, fever to 104°F, and diarrhea. Blood cultures remained negative. However, the patient's condition deteriorated with the development of wound abscesses, intraabdominal and liver abscess, and disseminated intravascular coagulation. Central nervous system dysfunction and cardiac arrhythmias supervened and she died.

Autopsy disclosed multiple infections including cytomegalovirus, *Candida*, and *Aspergillus* involving lungs, kidneys, and gastrointestinal tract. Grossly, the thyroid showed several small yellow nodules (ranging from 3 to 8 mm diameter). Sections showed these were *Aspergillus* abscesses (Figures 1 and 2). Intra- and perithyroidal vessels were involved by this organism, producing thrombosis and foci of necrosis within the gland as well.

III. CLINICAL FEATURES

The past few decades have witnessed the success of organ transplantation and the growth of the subspecialty of oncology. Successful transplantation of various organs has been dependent upon immunosuppression of the recipient. Widespread use of steroids in these patients, as well as for a variety of disorders, has produced a large population susceptible to various infections.[19,20]

Many cancer treatment modalities including radiation and chemotherapeutic drugs suppress the immune system.[19] In addition, some malignancies, especially those of the lymphoma-leukemia group, depress natural immunity.[20] Severe suppression of immunologic parameters may be noted also in congenital or acquired immunodeficiency states.[21]

Aubertin et al.[22] have recently outlined the factors which favor infections in cancer patients. Thus, local disorders in the vicinity of the tumor enhance infection: (a) ulceration and necrosis produce excellent culture media for organisms, (b) obstruction and compression of ducts and natural passages induce stasis which again favors the microbes (hence in a prostatic carcinoma, obstruction of the bladder neck would lead to

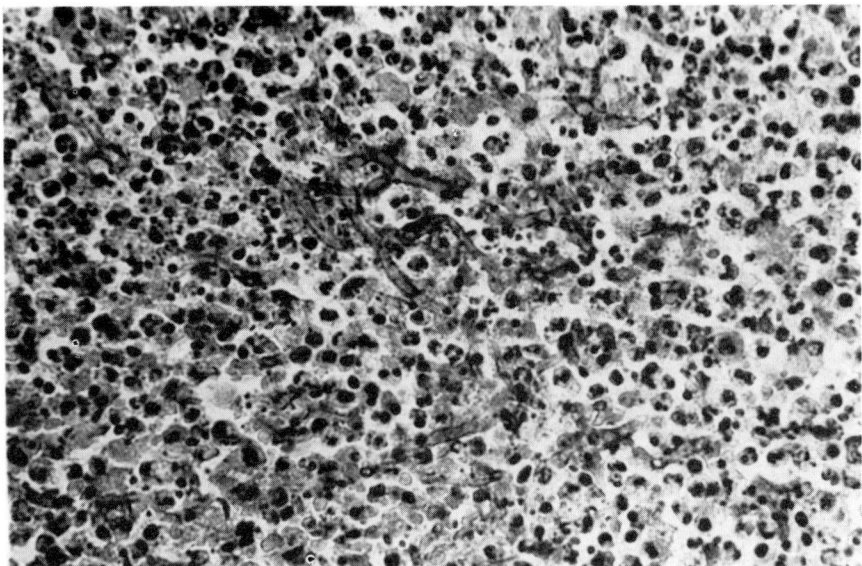

FIGURE 1. In the midst of numerous leukocyte fragments and necrotic debris, septate fungal forms can be seen (center). (Hematoxylin-eosin; magnification × 250.)

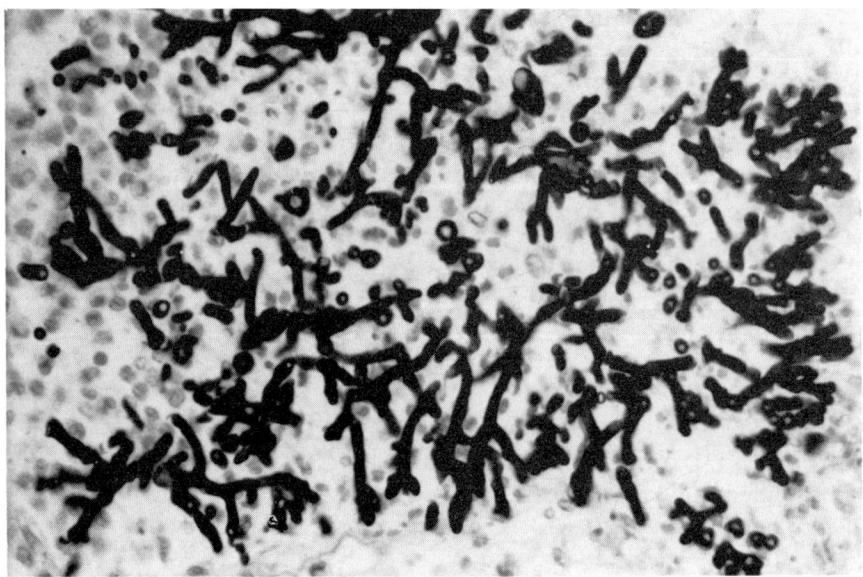

FIGURE 2. Grocott silver stain demonstrates many more of the organism (*Aspergillus*) than could be appreciated on the routine stain. (Magnification × 250.)

urinary retention and bacterial growth; pneumonia is found commonly distal to an obstructing bronchial tumor), and (c) production of a pathologic fracture or spinal cord compression by the neoplasms leads to immobilization and the formation of decubiti — another nidus in which organisms can thrive.[22]

Systemic consequences favoring infection include malnutrition (especially in head and neck and gastrointestinal cancer) and generalized depression of immunity (as discussed above).[22] Disturbances in phagocytosis, abnormalities of the complement system,[23] and impaired interferon production[24] may all contribute to the susceptibility of the cancer patient to infection.[22]

In addition, therapy of cancer which includes chemotherapy and radiation therapy not only affects bone marrow, but may lead to mucosal alterations enhancing invasion by low virulence or opportunistic organisms.[22] Transfusions may transmit hepatitis virus, intravenous or arterial lines are susceptible to infection[25] and, finally, antibiotic therapy may alter normal flora to such an extent as to allow for superinfection.[22]

Armstrong et al.[19] and Neu[20] have summarized a convenient scheme for understanding the interrelationships between the arm of the immune system affected and the type of organism most likely to be encountered as infectious agents. Hence, in conditions in which leukocyte function or number is depressed (acute myelogenous leukemia, radiation), the afferent arm of the immune system is affected and bacterial infections would be expected.[19,20] Therefore, one might see acute suppurative thyroiditis in such an individual.

Impaired cellular (lymphocyte) immunity, as occurs in lymphomas, often results in infection with intracellular parasites (mycobacteria, fungi).[20] Decreased immunoglobulin concentration (as in myeloma and chronic lymphocytic leukemia) may lead to susceptibility to bacterial infections.[20]

In the modern era, the major clinical settings in which the unusual mycobacterial and fungal infections of the thyroid are those associated with immunocompromised circumstances. Patients at risk for these infections include those with congenital immunodeficiencies, individuals with neoplasms of various types, patients receiving radiation and/or chemotherapy, or subjects who are being prepared for (or have undergone) transplantation.

Many of these cases of thyroiditis will be diagnosed only at autopsy, indicating a subclinical thyroid infection. When the infection is clinically overt, the patient may present as someone with acute thyroiditis (neck swelling, erythema, tenderness, fever, tachycardia).[8,9,14,17,18] Occasionally, a more indolent presentation may occur; the patient may complain of neck tenderness and swelling, but fever and tachycardia may not be obvious.[8] In most of these patients, the thyroid lesion is associated with evidence of infection elsewhere (especially lungs) and with a history of an immunocompromised state. Weight loss, pallor, and other signs of chronic disease may be noted.

IV. LABORATORY FINDINGS

Usually the patient remains euthyroid although occasionally mild increases in PBI, T_3 and T_4 may be found.[8,9,17,18] Radioiodine uptake may be decreased, especially in the area of maximum involvement. Indeed Loeb et al.[18] diagnosed their patients initially as having subacute thyroiditis because of mild hyperthyroidism and low radioiodine uptake. Scans of the thyroid may show a cold nodule[9] suggesting the possibility of a neoplasm. In immunodepressed patients, anemia, thrombocytopenia, and white cell abnormalities may be noted.

V. DIAGNOSIS

The diagnosis of a specific infectious thyroiditis requires demonstration of the organism by culture, smear, or histology of the thyroid tissue.[1,7-9,14-18] Needle biopsy of the gland may prove very useful here,[18] especially in the immunosuppressed patient, when formal surgical intervention may be contraindicated.

VI. DIFFERENTIAL DIAGNOSIS

A. Clinical
These types of thyroiditis, if they follow an acute course, may be confused with acute bacterial thyroiditis of the more common varieties (see Chapter 2), with hemorrhage into the thyroid or into a cyst or adenoma, or with an infected thyroglossal duct cyst.[26,27]

The more indolent forms of this disease, especially tuberculosis, must be distinguished from intrathyroidal masses of various types, especially neoplasms. Since thyroid function tests, and even scans, may not provide useful data, biopsy or surgery is often needed to make a correct diagnosis.

B. Pathological
Tuberculous thyroiditis may be confused with other forms of granulomatous inflammation involving the thyroid. Most commonly encountered is palpation thyroiditis[28] (Chapter 5) and subacute thyroiditis[1] (Chapter 4). Rarely, sarcoidosis will involve the thyroid.[29,30]

Microscopically, the granulomata of tuberculosis exhibit central caseation necrosis, a finding rarely, if ever, encountered in mimicker lesions. The diagnosis of tuberculosis in the thyroid as elsewhere demands the finding of organisms in sections or by culture. Similarly, the acute and focally histiocytic reaction found in fungal infections of the gland may be confused with acute thyroiditis. Demonstration of the organisms, especially with the use of silver stains, will clinch the diagnosis (Figure 2).

An important point should be made here. The patient who is susceptible to fungal thyroiditis will be an immunocompromised individual. Various types of immunosuppression will interfere with and alter the host's inflammatory response. Hence, although a granulomatous reaction might be expected in a fungal infection, depression of lymphocyte and macrophage function by therapy of the underlying disease process may prevent such a response. On the other hand, severe bone marrow depression may elicit minimal reaction or none at all. Therefore, if the pathologist is faced with an abnormal thyroid in which a peculiar inflammatory reaction is seen, or in which focal necrosis of the gland is noted (especially in appropriate clinical situations), the possibility of a fungal infection should be entertained and appropriate stains should be performed and examined.

VII. COURSE AND PROGNOSIS

The course of mycobacterial and fungal thyroiditis tends to be more protracted than the more common acute bacterial thyroid infections.[8,9,16,17] Relative antibiotic insensitivity may account for this.

The prognosis of this disease is dependent upon the underlying condition of the host. Since most of these individuals will show pulmonary or other systemic infection, the outcome depends upon successful therapy of the whole patient, not merely the thyroid lesion. Mortality rates of over 50% have been recorded, but only a minority of the deaths have been atttributed to the thyroiditis.[8,9,14-17]

VIII. TREATMENT

If this form of thyroiditis presents itself as acute disease, often as an abscess, drainage of the lesion for diagnosis and therapy should be accomplished; rarely, lobectomy may be needed.[8,9,14-16] After identification of the responsible organism, appropriate antibiotic or antifungal therapy should be instituted.[16-18] Drug sensitivities should be obtained and, subsequently, therapy may need to be altered.

REFERENCES

1. Hazard, J. B., Thyroiditis: a review, *Am. J. Clin. Pathol.*, 25, 289, 1955.
2. Pacheo, G. and Andrade, M., Tireodite supurada Brucelosa, *Rev. Bras. Med.*, 20, 127, 1963.
3. Laird, S. M., Gumma of the thyroid gland, *Br. J. Vener. Dis.*, 21, 162, 1945.
4. Skarapora, G. I., Specific thyroiditis in a syphilitic woman, *Sov. Med.*, 27, 120, 1964.
5. Leers, W. D., Dussault, J., Mullens, J. E., and Volpe, R., Suppurative thyroiditis: an unusual case caused by *Actinomyces naeslundi*, *Can. Med. Assoc. J.*, 101, 714, 1969.
6. Shaw, H. M., A case of hydatid disease of the thyroid gland, *Med. J. Aust.*, 2, 413, 1946.
7. Jaffe, R. H., Tubercle-like structures in human goiters, *Arch. Surg. Chicago*, 21, 719, 1930.
8. Klassen, K. P. and Curtis, G. M., Tuberculous abscess of the thyroid gland, *Surgery*, 17, 552, 1945.
9. Goldfarb, H., Schifrin, D., and Graig, F. A., Thyroiditis caused by tuberculous abscess of the thyroid gland, *Am. J. Med.*, 38, 825, 1965.
10. Rundle, F. F., *Joll's Diseases of the Thyroid Gland*, Heinemann, Ltd., London, 1951, 325.
11. Torri, O., La tiroide nei morbi infettivi, *Policlinico Sez. Chir.*, 7, 145, 1900.
12. Roger, H. and Garnier, M., Des lesions de la glande thyroide dans la tuberculose, *Arch. Gen. Med. Paris*, 185, 385, 1900.
13. Shimodiara, Y., Experimentelle Untersuchungen uber die tuberkulose Infection der Schilddruse, *Dtsch. Z. Chir.*, 109, 443, 1911.
14. Olin, R., LeBien, W. E., and Leigh, J. E., Acute suppurative thyroiditis, Report of two cases including one caused by *Mycobacterium intracellulare*, *Minn. Med.*, 56, 586, 1973.
15. Gutman, L. T., Handwerger, S., Zwadyk, P., Abramowsky, C. R., and Rodgers, B. M., Thyroiditis due to *Mycobacterium chelonei*, *Am. Rev. Respir. Dis.*, 110, 807, 1974.
16. Robinson, M. F., Forgan-Smith, W. R., and Craswell, P. W., *Candida* thyroiditis treated with 5-fluoro-cytosine, *Aust. N. Z. J. Med.*, 5, 472, 1975.
17. Halazun, J. F., Anast, C. S., and Lukens, J. N., Thyrotoxicosis associated with *Aspergillus thyroiditis* in chronic granulomatous disease, *J. Pediatr.*, 80, 106, 1972.
18. Loeb, J. M., Livermore, B. M., and Wofsy, D., Coccidioidomycosis of the thyroid, *Ann. Intern. Med.*, 91, 409, 1979.
19. Armstrong, D., Young, L. S., Meyer, R. D., and Blevins, A. H., Infectious complications of neoplastic disease, *Med. Clin. North Am.*, 55, 729, 1971.
20. Neu, H. C., The role of cellular and humoral factors in infections, *Clin. Hematol.*, 5, 449, 1976.
21. Gehrz, R. C., Marker, S. C., Knorr, S. O., Kalis, J. M., and Balfour, H. H., Specific cell mediated immune defect in active cytomegalovirus infection of younger children and their mothers, *Lancet*, 2, 844, 1977.
22. Aubertin, J., Hoerni, B., Lacut, J. Y., and Durand, M., *Opportunistic Infections in Cancer Patients*, Masson Publ. Co., New York, 1978.
23. Audran, R., Notions actuelles concernant de complement, *Rev. Eur. Etud. Clin. Biol.*, 15, 610, 1970.
24. Rassiga-Pidot, A. L. and McIntyre, O. R., In vitro leucocyte interferon production in patients with Hodgkin's disease, *Cancer Res.*, 34, 2995, 1974.
25. Copeland, E. M., MacFadyen, B. V., McGown, C., and Dudrick, S. J., The use of hyperalimentation in patients with potential sepsis, *Surg. Gynecol. Obstet.*, 138, 377, 1974.
26. Adler, M. E., Jordan, G., and Walter, R. M., Acute suppurative thyroiditis, *West. J. Med.*, 128, 165, 1978.
27. Hurley, J. R., Thyroiditis, *Disease-A-Month*, December, 1977.
28. Carney, J. A., Moore, S. B., Northcutt, R. C., Woolner, L. B., and Stillwell, G. K., Palpation thyroiditis (multifocal granulomatous folliculitis), *Am. J. Clin. Pathol.*, 64, 639, 1975.
29. Thompson, W. B., McGrouther, D. A., and Stockdill, G., Thyrotoxicosis with sarcoid-like granulomata, *J. Pathol.*, 111, 289, 1973.
30. von Knorring, J. and Selroos, O., Sarcoidosis with thyroid involvement, polymyalgia rheumatica and breast carcinoma, *Scand. J. Rheumatol.*, 5, 77, 1976.

Chapter 4

SUBACUTE THYROIDITIS

Hannibal Edwards and Virginia A. LiVolsi

TABLE OF CONTENTS

I.	Introduction	22
II.	Incidence	22
III.	Sex, Age	23
IV.	Etiology	23
	A. Old Theories	23
	B. Viral Causation	24
	C. Genetics	25
	D. Autoimmunity Theory	25
V.	Pathophysiology and Course of Subacute Thyroiditis	26
VI.	Illustrative Case Report	26
VII.	Clinical Features	27
	A. Symptoms	27
	B. Physical Findings	29
VIII.	Laboratory Data	29
IX.	Pathologic Features	31
	A. Gross Pathology	31
	B. Microscopic Features	31
	C. Cytology	31
	D. The Giant Cell	32
	E. Ultrastructural Observations	32
X.	Painless Thyroiditis	33
XI.	Diagnosis and Differential Diagnosis	34
	A. Clinical	34
	B. Pathological	34
XII.	Therapy	34
XIII.	Outcome and Prognosis	35
XIV.	Associations with Other Diseases	35
	A. Thyroidal	35
	B. Extrathyroidal	35

XV. Summary...36

References...36

I. INTRODUCTION

Subacute thyroiditis describes nonsuppurative inflammation of the thyroid gland characterized by certain clinical features and a distinctive histologic picture.[1-21] Volpe[20] points out that although the term "subacute" implies a temporal meaning and could be applied to certain bacterial and fungal thyroiditides, this descriptive phase is used to connote a specific clinicopathologic syndrome (Table 1).

Various names have been given to this entity: pseudotuberculous thyroiditis, giant cell thyroiditis, migrating "creeping" thyroiditis, nonsuppurative thyroiditis, and struma granulomatosa.[1,2,5,7,9,13-16,19,20] The most popular and widely recognized terms used by pathologists in the modern era include granulomatous thyroiditis or de Quervain's thyroiditis, although clinicians prefer "subacute thyroiditis" since this phrase defines a rather specific syndrome, implying a self-limited disorder.[5,7,10,12,13,15,19-21]

Although first reported by Mygind in 1895,[22] it was de Quervain in 1904[23] and de Quervain and Giordenengo in 1935[1] who described the clinical and pathological features of subacute thyroiditis, and separated this lesion from other forms of thyroid inflammation. In his initial report, de Quervain summarized his own cases and 57 from the literature. Before the redefinition of this disease in 1935[1] based on a larger series, confusion existed regarding the relationship of acute and subacute thyroiditis on the one hand and between subacute and chronic thyroiditis on the other. Jaffe[2] and Crile[3,4] emphasized the importance of separating subacute thyroiditis as a distinct entity. Jaffe[2] is attributed with supporting a nontuberculous, indeed, non-infectious etiology for this disorder.

Modern authors[5-10,12-14,16-21] have supported this concept of subacute thyroiditis and define it as a self-limited disease of unknown (possibly viral) etiology characterized by neck pain, fever, and other mild systemic symptoms with a course of weeks to months of thyroid dysfunction, and with complete recovery in the overwhelming majority of cases. The identification of a related disorder, "painless" thyroiditis[20] has evoked some controversy as will be discussed below.

II. INCIDENCE

Subacute thyroiditis has been reported from all areas of the globe.[17,21] The true incidence of the disease, however, is unknown, since (a) it has been confused with other thyroiditides and (b) many mild cases may never be diagnosed.[20] Giordenengo, in 1938,[24] claimed that only 54 documented cases had been recorded since the 1904 de Quervain paper. Initial reports described only cases sufficiently severe to necessitate surgery.[1,4,9,14]

Incidence rates vary and reflect surgical or medical series. Thus, Stalker and Walther[25] reported an incidence of 1.4% of all thyroid disorders, and Osmond and

Table 1
FEATURES OF SUBACUTE THYROIDITIS

Classically occurs as painful thyroid swelling associated with fever and systemic symptoms
    Degree of severity of symptoms variable from case to case
    More common in women
    Possible viral association
    Clinically, hyperthyroid, hypothyroid, and recovery phases
Laboratory values show elevated PBI and thyroid hormones but low to absent radioactive iodine uptake. These results are diagnostic early on in the course and distinguish subacute thyroiditis from mimickers. Antithyroid antibodies present in low titer and disappear on recovery
Pathologically, granulomatous inflammation with central fibrosis are classic findings. Few reports suggest some of the giant cells are derived from follicular epithelium and the rest from histiocytes
Course usually of few months with recovery; no functional residua. Permanent hypothyroidism very rare
Recent evidence suggests that painless thyroiditis with hyperthyroidism is a form of subacute disease

Portman found only an 0.04% incidence.[26] Surgical incidences of 0.31% to 2% of all thyroid resections have been noted.[3,5] Werner[27] estimates that 0.5 to 2% of all thyroid diseases represent subacute thyroiditis.

Comparing the incidence of subacute thyroiditis with other thyroiditides indicates that this disease is 1/5 to 1/10 as common as Hashimoto's thyroiditis and 10 to 50 times more frequent than Riedel's struma.[3,5,9,28-36] It is estimated to be 1/8 to 1/10 as common as Graves' disease.[9] In the report of Marshall et al.,[37] subacute thyroiditis comprised 1/5 of the operative series on thyroiditis.

This condition is diagnosed more frequently in recent years (since its separation from other thyroiditides) since the use of radioiodine scans[38-45] and thyroid needle biopsy[15,17,19,26,46,47] is becoming widespread, and since the recognition of a "painless" variant.[9,15-20,27,48-51] Probably, subacute thyroiditis occurs more commonly than reported, because, as a self-limited and spontaneously resolving disorder, it is underdiagnosed.[15-20,26]

III. SEX, AGE

Most studies document a female predominance (ratios 2:1 to 6:1) for subacute thyroiditis.[5,7,9,10,12-20,26] Almost all affected individuals are adults ranging from 20 to 71 years of age. The most common age of occurrence is the third to sixth decades.[5,7,12-20]

IV. ETIOLOGY

The cause of subacute thyroiditis remains unknown.

A. Old Theories

Clinical features of a systemic illness, milder but showing some similarity to acute thyroiditis, led early investigators to postulate an infectious etiology. The pathologic finding of granulomata encouraged the proponents of a mycobacterial causation.[2,25] However, cultures and stains of tissues for various organisms gave uniformly negative results.[2,7,9-17,19]

Because of this failure to isolate a specific organism, other theories were proposed. DeCourcy suggested a relationship to Riedel's disease,[52,53] considering subacute thyroiditis as a phase of Riedel's struma. Another case suggesting this relationship has been reported recently.[54] However, these two entities appear distinct in their clinical and pathological characteristics in most instances. In addition, since the cause of neither condition is known, proposed interrelationships seem tenuous, at best.[5,7,9-20]

Chesky et al.[32] believed that the pathogenesis of subacute and other forms of thyroiditis could be explained by a change in colloid composition, resulting in an inflammatory reaction. Crile[3,4] supported the experimental work of Ferguson[55] and considered subacute thyroiditis as a disorder reflecting reaction of macrophages to released colloid. Ferguson[55] produced foreign-body reactions by injecting colloid into guinea pigs. However, this latter reaction more closely simulates palpation thyroiditis than the subacute variety (see Chapter 5).

Certain clinical features of subacute thyroiditis, however, point to altered colloid as one aspect of the disease. Thus, radioactive iodine is not taken up in the usual manner, but in the fashion of an individual on propylthiouracil drugs.[6,32,56] The capacity to form thyroglobulin is impaired, but not its release. Whether this inability to concentrate radioiodine is produced by a primary thyroid abnormality, or by a pituitary reaction, is unclear.[4,5,57]

Typically, the thyroid-stimulating hormone levels are low during the initial phase of subacute thyroiditis. In addition, the response of thyroid hormone output to stimulation by thyrotropin-releasing hormone is severely diminished.[58] Diminished or absent radioiodine uptake and low thyrotropin levels suggest that high levels of circulating iodoproteins (released via colloid leakage following follicular damage) may suppress the pituitary. Another explanation, certainly not mutually exclusive with the first, is that in subacute thyroiditis, thyroid resistance to thyrotropin may occur. If only high circulating iodoprotein levels were the cause of decreased thyroid-stimulating hormone and radioiodine uptake, administration of exogenous thyrotropin should correct the iodine concentrating abnormality. Indeed, this is not the case.[59] Hence, this failure of exogenous thyrotropin to affect radioiodine uptake supports a component of thyroid glandular (follicular epithelial cell) resistance to thyroid-stimulating hormone. The pathologic finding of follicular destruction indicates interference with function and hence these abnormalities would not be unexpected.

B. Viral Causation

Fraser and Harrison suggested a relationship between viruses and subacute thyroiditis as early as 1952.[6] Most modern investigators believe that a viral causation will emerge for subacute thyroiditis, although association of this disorder with malaria,[68] Q-fever,[61] and cat-scratch disease[62] do not fit in this scheme. Hurley,[17] Bastenie,[14] and Volpe[19] have summarized the evidence suggesting a viral etiology:

1. Subacute thyroiditis is often preceded by either an upper respiratory infection or a prodrome phase of pains, aches, fatigue, and malaise. Fifty to ninety percent of patients show this prodrome.[12-21] Fever and other systemic manifestations suggest an infectious origin.[14,17]
2. No leukocytosis is noted, which would be expected in a bacterial infection.[14,17]
3. Antibiotics have no effect on the disease.[14-21]
4. Complete recovery, even without therapy, is the rule.[14-21]
5. Epidemiologic studies have shown outbreaks of subacute thyroiditis at times when a specific virus is epidemic in a certain population.[13,14] Thus, the study of Eylan et al. in 1957[63] showed that, during a mumps epidemic in Israel, 2 of 11 patients who developed subacute thyroiditis had mumps virus isolated from their thyroids. In addition, complement fixation antibodies to mumps were identified in 10 of these subjects. Greene,[13] in his review, summarized reports of subacute thyroiditis associated with infections with many viruses: mumps,[64-69] measles,[59,70,71] influenza,[72] Coxsackie,[73] mononucleosis,[74-77] adenovirus,[75,78] St. Louis encephalitis virus,[79] and the "common cold" virus.[74]

The epidemiologic study of Hintze et al.[74] showed a relationship between upper respiratory tract infection (common cold) and the outbreak of subacute thyroiditis in individuals employed by one factory in Helsinki. Attempts to isolate a specific agent were unsuccessful, however.

Volpe et al.[80] studied 72 cases of subacute thyroiditis and found elevated complement fixing antibodies to a variety of viruses in about 50%. The implicated agents included influenza, Coxsackie, adenovirus, ECHO-virus, and mumps. Eylan et al.[63] documented a rising titer of mumps antibodies in the sera of some patients with subacute thyroiditis. Whether these reactions reflect specific infection or whether they indicate merely a generalized anamnestic response to inflammation of the thyroid remains unclear.[14,80]

In 1976, Stancek et al.[81-83] isolated a previously unknown virus from the serum, urine, and thyroid of 5 of 28 individuals with subacute thyroiditis. This cytopathic agent (termed MGI virus) when grown in rat lung culture, produced changes identical to those seen in thyroids of affected patients. In addition, these patients' sera contained antibodies to this agent as shown by immunofluorescence. Ultrastructural analysis of these organisms have disclosed rod-shaped and oval forms.[81] This exciting work awaits confirmation by other studies.

C. Genetics

Nyulassy et al.[84-86] addressed the question of genetic predisposition to subacute thyroiditis. In comparing the frequency of HLA antigens in thyroiditis patients and normals, 70% of the individuals with subacute thyroiditis had an association with HLA-BW35, whereas only 9% of controls showed this. This dramatically significant difference was noted again by Majsky and Feix[87] who identified HLA-BW35 in 65% of test subjects and only 14% of controls.

In addition, Nyulassy et al.[84-86] identified mild immunologic abnormalities in patients with subacute thyroiditis; these individuals showed decreased serum Clq, C4, and C3 activator and increased C3, IgM, and alpha-1-antitrypsin levels.

D. Autoimmunity Theory

The role of autoimmunity in the pathogenesis of subacute thyroiditis has been evaluated extensively. Felix-Davies[65] demonstrated antithyroid antibodies in an affected patient and suggested that thyroid damage may result in part from an autoimmune mechanism. This particular individual also showed evidence of mumps antibodies; indeed, the mumps virus titer reached 1:900 (hemagglutination), whereas the antithyroid antibody peaked at 1:16.

Solmo et al.[61] demonstrated high (1:2500) antithyroid antibody titers in a patient with subacute thyroiditis who also had Q fever; antibodies to the causative agent, *Coxiella burnetti*, rose during the acute phase of the illness (titer 1:64). Hintze et al.[74] recognized rising antithyroid antibody titers in some of their cases during the Helsinki epidemic associated with the common cold virus.

Antibodies to thyroid antigens can be detected in some patients with subacute thyroiditis, but these are of low titer, correlate poorly with course of the disease, and disappear as the disease resolves;[10,12-20] an autoimmune disorder appears unlikely. In addition, a few authors have identified thyroid-stimulating immunoglobulins in the early phase of subacute thyroiditis,[20,88-91] which was considered related to the hyperthyroidism seen in this phase. However, Sugenoya et al.[91] showed that this antibody did not stimulate thyroid cells, disappears rapidly, and is considered a nonspecific response.[90,91] Similarily, tests of cell-mediated immunity have shown transitory changes and are also considered nonspecific.[20,92,93] These features of subacute thyroiditis do not hint to etiology, however, and appear to represent functional manifestations of thyroid damage.

Volpe's[20,80] studies of subacute thyroiditis seemed to lay the autoimmune theory to rest. He found elevated antithyroid antibodies in 20% of cases of proven subacute thyroiditis; 3% of control sera showed similar titers. In general, these titers are low and follow the course of the disease, i.e., they disappear after resolution of the illness. This author concluded that the antithyroid antibodies do not cause the thyroiditis, but represent a response to products released from the damaged gland during the course of the disease.[14,20,60-65,80]

Hence, evidence from multiple sources implicates a virus (not necessarily one specific type) as the cause of subacute thyroiditis. The pathogenesis of the disorder may be postulated as follows: the virus, especially in genetically susceptible hosts, infects thyroid epithelial cells leading to their destruction. Subsequent inflammation and follicular damage produces colloid leakage. This, in turn, elaborates thyroid antigens into the serum, eliciting the production of antibodies. In addition, early on, formed, stored thyroid hormone is released, causing chemical and sometimes clinical hyperthyroidism. Later in the course of the disease, as follicular damage has not yet given way to regeneration, hypothyroidism may occur. Resolution follows with return of normal function and histology and disappearance of thyroid antibodies.

Whether one specific virus or, as seems more likely, several agents may initiate the process, the clinical, chemical, and pathological final, common pathway is followed.

V. PATHOPHYSIOLOGY AND COURSE OF SUBACUTE THYROIDITIS

To better understand the clinical spectrum and laboratory data associated with subacute thyroiditis, division of this disorder into stages or phases is useful. The course of the disorder can be divided readily into four stages.[8,13,19,94]

The first stage (thyrotoxic phase), lasting up to 2 months, is characterized by a painful, swollen thyroid and mild systemic symptoms, and is associated with elevation of serum thyroid hormone levels. Disruption of thyroid follicles with colloid leakage corresponds to this histologically.

In the second (euthyroid or transition) stage, the gland is firm and large; thyroid function tests return to normal, although radioiodine uptake is depressed. Areas of follicular disruption and colloid depletion coexist with areas of repair and granulomatous inflammation. This phase lasts about 4 to 6 weeks.

The third phase (hypothyroid) begins 2 to 4 months after onset, is characterized by decreased serum thyroid hormone levels, and microscopically corresponds to reparative changes and granulomatous inflammation in the gland. At the end of this stage, regeneration of follicles occurs with the resumption of hormone synthesis and entry into the fourth phase.

Phase four (stage of resolution) is characterized by recovery of thyroid function and regression of symptoms. Although the gland may remain larger and firmer than normal, almost all patients finally recover.

VI. ILLUSTRATIVE CASE REPORT

A 60-year-old woman noted a nodule in the right side of her neck for 8 months. The mass was palpable intermittently for 6 months and then it enlarged rapidly. The latter was associated with right neck pain, which radiated to the right ear. There were no associated symptoms, specifically, no dysphasia, dyspnea, hoarseness, or evidence of hyperthyroidism. The mass measured 3 × 1.5 cm and was tender to palpation. No lymphadenopathy was noted.

Laboratory data showed a normal protein-bound iodine and a low normal-radioiodine uptake (17% at 24 hr). Scan showed an area of decreased uptake in the right lobe, interpreted as a "cold nodule".

With a clinical diagnosis of carcinoma, right thyroid lobectomy was performed. No enlarged lymph nodes were seen. The specimen, on cut section, showed a yellow-white appearance and was very firm. This tissue freely interdigitated with the relatively spared thyroid at the periphery of the lobe and was grossly mistaken for carcinoma. Frozen section and, subsequently, permanent sections disclosed a granulomatous thyroiditis occupying the major portion of the right lobe. Follicular destruction, fibrosis and numerous giant cells were identified (Figures 1 to 3). Postoperatively, the patient recuperated satisfactorily and was clinically and chemically euthyroid 2 months after surgery without thyroid supplements.

The patient died of widely metastatic pancreatic adenocarcinoma 13 years following the episode of thyroiditis. At autopsy, the residual thyroid was described as grossly normal. Microscopically, the thyroid architecture was entirely normal — no evidence of inflammation was seen. Rare focal scars were noted as the only trace of the prior thyroiditis.

VII. CLINICAL FEATURES

The above case illustrates many of the clinical and pathological aspects of subacute thyroiditis. In this section, symptoms and physical findings of the disorder will be described.

A. Symptoms

The presentation of subacute thyroiditis may be variable. Acute toxicity with exquisite tenderness of the gland, high fever, and a septic picture resembling acute bacterial thyroiditis may be seen, but is rare.[5,7-10,13-21,27] At the other end of the spectrum, a chronic illness with minimal thyroid enlargement and no pain or fever may be found, so-called "painless" thyroiditis.[9,12,17,44,48,50,51,95-97] Typically, the patient with subacute thyroiditis lies somewhere between these two extremes.[5,8-20,27,98-101]

Subacute thyroiditis is usually ushered in by a prodrome of fatigue, malaise, and weakness.[8-20,27,98-101] This prodrome occurs in 50 to 90% of the cases. Less often, patients note also myalgias, arthralgias, anorexia, headaches, nausea, and increased salivation.[13,14,17,19-21] Hearing loss, tinnitus, and facial parasthesias have also been reported.[13,17,19,102,103]

Thyroid pain is a common complaint elicited in 90 to 100% of patients with typical subacute thyroiditis.[5,8-21,27,98-101,104-106] Swelling and tenderness are associated commonly with the pain.[5,8-21,27,98-101] In 2/3 of patients, the pain radiates to the side of the neck or the ear.[5,8,9,13,14,17,20,49,107] Of these, about half will manifest unilateral neck pain and others will complain of pain alternating from side to side. Less frequently, the pain radiates to the low neck or anterior chest[9,13,17,19] simulating cardiac disease. Jaw pain is noted in 15 to 20% of cases.[9,13,14,17,19-21,27,102,103] Although pain is a common presenting symptom, some series show it to occur in less than 50% of cases.[28,49] Indeed, thyroid enlargement without pain may simulate a neoplasm.[20,28,49]

Thyrotoxicosis, without associated thyroid pain, may represent so-called "painless" or "silent" subacute thyroiditis.[17,19,20,48,50,51,95-97,108-110] In such patients, needle or open biopsy may disclose lymphocytic thyroiditis only[108-110] or granulomatous inflammation. The latter finding has convinced Volpe[19,20] that most patients with painless thyroiditis are suffering from the subacute variety.

A sore throat has been reported in 40 to 90% of patients at some point during the

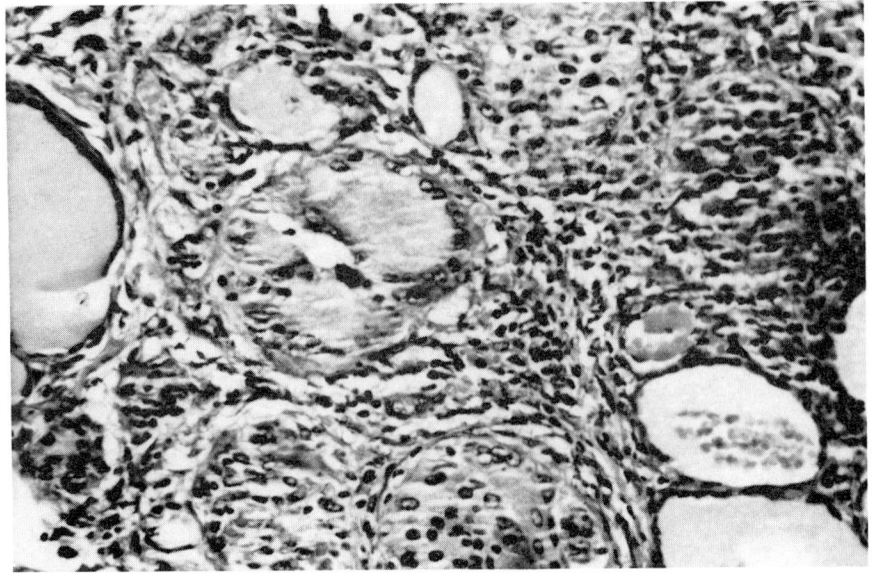

FIGURE 1. Granulomatous thyroiditis showing numerous giant cells, inflammatory cells, and fibrosis. (Hematoxylin-eosin; magnification × 125.)

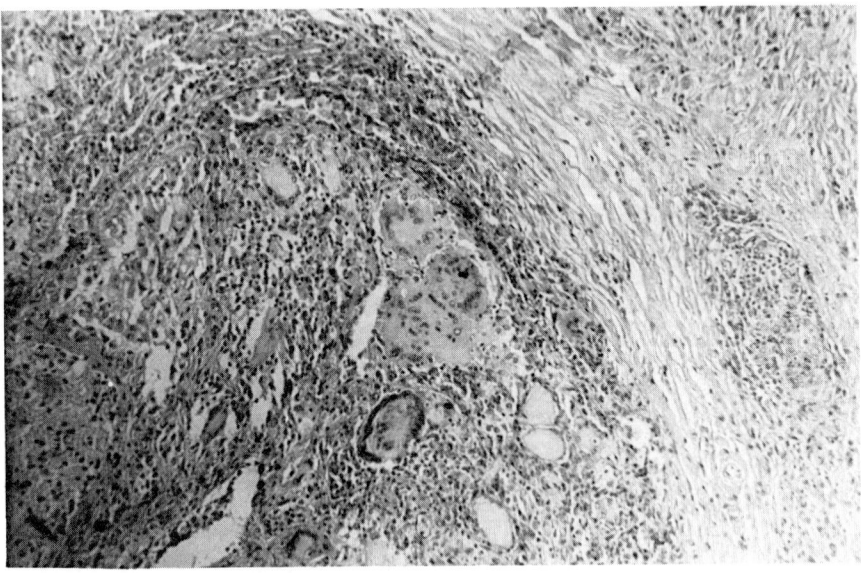

FIGURE 2. Another view of the granulomatous reaction at the edge of a fibrotic area (right). (Hematoxylin-eosin; magnification × 100.)

course of the disease. This symptom is caused most likely by the enlarged and inflamed thyroid.[5,8-21,98-101,104-108] However, up to 30% of patients with subacute thyroiditis may have as associated pharyngitis.[8,14,17,19,20,107,111,112]

Low grade fever (up to 40°C) is reported in 70% of patients with subacute thyroiditis[4-20,57,98-101,104,107,113] and chills may accompany the fever.[104] Erythema may be noted over the gland.[4-21,98-101,107] Fatigue, weakness, muscle aches, irritability, nausea, and

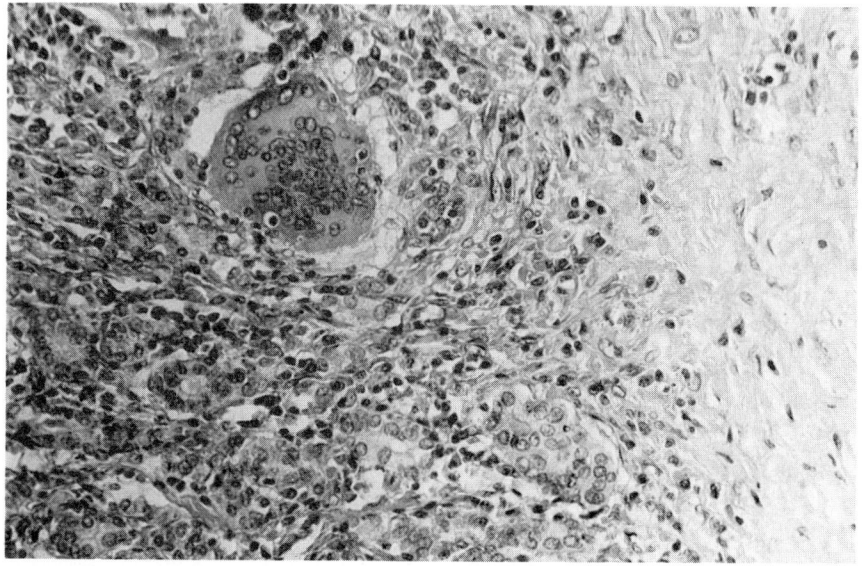

FIGURE 3. High power illustrates giant cell which resembles foreign body type macrophagic cell here. (Hematoxylin-eosin; magnification × 250.)

nervousness have been recorded in 60 to 100% of the cases.[9,17,19,101,105] Weight loss frequently accompanies these symptoms.[28,98,106,114,115]

Other symptoms in any given patient may reflect the stage of the disease and its severity. Thus, a patient in the first stage may exhibit symptoms of hyperthyroidism: nervousness, irritability, weight loss, diaphoresis, palpitations, tremors, and diarrhea. These symptoms correspond to the increase in circulating thyroid hormones.[8,49,107] Similarly, an individual in the hypothyroid phase may show weight gain, dyspnea, hair loss, and other evidence of an underactive gland.[8,29,104] Menstrual irregularities have been described.[104] Green[13] emphasizes that "0 to 46% of patients have been reported to manifest all or part of this syndrome"[4,8,9,57,63,98,107,116-118] reflecting variable diagnostic criteria.

B. Physical Findings

General physical examination usually discloses low-grade fever and mild tachycardia.[4-20,26,93-95,101] The thyroid is usually enlarged and tender to palpation. Disparity in size of the lobes is found often in 20 to 30% of cases having unilateral swelling,[4,5,8,13,14,19,20,62,98-101,107,119] easily mistaken for tumor (as occurred in the illustrative case above). The right lobe is affected more often than the left.[8,9]

VIII. LABORATORY DATA

The laboratory findings in subacute thyroiditis will reflect the clinical stage of the disease.[13,19] During the thyrotoxic stage, thyroid function tests show a characteristic change.[32,40,59] Protein-bound iodine (PBI) is usually markedly increased (8 to 15 mg/dℓ).[56] Butanol-extractable iodine level in the serum is elevated, but to a lesser degree. The basal metabolic rate is elevated into the +20% to +40% range, but is too variable to be of specific use.[13,98-101,107] Usually, thyroid hormone levels (T_3 and T_4) are raised to slightly above the normal range.[4-20,40,98-101,107]

Typically, the thyroid-stimulating hormone (TSH) is low (less than 1 ng/dℓ). Response to thyrotropin-releasing hormone is severely diminished.[58,120-126] Radioiodine uptake is low to markedly depressed and may be less than 1% at 24 hr.[5,6,8,9,13,14,17,20,38,42,44,56,58,98,99,107,114,127-130] This diminished or absent radioiodine uptake and low TSH suggests that high levels of circulating iodoproteins are responsible. High levels of the latter may be acting to suppress TSH output from the pituitary.[5]

An alternative explanation for these findings suggests thyroid resistance to TSH. If high iodoproteins were responsible for the laboratory results, the problem would be corrected by administration of exogenous TSH.[59] However, iodine uptake remains low despite exogenous TSH.[19,59] This failure strongly supports the thyroid resistance theory. Probably thyroid follicular epithelial damage makes iodine uptake impossible and explains resistance to TSH;[39,40] the excess serum iodoproteins depress TSH output concomitantly.

In the second phase, serum T_3, T_4, and PBI return to normal, although radioiodine uptake remains depressed. This corresponds histologically to areas of inflammation coexisting with zones of repair. Leakage of the colloid from the follicles becomes less apparent. This decreased leakage may be due to two factors which may occur either independently or may act concomitantly. Firstly, colloid content of the thyroid may be at a nadir; secondly, the effect of regeneration and repair may be acting to seal off the leak. The ensuing clinical course is determined by which of these mechanisms dominates. For example, the patient who experiences a depletion in the colloid content will inevitably progress to the next stage of hypothyroidism, whereas one whose primary mechanism is that of repair and regeneration will experience minimal or no hypothyroidism.[17,19,131-135]

Stage three, or hypothyroid phase, is characterized by decreased PBI, T_3, and T_4 levels into the hypothyroid range. This corresponds to colloid depletion and early regeneration prior to new hormone synthesis.[19,58,130-132]

Finally, normalization of thyroid function tests, including normal radioiodine uptake, characterize the fourth or resolution phase.

Although the course of subacute thyroiditis is divided into four stages for easier understanding of its pathogenesis, it should be remembered that this is an artificial separation. The course of subacute thyroiditis is a smooth one, with phases blending one into the other. In many cases, division into stages is not possible. Some patients proceed directly from the hyperthyroid stage to recovery, bypassing the hypothyroid phase. Obviously, laboratory findings of thyroid function will reflect these changes.[5,6,14,19,58,99,107,114,129-134]

Other laboratory findings in subacute thyroiditis reflect a generalized systemic illness.[4-21,98-101,107,130,135-137] Thus, a mild anemia has been documented in 30 to 40% of patients.[8,9,13,14,17,19,20,135,137] Although a leukocytosis may occur, this is usually not marked; indeed, if leukocytosis is prominent, the diagnosis of subacute thyroiditis should be doubted.[4-21] Some authors have described a lymphocytosis.[14] The erythrocyte sedimentation rate is always elevated (mean values 40 to 70 mm/hr), but is rarely as high as in acute suppurative thyroiditis.[6,8-10,12-14,17,19,99,130,139] Liver function abnormalities have been described in subacute thyroiditis. These are mild with transaminases of 40 to 150 IU/dℓ and alkaline phosphatases of 4.5 to 5 IU/dℓ.[139]

Stemmerman[140] found a change in serum electrophoretic pattern reflecting an increase in alpha-2-macroglobulin.[100,135,139,140] This was thought to represent an increase in circulating thyroglobulin,[140] but now is believed to reflect a nonspecific response to inflammation.[137,141]

All of these changes in laboratory values are considered nonspecific and are recognized most frequently in the first two stages of the disease. After the thyroiditis has run its course, these laboratory values return to normal.

Hamburger et al.[44] followed the evaluation of subacute thyroiditis using I^{131} scintigrams. These authors showed a decrease in iodine uptake to as low as 1% during the initial phase of the disorder. Since the disease may not be diffuse initially, decreased uptake may appear focal resembling a cool or cold nodule. Usually after 1 to 2 months, a generalized decrease in uptake is noted as the disorder becomes more diffuse.

Significant negative laboratory findings include the absent or very low titers of antithyroid antibodies of various types in patients with subacute thyroiditis.[10,12-20] Those individuals who manifest antibody production have low levels, usually in the early phases of their disease only; these antibodies disappear after recovery.[10,12-20,88-93,142] The swollen gland may show nodularity on palpation.[9,49,107] Tenderness is variable, usually of moderate degree; exquisite tenderness is rare and when present is associated with visible erythema and warmth.[98,106,120,136,143,144] (As the disease progresses, the abnormalities spread to the contralateral side as the original lesion begins to subside.) Cervical lymphadenopathy has been noted only rarely.[106,107,121,142,145]

The physical findings vary according to the phase of the disease. During the hyperthyroid stage, widened pulse pressure, lid lag, and hyperreflexia can be seen, while in the hypothyroid stage, hyporeflexia, hoarseness, and narrow pulse pressure may be found.

IX. PATHOLOGIC FEATURES

A. Gross Pathology

The thyroid gland affected by subacute thyroiditis may be loosely adherent to trachea and strap muscles. However, unlike the thyroid in Riedel's disease, the former is easily shelled out from the surrounding tissue. The thyroid capsule remains intact and the outline of the gland is preserved; this distinguishes this lesion from Riedel's struma.[1,9,14,17,19]

The gland may be grossly enlarged, but not strikingly so; assymetry is found frequently with one lobe obviously bigger than the other.[1,5,9,14,17,19,146] The uninvolved gland may appear normal or may show associated adenomatous nodules.[146]

Upon section, the involved areas are very firm, yellow-white, and poorly defined, without precise demarcation from the surrounding, uninvolved gland. These features resemble carcinoma,[5,9,14,17,19,146] especially if the disease process is localized to one area of the gland. Woolner[146] describes these foci as tumorlike.

B. Microscopic Features

The histologic picture varies with the stage of the disease.[1,146] de Quervain and Giordenengo summarized the histologic features of subacute thyroiditis. The initial process affects the follicular epithelium which degenerates and desquamates.[1,5,9,146] This is followed by alteration and depletion of colloid with apparent leakage of stored hormones and thyroglobulin into the circulation.[80] An inflammatory response ensues and this is composed of leukocytes, lymphocytes, plasma cells, and histiocytes. The formation of giant cells (foreign-body type) occurs around remnants of colloid.[34,146] This granulomatous reaction resembles tubercles although caseous necrosis is not found. Microabscesses are noted in half the cases.[146] Simultaneously and subsequently, fibrosis occurs; the latter is found diffusely, both in interfollicular and interlobular areas.[146] Woolner[146] emphasizes the characteristic central fibrotic zone of healing surrounded by active disease with granulomatous reaction and follicular destruction. Finally, regeneration of follicles and complete histologic recovery take place.[1,5,9,14,146]

C. Cytology

Persson[147] described the cytologic appearance of subacute thyroiditis. At the height of the disease, degenerated follicular epithelial cells are seen. These contain paravacuolar granules[147] which probably represent lipid[14] and reflect degenerative change.

Numerous inflammatory cells (lymphocytes, plasma cells, macrophages, leukocytes) are noted; giant cells are readily identified.[147-149] The lymphocytes in subacute thyroiditis consist predominantly of T-cells, suggesting to Totterman et al.[150] a reaction to a viral disorder.

Wall et al.[93] tested seven patients with subacute thyroiditis for cell-mediated immunity and found in five of these evidence of lymphocyte transformation when exposed to human thyroid extract. These investigators reported that these abnormalities reversed upon recovery, suggesting a temporary T-cell abnormality different from the permanent alterations noted in Hashimoto's and Graves' disease.

D. The Giant Cell

What is the histogenesis of the giant cell in subacute thyroiditis? Many authors consider it to represent a macrophage or histiocyte which is functioning as a scavenger of destroyed follicular cells and extruded colloid.[9,14,19,146] In support of this view are (a) the resemblance of these cells to the epithelioid histiocytes of tuberculous and fungal granulomata,[134,151] (b) the presence within their cytoplasm of PAS-positive material (phagocytized colloid),[5] and (c) ultrastructural evidence of nonepithelial nature.[14,152,153]

Other authors believe these giant cells represent fused, multinucleated, follicular epithelial cells.[1,81-83,154-156] These workers cite (a) ultrastructural evidence suggesting these cells are epithelial[81,155,156] and (b) resemblance to virally infected epithelial cells in tissue culture. Some studies showing viral particles in the cytoplasm of these giant cells[81,155,156] and the aforementioned epidemiologic and serologic data for a viral etiology for this disorder[8,80,81] support this view also.

Lindsay and Dailey[5] suggest dual origin for the giant cells. Those peripherally located (abut follicular basement membrane), they believe, represent altered epithelial cells, since they are smaller and appear focally continuous with recognizable follicular cells. These workers suggest that regeneration of the thyroid originates from these elements. The central ones are macrophages capable of colloid phagocytosis.[5]

The present authors concur with this dual histogenesis theory. There appear to be two distinctive types of giant cell, one obviously histiocytic and the other most likely of epithelioid nature. Resemblance of the former type to those elements seen in palpation thyroiditis,[157] (see Chapter 5) in which these cells are definitely histiocytic, supports this view. Cells of the second variety, the epithelial ones, do not appear in palpation or traumatic thyroiditis (Figure 4).

E. Ultrastructural Observations

Bastenie[14] described a case of subacute thyroiditis studied by electron microscopy. Some of the ultrastructural features suggested increased activity with apical cytoplasmic protrusions, dilated rough endoplasmic reticulum, and well-developed Golgi apparatus. Lipid inclusions were noted in the epithelial cells. The giant cells resembled epithelioid histiocytes, rather than epithelial cells, and these were believed to represent fusion of mononuclear cells. The cytoplasm contains lipid and cellular debris, although colloidophagy was not documented. No viral particles were identified in this study or by other authors.[80,152] Reidbord and Fisher[152] did note lipofusccin and colloid-like material in follicular epithelial cells, but not in the giant cells.

These ultrastructural studies seem to lay to rest the theory that the giant cells represent syncytia of epithelial elements. However, two separate groups of workers[81,155,156] have demonstrated viral particles (? respiratory syncytial virus) resembling known RNA type viruses within the giant cells that appear epithelial. Indeed, Satoh's[155,156]

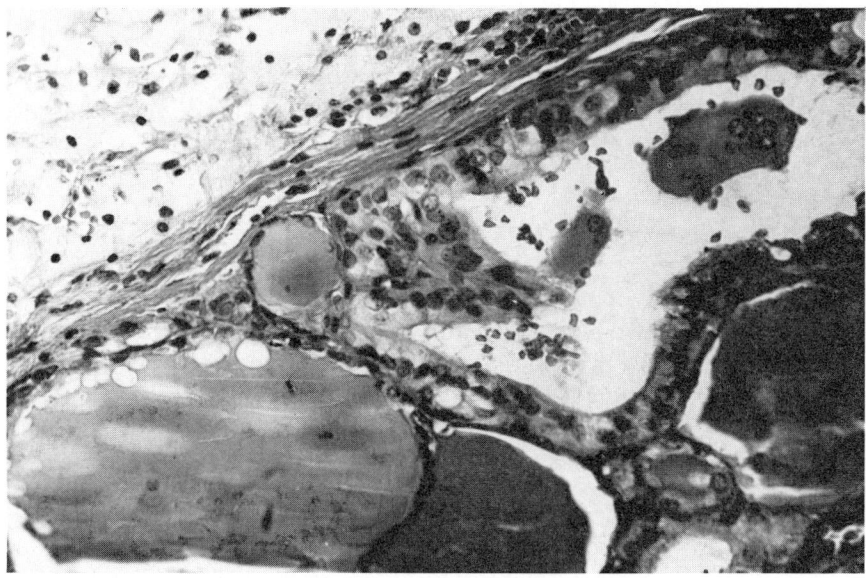

FIGURE 4. One follicle lined by histiocytic cells in case of palpation thyroiditis associated with nodular goiter. Obviously this unifollicular pattern differs from subacute thyroiditis pattern. (Hematoxylin-eosin; magnification × 250.)

studies showed numerous desmosomes in these cells. Further studies appear necessary to resolve this question of giant cell origin.

X. PAINLESS THYROIDITIS

The incidence of painless thyroiditis is estimated at 40% of all cases of the subacute form of the disease,[20] although the true incidence is unknown since patients with painless thyroiditis without goiter or with minimal symptoms do not come to medical attention. This form of the disease is postulated to occur in three settings: (a) painless thyroiditis, goiter and dominant mass, in which the diagnosis is made after surgery for suspected tumor,[9,28,158] (b) painless thyrotoxic thyroiditis,[20,95-97,109,110] and (c) painless nontoxic disease, a clinically unrecognizable disorder, the incidence of which remains unknown.[20]

Laboratory values separate subacute thyroiditis from Graves' disease, and in the former, divide painful from painless types.[20] Thus, although clinical evidence of hyperthyroidism is supported by serum thyroid function tests, radioiodine uptake is very low in subacute thyroiditis.[128,130-134] Weihl et al.[131] noted that T_3 levels are less elevated in either form of subacute thyroiditis than in classical Graves' disease. This distinction is essential for proper therapy.[20] Sedimentation rate is mildly elevated in the painless form but much more so in the classic form.[8,13,14,20,96,134] Thyroid autoantibodies are unmeasurable in painless thyroiditis by usually employed methods,[110] but are recognized in low titer in some patients with the classic disease.[20,129-134]

Since pathologic examination of such cases, limited to needle biopsy, has disclosed lymphocytic, not granulomatous inflammation, the possibility of painless thyroiditis representing a form of Hashimoto's disease was raised.[20,95-97,109] However, since lymphoid infiltration can be found in subacute thyroiditis especially late in the course and since no germinal center formation or Hurthle cell metaplasia is recognized in these biopsies, Volpe[20] maintains that they represent subacute thyroiditis. Support for this is obtained by the subsequent clinical course, lasting weeks to months, and final recovery without associated thyroid dysfunction. Additionally, no autoimmune paraphenomena have been described for painless thyroiditis as have been with Hashimoto's (chronic lymphocytic) thyroiditis, lending further credence to the opinion relating painless thyroiditis to the subacute variety.[20] However, the question continues to be unresolved.

XI. DIAGNOSIS AND DIFFERENTIAL DIAGNOSIS

A. Clinical

Usually, the difficulty in the diagnosis of subacute thyroiditis lies in the confusion between it and other types of thyroiditis, or between it and some nonthyroid condition. Volpe et al.[8] reviewed 56 patients with thyroiditis and found that a correct diagnosis was made initially in under 50%. Most often, subacute thyroiditis was mistaken for pharyngitis. Less common misdiagnoses included acute thyroiditis, hemorrhage into a nodular goiter or an adenoma, Hashimoto's disease, myxedema, and thyroid carcinoma.[4-21,39,44,49,98-101,104,107,159] Tonsillitis, Graves' disease, and globus hystericus may be mistaken as subacute thyroiditis.[98-103,107]

Subacute thyroiditis should be considered in anyone with dysphagia, soreness in the neck, or a lump in the thyroid. In thyroiditis, the sore throat is localized over the thyroid; this distinguishes this entity from true pharyngitis. Helpful hints pointing to thyroiditis include, absence of pharyngeal injection, absence of lymphadenopathy, and precise localization of the pain (point tenderness) by the patient.[14,20]

The history may serve as a useful guide to differentiate subacute thyroiditis from its mimickers. A prodrome may help distinguish the lesion from carcinoma, nodular goiter, idiopathic myxedema, or acute thyroiditis. Carotid body tumors and lymphadenopathy due to metastatic tumors or lymphoma usually have a more prolonged history, are rarely painful, and tend to produce extrathyroidal masses, predominantly.

Laboratory values may prove helpful also. Markedly depressed iodine uptake, elevated PBI, T_3, and T_4 point to subacute thyroiditis. Severe leukocytosis, marked increased erythrocyte sedimentation rate, and evidence of suppuration distinguish acute from subacute thyroiditis.[4-20,98-101,105,107,159,160] When the history, examination and laboratory data fail to clarify the diagnosis, needle or open biopsy will often yield diagnostic material.[46,47]

B. Pathological

The histologic picture of granulomatous inflammation is characteristic (Figures 1 to 4). Confusion with tuberculous or fungal infection should be eliminated by demonstration of organisms in the tissues[161-163] (see Chapter 3). Sarcoidosis rarely involves the thyroid, but if it does, the granulomas affect the interstitium, not the follicles; often lymph node, lung, and liver involvement is also present.[164-167]

Palpation thyroiditis[157] (see Figure 5 in Chapter 5) can be confused with subacute thyroiditis but in the former, the lesions are isolated and focal, whereas in the subacute disease, the lesion is zonal or diffuse. In the latter, inflammatory cells other than histiocytes are prominent as is fibrosis.

XII. THERAPY

Early forms of treatment for subacute thyroiditis involved the use of antibiotics, thyroid hormone, and thyrotropin. None of these modalities has been efficacious.[4-20] The rationale for the use of antibiotics is wanting since it is known that the disease is not of bacterial etiology.[18,19] Thyroid hormones were instituted on the basis that they would suppress pituitary thyrotropin.[168] However, it seems that thyrotropin is already suppressed by the elevated level of circulating thyroid hormone.

Radiation therapy came into vogue in the 1950s.[13,14,169,170] Hazard[7] and Volpe[169] were supporters of this mode of treatment. Volpe advocated the use of relatively low doses of radiation (200 to 400 rads). Most authors, including Volpe,[8,169] admitted to at least a 25% failure rate with the use of radiotherapy. In recent years there is an understandable reluctance to use radiation in treating a benign self-limiting disease;[19,29] permanent hypothyroidism may occur[13,29] and the danger of the subsequent development of carcinoma must also be considered.[171]

Mild cases of subacute thyroiditis may respond to the usual antiinflammatory agents: aspirin, indomethacin, and phenylbutazone[4-21,107,172] have been used with good results in some patients, especially in mild and painless forms. The use of triodothyronine may relieve symptoms in some cases[131,173] although many authors disagree.[20] Volpe[20] and others[13,14,170] suggest its use in preventing recurrences in those cases where reexacerbation occurs.

For symptomatic relief in severe cases, the therapy of choice today is corticosteroids.[13,14,17,19,20,107,143,151,168] These drugs provide rapid relief of symptoms. Within 24 hr, the gland may no longer be tender or painful. The general feeling of malaise that makes up part of the symptom complex of this disease also disappears. The usual starting dosage is 10 mg prednisone every 6 hr; this dosage is maintained for a week, after which tapering can begin. Usually this therapy must be maintained for a period of several months to prevent rebound.[20] Surgery is rarely needed in treatment of this disorder. The place of surgery appears to lie in those cases where the diagnosis is doubtful and a tumor is suspected.[5,7-9,13,14,17,19,28,36]

XIII. OUTCOME AND PROGNOSIS

Full recovery is the rule in most cases (over 95%) of subacute thyroiditis with return of normal thyroid function clinically and chemically.[15,20] Even with minimal or no therapy, the disease is self-limited. Rarely, permanent hypothyroidism may ensue.[15,173] Much less often, hyperthyroidism may occur.[9,114,174,175]

XIV. ASSOCIATIONS WITH OTHER DISEASES

A. Thyroidal

Some authors have described subacute thyroiditis as a precursor lesion to Hashimoto's or Riedel's disease.[14,54,176-178] However, recent work delineating and defining these disorders as distinct clinicopathologic entities has indicated that these conditions are unrelated and separate.[13,14,17-19,98-101,107,114] Rare instances of hypothyroidism following subacute thyroiditis may occur after severe cases and probably reflect extensive glandular scarring.[9,173]

B. Extrathyroidal

No specific nonthyroid disorder has been associated with subacute thyroiditis. Unlike Hashimoto's disease in which associated "autoimmune phenomena" in organs such as adrenal, stomach, and liver, may be found, subacute thyroiditis shows no consistent associations.[14,17,19]

XV. SUMMARY

Subacute thyroiditis is a benign self-limited disorder often following a viral upper-respiratory infection and suspected of having a viral etiology. Recent work has shown antibodies to various viral species in the majority of patients with this disease. A preponderance of a certain HLA-haplotype has been recognized (BW 35), suggesting a certain genetic composition predisposing the host's response to a specific pathogen.

The pathologic features of this disorder are characteristic. Clinically, the disorder which ranges from classic to mild and even painless or silent forms, shows four phases of varied degrees of severity.

Diagnosis by clinical or laboratory features is often not difficult; needle biopsy or cytology may be diagnostic. Therapy reflects the severity of the disease with salicylates or other antiinflammatory agents sufficient for most patients; steroids can be used for severe cases.

REFERENCES

1. de Quervain, F. and Giordanengo, G., Die akute und subakute thyreoditis, *Mitt Grenzgeb. Med. Chir.*, 44, 538, 1935.
2. Jaffe, R. H., Tubercle-like structures in human goiters, *Arch. Surg. Chicago*, 21, 717, 1930.
3. Crile, G., Thyroiditis, *Ann. Surg.*, 127, 640, 1948.
4. Crile, G. and Rumsey, E. W., Subacute thyroiditis, *JAMA*, 142, 458, 1950.
5. Lindsay, S. and Dailey, M. E., Granulomatous or giant cell thyroiditis; clinical and pathologic study of 37 patients, *Surg. Gynecol. Obstet.*, 98, 197, 1954.
6. Fraser, R. and Harrison, R. J., Subacute thyroiditis, *Lancet*, 1, 382, 1952.
7. Hazard, J. B., Thyroiditis: a review, *Am. J. Clin. Pathol.*, 25, 289, 399, 1955.
8. Volpe, R. and Johnson, M. W., Subacute thyroiditis: a disease commonly mistaken for pharyngitis, *Can. Med. Assoc. J.*, 77, 297, 1957.
9. Woolner, L. B., McConahey, W. M., and Beahrs, O. H., Granulomatous thyroiditis (de Quervain's thyroiditis), *J. Clin. Endocrinol. Metab.*, 17, 1202, 1957.
10. Steinberg, F. V., Subacute granulomatous thyroiditis: a review, *Ann. Intern. Med.*, 52, 1014, 1960.
11. Skillern, P. G., Thyroiditis, in *The Thyroid Gland*, II, Pitt-Rivers, R. and Trotter, W. R., Eds., Butterworths, Inc., Washington, 1964, 130.
12. Furszyfer, J., McConahey, W. M., Wahner, H. W., and Kurland, L. T., Subacute (granulomatous) thyroiditis in Olmsted county, *Mayo Clin. Proc.*, 45, 396, 1970.
13. Green, J. N., Subacute thyroiditis, *Am. J. Med.*, 51, 97, 1971.
14. Bastenie, P. A., Bonnyns, M., and Neve, P., Subacute and chronic granulomatous thyroiditis, in *Thyroiditis and Thyroid Function, Clinical, Morphological and Physiological Studies*, Bastenie, P. A. and Ermans, A. M., Eds., Pergamon Press, Oxford, 1972, 69.
15. Volpe, R., Thyroiditis: current views of pathogenesis, *Med. Clin. North Am.*, 59, 1163, 1975.
16. DeGroot, L. J. and Stanbury, J. B., *The Thyroid and Its Diseases*, John Wiley and Sons, New York, 1975, 572.
17. Hurley, J. R., Thyroiditis, *Disease-a-Month*, December 1977.
18. Volpe, R., Acute and subacute thyroiditis, *Pharmacol. Ther. C.*, 1, 171, 1976.
19. Volpe, R., Subacute (nonsuppurative) thyroiditis, in *The Thyroid*, Werner, S. C. and Ingbar, S. H., Eds., Harper and Row, New York, 1978, 986.
20. Volpe, R., Subacute (de Quervain's) thyroiditis, *Clin. Endocrinol. Metab.*, 8, 81, 1979.
21. DePauw, B. E. and DeRooy, H. A. M., de Quervain's subacute thyroiditis, *Neth. J. Med.*, 18, 70, 1975.
22. Mygind, H., Thyroiditis akuta simplex, *Hosp. Tjbenk.*, 2, 1181, 1895.

23. de Quervain, F., Die akute, nicht eiterige Thyreoditis und die Beteilgung der Schilddruse an akuten Intoxikationen und Infektionen uberhaupt, *Mitt. Grenzgeb. Med. Chir.*, 2, (Suppl.), 1, 1904.
24. Giordenengo, G., Acute non-suppurative thyroiditis, *Lancet*, 1, 1144, 1938.
25. Stalker, L. K. and Walther, C. D., Thyroiditis, *Am. J. Surg.*, 82, 381, 1951.
26. Osmond, J. D. and Portman, U. V., Subacute (pseudotuberculous giant cell) thyroiditis and its treatment, *Am. J. Roentgenol.*, 61, 826, 1949.
27. Werner, S. C. and Ingbar, S. H., *The Thyroid,* Harper and Row, New York, 1978.
28. Harland, W. A. and Frantz, V. K., Clinicopathologic study of 261 surgical cases of so-called thyroiditis, *J. Clin. Endocrinol.*, 17, 1202, 1957.
29. Hendrick, J. W., Diagnosis and management of thyroiditis, *JAMA,* 164, 127, 1967.
30. Kinney, F. J. and Herrmann, R. E., Increasing occurrence of thyroiditis in Rocky Mountain area, *Rocky Mount. Med. J.*, 59, 35, 1962.
31. Jackson, A. S. and Gilman, L. C., Thyroiditis, *Am. J. Surg.*, 88, 891, 1954.
32. Chesky, V. E., Dreese, W. C., and Hellwig, C. A., Chronic thyroiditis. Supravital studies of surgical goiter specimens, *Surg. Gynecol. Obstet.*, 93, 575, 1957.
33. Lindsay, S., Dailey, M. E., Friedlander, J., Yee, G., and Soley, M. H., Chronic thyroiditis. A clinical and pathological study of 354 patients, *J. Clin. Endocrinol.*, 12, 1578, 1952.
34. Meachim, G. and Young, M. H., de Quervain's subacute granulomatous thyroiditis: histological identification and incidence, *J. Clin. Pathol.*, 16, 189, 1963.
35. Young, M. H. and Meachim, G., Surgical pathology of thyroid disease — a 7 year survey in Sheffield, *Br. J. Surg.*, 51, 497, 1964.
36. Woolner, L. B., McConahey, W. M., and Beahrs, O. H., The surgical aspects of thyroiditis, *Am. J. Surg.*, 104, 666, 1962.
37. Marshall, S. F., Meissner, W. A., and Smith, D. C., Chronic thyroiditis, *N. Engl. J. Med.*, 238, 758, 1948.
38. Marchetta, F. C. and Bender, M. A., Radioactive iodine uptake and localization studies with a scintiscanner in subacute thyroiditis, *N.Y. State J. Med.*, 56, 1951, 1956.
39. Lewitus, Z., Rechnic, J., and Lubin, E., Sequential scanning of the thyroid as an aid in diagnosis of subacute thyroiditis, *Isr. J. Med. Sci.*, 3, 847, 1967.
40. Dorta, T. and Beraud, T., New studies on the subject of subacute thyroiditis, *Helv. Med. Acta*, 28, 19, 1961.
41. Rechnic, J. and Lewitus, Z., The value of scintigraphy of the thyroid in subacute thyroidits, *Proc. Beilinson Hosp.*, 8, 8, 1965.
42. Hintze, G., Lamberg, B. A., Wahlberg, P., and Malm, P., Radioiodine thyroid scanning as applied to thyroid problems in an endemic goiter region, *Acta Med. Scand.*, 171, 99, 1962.
43. DeWind, L. T., Reversible manifestations of thyroiditis, *JAMA,* 172, 158, 1960.
44. Hamburger, J. I., Kadian, G., and Rossin, H. W., Subacute thyroiditis — evaluation depicted by serial ^{131}I scintigrams, *J. Nucl. Med.*, 6, 560, 1965.
45. Blum, M., Passalagua, A. M., Sackler, J. P., and Pudlowski, R., Thyroid echography of subacute thyroiditis, *Radiology,* 125, 795, 1977.
46. Crile, G. and Hazard, J. B., Classification of thyroiditis with special reference to the use of needle biopsy, *J. Clin. Endocrinol.*, 11, 1123, 1951.
47. Wang, C., Vickery, A. L., and Maloof, F., Needle biopsy of the thyroid, *Surg. Gynecol. Obstet.*, 143, 365, 1976.
48. Blonde, L., Witkin, M., and Harris, R., Painless subacute thyroiditis simulating Graves' disease, *West. J. Med.*, 125, 75, 1976.
49. Stein, A. A., Hernandez, I., and McClintock, J. C., Subacute granulomatous thyroiditis: a clinicopathologic review, *Ann. Surg.*, 153, 149, 1961.
50. Hamburger, J. I., Occult subacute thyroiditis — diagnostic challenge, *Mich. Med.*, 70, 1125, 1971.
51. Woolf, P. D. and Daly, R., Thyrotoxicosis with painless thyroiditis, *Am. J. Med.*, 60, 73, 1976.
52. DeCourcy, J. L., Perithyroiditis. A distinct entity, *JAMA,* 123, 397, 1943.
53. DeCourcy, J. L., Etiologic factors in Riedel's struma: possible roles of perithyroiditis and ischemia, *Trans. Am. Goiter Assoc.*, 225, 1949.
54. Chopra, D., Wool, M. S., Crosson, A., and Sawin, C. T., Riedel's struma associated with subacute thyroiditis, hypothyroidism and hypoparathyroidism, *J. Clin. Endocrinol. Metab.*, 46, 869, 1978.
55. Ferguson, J. A., Tissue reaction to colloid and lipoids from the human thyroid gland, *Arch. Pathol.*, 15, 244, 1933.
56. Hamilton, H. E., Kirkendall, W. M., and Barker, S. B., Radioactive iodine uptake of thyroid and protein bound iodine in subacute thyroiditis, *J. Clin. Invest.*, 29, 819, 1950.
57. Robbins, J., Rall, J. E., Trunnell, J. B., and Rawsson, R. W., Effect of thyroid stimulating hormone in acute thyroiditis, *J. Clin. Endocrinol.*, 11, 1106, 1951.

58. **Larson, P. R.,** Serum triiodothyronine, thyroxine, and thyrotropin during hyperthyroid, hypothyroid and recovery phases of subacute, non-suppurative thyroiditis, *Metabolism,* 23, 467, 1974.
59. **McQuillan, A. S.,** Thyroiditis, Trans Third International Goitre Conference, Washington, D.C., 212, 1939.
60. **Sein, M.,** Acute nonsuppurative thyroiditis, *Lancet,* 2, 673, 1938.
61. **Somlo, F. M. and Kovalik, M.,** Acute thyroiditis in a patient with Q fever, *Can. Med. Assoc. J.,* 95, 1091, 1966.
62. **Shumway, M. and Davis, P. L.,** Catscratch thyroiditis treated with thyrotropic hormone, *J. Clin. Endocrinol. Metab.,* 14, 742, 1954.
63. **Eylan, E., Zmucky, R., and Sheba, C.,** Mumps virus and subacute thyroiditis — evidence of a causal association, *Lancet,* 1, 1062, 1957.
64. **Eyquem, A., Calmattes, C., and Decourt, J.,** Etude immunologique d'un goitre de Hashimoto consecutif a une thyuroidite ourlienne, *Rev. Fr. Etud. Clin. Biol.,* 4, 823, 1959.
65. **Felix-Davies, D.,** Auto-immunization in subacute thyroiditis, *Lancet,* 1, 880, 1958.
66. **Hung, W.,** Mumps thyroiditis and hypothyroidism, *J. Pediatr.,* 74, 611, 1969.
67. **Lyon, E.,** Die subakut mumps Thyreoiditis und ihre Behandlung, *Med. Klin. Munich,* 62, 208, 1967.
68. **McArthur, A. M.,** Subacute giant cell thyroiditis associated with mumps, *Med. J. Aust.,* 1, 116, 1964.
69. **Sheba, C. and Bank, H.,** Prevention of mumps thyroiditis, *N. Engl. J. Med.,* 279, 108, 1968.
70. **Candel, S.,** Acute non-suppurative thyroiditis following measles, *U.S. Nav. Med. Bull.,* 46, 1109, 1946.
71. **Robertson, W. S.,** Acute inflammation of the thyroid gland, *Lancet,* 1, 930, 1911.
72. **Saito, S.,** Clinical studies on subacute thyroiditis, *Gumma J. Med. Sci.,* 8 (Suppl. 17), 1, 1959.
73. **Liberman, U., Djaldetti, M., and deVries, A.,** A case of herpangina, pleurodynia and subacute thyroiditis, *Harefuah,* 67, 343, 1964.
74. **Hintze, G., Fortelius, P., and Railo, J.,** Epidemic thyroiditis, *Acta Endocrinol.,* 45, 381, 1964.
75. **Mosonyi, L.,** Thyroiditis, *Br. Med. J.,* 1, 1132, 1960.
76. **Swann, N. H.,** Acute thyroiditis: five cases associated with adenovirus infection, *Metabolism,* 13, 908, 1964.
77. **Fennell, J. S. and Tomkin, G. H.,** Subacute thyroiditis and hepatitis in a case of infectious mononucleosis, *Postgrad. Med. J.,* 54, 351, 1978.
78. **McWhinney, I. R.,** Incidence of de Quervain's thyroiditis: ten cases from one general practice, *Br. Med. J.,* 1, 1225, 1964.
79. **Goldman, J., Bockna, A. J., and Becker, F. O.,** St. Louis encephalitis and subacute thyroiditis, *Ann. Intern. Med.,* 87, 250, 1977.
80. **Volpe, R., Row, V. V., and Ezrin, C.,** Circulating viral and thyroid antibodies in subacute thyroiditis, *J. Clin. Endocrinol. Metab.,* 27, 1275, 1967.
81. **Stancekova, M., Stancek, D., Ciampor, F., Mucha, V., and Hnilica, P.,** Morphological, cytological and biological observations on viruses isolated from patients with subacute thyroiditis of de Quervain, *Acta Virol. Praha,* 20, 183, 1976.
82. **Stancek, D. and Gressnerova, M.,** A viral agent isolated from a patient with subacute de Quervain type thyroiditis, *Acta Virol. Praha,* 18, 365, 1974.
83. **Stancek, D., Stancekova-Gressnerova, M., Janotka, M., Hnilica, P., and Oravec, D.,** Isolation and some serological and epidemiological data on the viruses recovered from patients with subacute thyroiditis de Quervain, *Med. Microbiol. Immunol.,* 161, 133, 1975.
84. **Nyulassy, S., Hnilica, P., Buc, M., Guman, M., Hirschova, V., and Stefanovic, J.,** Subacute (de Quervain's) thyroiditis: association with HLA-BW 35 antigen and abnormalities of the complement system, immunoglobulins and other serum proteins, *J. Clin. Endocrinol. Metab.,* 45, 270, 1977.
85. **Buc, M., Nyulassy, S., Hnilica, P., and Stefanovic, J.,** HLA-BW 35 and subacute de Quervain's thyroiditis, *Diabete Metab.,* 2, 163, 1976.
86. **Nyulassy, S., Hnilica, P., and Stefanovic, J.,** The HL-A system and subacute thyroiditis. A preliminary report, *Tissue Antigens,* 6, 105, 1975.
87. **Majsky, A. and Feix, C.,** HLA-BW 35 antigen and subacute thyroiditis, *Tissue Antigens,* 9, 173, 1977.
88. **Mukhtar, E. D., Smith, B. R., Pyle, G. A., Hall, R., and Vici, P.,** Relation of thyroid-stimulating immunoglobulins to thyroid function and effects of surgery, radioiodine and antithyroid drugs, *Lancet,* 1, 13, 1975.
89. **Hashizume, K., Roudebush, C. P., Fenzi, G., and DeGroot, L. J.,** Effect of antithyroid therapy on thyroid stimulating immunoglobulin (TSI) in Graves' disease, Abstr. presented at Proc. Am. Thyroid Assoc. 53rd Meeting, Cleveland, September 1977.
90. **Strakasch, C. R., Joyner, D., and Wall, J. R.,** Thyroid stimulating antibodies in patients with subacute thyroiditis, *J. Clin. Endocrinol. Metab.,* 46, 345, 1978.

91. Sugenoya, A., Kidd, A., Silverberg, J., Row, V. V., and Volpe, R., A comparison of the radioligand technique and the cellular stimulation technique for the demonstration of thyroid stimulating immunoglobulins, Abstract presented at Proc. Endocrinol. Soc., Miami, Fla., June 1978.
92. Delespesse, G., Duchateau, J., Kennes, B., Govaerts, A., and Bastenie, P. A., The leukocyte migration test in human thyroid autoimmunity, *Horm. Metab. Res.*, 5, 176, 1973.
93. Wall, J. R., Fang, S. L., Ingbar, S. H., and Braverman, L. E., Lymphocyte transformation in response to human thyroid extract in patients with subacute thyroiditis, *J. Clin. Endocrinol. Metab.*, 43, 587, 1976.
94. Czernick, P. and Steinberg, A. H., The chronology of events in the development of subacute thyroiditis studied by radioactive iodine, *J. Clin. Endocrinol.*, 17, 1448, 1957.
95. Papapetrou, P. D. and Jackson, I. M., Thyrotoxicosis due to "silent" thyroiditis, *Lancet*, 1, 361, 1975.
96. Morrison, J. and Caplan, R. H., Typical and atypical ('silent') subacute thyroiditis in a wife and husband, *Arch. Intern. Med.*, 138, 45, 1978.
97. Gegick, C. G. and Herring, W. B., Painless subacute thyroiditis, *N. C. Med. J.*, 38, 387, 1977.
98. Bergen, S. S., Acute nonsuppurative thyroiditis. A report of 12 cases and review of the literature, *Arch. Intern. Med.*, 102, 747, 1958.
99. Guerrero, R. A., Subacute diffuse thyroiditis, *Minn. Med.*, 47, 585, 1964.
100. Lamberg, B. A., Hintze, G., Jussila, R., and Berlin, M., Subacute thyroiditis, *Acta Endocrinol.*, 33, 457, 1960.
101. Brown, D. E., Subacute thyroiditis with a discussion of other types of thyroiditis, *Ann. Otol.*, 65, 595, 1956.
102. Tolman, D. E., Gibilisco, J. A., and McConahey, W. M., Subacute thyroiditis. A diagnostic possibility for the dentist, *Oral Surg.*, 15, 293, 1962.
103. Smith, M. J. and Myall, R. W., Subacute thyroiditis as a cause of facial pain, *Oral Surg.*, 43, 59, 1977.
104. Saito, S., Studies on subacute thyroiditis, *Endocrinol. Jpn.*, 11, 119, 1964.
105. Frid, G. and Wijnbladh, H., Subacute thyroiditis, struma lymphomatosa, and chronic invasive goiter (Riedel's disease). A clinical study based on a 20 year series of 83 cases, *Acta Chir. Scand.*, 12, 170, 1957.
106. Lasser, R. P. and Grayzel, D. M., Subacute thyroiditis, struma fibrosa, struma lymphomatosa: a clinicopathologic study, *Am. J. Med. Sci.*, 217, 518, 1949.
107. Schultz, A. L., Subacute diffuse thyroiditis. Clinical and laboratory findings in 24 patients and the effect of treatment with adrenal corticoids, *Postgrad. Med.*, 29, 76, 1961.
108. Jackson, I. M. D., "Hyper-thyroiditis" — a diagnostic pitfall, *N. Engl. J. Med.*, 293, 661, 1975.
109. Gluck, F. B., Nusynowitz, M. L., and Plymate, S., Chronic lymphocytic thyroiditis, thyrotoxicosis and low radioactive iodine uptake, *N. Engl. J. Med.*, 293, 624, 1975.
110. Dorfman, S. G., Cooperman, M. T., Nelson, R. L., Depuy, H., Peake, R. L., and Yonge, R. L., Painless thyroiditis and transient hyperthyroidism without goiter, *Ann. Intern. Med.*, 86, 24, 1977.
111. Jensen, D. R., Acute thyroiditis complicating scarlet fever, *Am. J. Surg.*, 60, 301, 1946.
112. Beckman, H., Subacute thyroiditis, *Wis. Med. J.*, 68, 302, 1969.
113. Danowsi, T. S., Mateer, F. M., Weigle, W. O., Borecky, D. C., and Moses, C., Thyroiditis following administration of thyroid stimulating hormone, *J. Clin. Endocrinol.*, 20, 1521, 1960.
114. Perloff, W. H., Thyrotoxicosis following acute thyroiditis, *J. Clin. Endocrinol.*, 16, 542, 1956.
115. St. John, J. H. and Nicholson, W. M., An evaluation of the treatment of thyroiditis, *South. Med. J.*, 44, 1059, 1951.
116. Thomas, W. C., Anderson, R. M., Jurkiewicz, M. J., Araujo, J. D., and Blizzard, R. M., Clinical studies in thyroiditis, *Ann. Intern. Med.*, 63, 808, 1965.
117. Weinstein, M., Soto, R. J., Flaster, H., and Brunengo, A. M., Radioiodine uptake in subacute thyroiditis developing in an environment of endemic goiter, *Acta Endocrinol. Copenhagen*, 56, 585, 1967.
118. McConahey, W. M. and Keating, F. R., Radioiodine studies in thyroiditis, *J. Clin. Endocrinol.*, 11, 1116, 1951.
119. Hagan, A. D., Goffinet, J., and Davis, J. W., Acute streptococcal thyroiditis, *JAMA*, 202, 842, 1967.
120. Schlicke, C. P., Hill, J. E., and Arguinchona, H. B., Thyroiditis, *Northwest Med.*, 64, 345, 1965.
121. Schlicke, C. P., Thyroiditis, *Arch. Surg.*, 63, 656, 1951.
122. Gordin, A. and Lamberg, B. A., Serum thyrotropin response to thyrotrophin releasing hormone and the concentration of free thyroxine in subacute thyroiditis, *Acta Endocrinol.*, 74, 111, 1973.
123. Ogihara, T., Yamamoto, T., Azukizawa, M., Miyai, K., and Kumahara, Y., Serum thyrotrophin and thyroid hormones in the course of subacute thyroiditis, *J. Clin. Endocrinol. Metab.*, 37, 602, 1973.

124. Staub, J. J., TRH test in subacute thyroiditis, *Lancet,* 1, 868, 1975.
125. Demeester-Mirkine, N., Brauman, H., and Corvilain, J., Delayed adjustment of the pituitary response in circulating thyroid hormones in a case of subacute thyroiditis, *Clin. Endocrinol.,* 5, 9, 1976.
126. Lebacq, E. G., Therasse, G., Schmitz, A., Delannoy, A., and Destailleurs, C., Subacute thyroiditis, *Acta Endocrinol.,* 81, 707, 1976.
127. Werner, S. C., Quimby, E. H., and Schmidt, C., The use of tracer doses of radioactive iodine, ^{131}I, in the study of normal and disordered thyroid function in man, *J. Clin. Endocrinol.,* 9, 342, 1949.
128. Jeffries, W. M., Kelly, L. W., Levy, R. P., Cooper, G. W., and Prouty, R. L., The significance of low thyroid reserve, *J. Clin. Endocrinol.,* 16, 1438, 1956.
129. Towerly, B. T., A study of idiopathic subacute thyroiditis, *J. Clin. Endocrinol.,* 16, 982, 1956.
130. Ingbar, S. H. and Freinkel, N., Thyroid function and the metabolism of iodine in patients with subacute thyroiditis, *Arch. Intern. Med.,* 101, 339, 1958.
131. Weihl, A. C., Daniels, G. H., Ridgway, E. C., and Maloof, F., Thyroid function tests during the early phase of subacute thyroiditis, *J. Clin. Endocrinol. Metab.,* 44, 1107, 1977.
132. Izumi, M. and Larsen, P. R., Correlation of sequential changes in serum thyroglobulin, triiodothyronine and thyroxine in patients with Graves' disease and subacute thyroiditis, *Metabolism,* 27, 449, 1978.
133. Ginsberg, J. and Walfish, P. G., Postpartum transient thyrotoxicosis with painless thyroiditis, *Lancet,* 1, 1125, 1977.
134. Volpe, R., Johnston, M. W., and Huber, N., Thyroid function in subacute thyroiditis, *J. Clin. Endocrinol.,* 18, 65, 1958.
135. Skillern, P. G. and Lewis, L. A., Fractionated plasma protein values in subacute thyroiditis, *J. Clin. Endocrinol.,* 18, 1407, 1958.
136. Giordanengo, G., Acute nonsuppurative thyroiditis, *Lancet,* 1, 1144, 1938.
137. Skillern, P. G., Nelson, H. E., and Crile, G., Jr., Some new observations on subacute thyroiditis, *J. Clin. Endocrinol.,* 16, 1422, 1956.
138. Crile, G., Thyroiditis, *Ann. Intern. Med.,* 37, 519, 1952.
139. Vogt, J. H., Subacute thyroiditis with elevated serum alkaline phosphatase level, *Acta Endocrinol.,* 34, 256, 1960.
140. Stemmermann, G. N., Serum protein changes in subacute thyroiditis, *JAMA,* 162, 31, 1956.
141. Weissman, N. and Perlmutter, M., An electrophoretic study of serum proteins in thyroiditis, *J. Clin. Invest.,* 36, 780, 1957.
142. Fui, S. N. T. and Jeffreys, D. B., Subacute autoimmune thyroiditis simulating de Quervain's thyroiditis, *Lancet,* 1, 622, 1979.
143. Izak, G. and Stein, Y., Subacute nonsuppurative thyroiditis. Treatment with cortisone and corticotrophin, *Lancet,* 1, 225, 1956.
144. Hunter, R. C. and Sheehan, D. J., Treatment of subacute thyroiditis with cortisone, *N. Engl. J. Med.,* 251, 174, 1954.
145. Danyluk, J. M., Stirrat, J. H., and Laskin, M. M., Subacute (granulomatous) thyroiditis associated with granulomatous changes in adjacent lymph nodes, *Can. Med. Assoc. J.,* 100, 388, 1969.
146. Woolner, L. B., Thyroiditis: classification and clinicopathologic correlation, in *The Thyroid,* Hazard, J. B. and Smith, D. E., Eds., Williams & Wilkins, Baltimore, 1964, 123.
147. Persson, P. S., Cytodiagnosis of thyroiditis: a comparative study of cytological, histological, immunological and clinical findings in thyroiditis, particularly in diffuse lymphoid thyroiditis, *Acta Med. Scand. Suppl.,* 483, 7, 1967.
148. Saito, S., Needle biopsy of thyroid, especially in thyroiditis, *Gumma J. Med. Sci.,* 12, 304, 1963.
149. Mahadev, V., Dharmalingam, S. K., Tan, D., Narasimba, L., Lob, C. W., and Tschang, T. T., Subacute (de Quervain's) thyroiditis — study of seven cases, *Med. J. Malay.,* 31, 331, 1977.
150. Totterman, V. H., Gordin, A., Hayry, P., Andersson, L. C., and Makinen, T., Accumulation of thyroid antigen-reactive T lymphocytes in the gland of patients with subacute thyroiditis, *Clin. Exp. Immunol.,* 32, 153, 1978.
151. Mariano, M. and Spector, W. G., The formation and properties of macrophage polykaryons (inflammatory giant cells), *J. Pathol.,* 113, 1, 1974.
152. Reidbord, H. E. and Fisher, E. R., Ultrastructural features of subacute granulomatous thyroiditis and Hashimoto's disease, *Am. J. Clin. Pathol.,* 59, 327, 1973.
153. Neve, P., Ultrastructure of the thyroid in de Quervain's subacute granulomatous thyroiditis, *Virch. Arch. B.,* 351, 87, 1970.
154. Goetsch, E., Origin, evolution and significance of giant cells in Riedel's struma, *Arch. Surg.,* 41, 308, 1940.
155. Satoh, M., Virus-like particles in the follicular epithelium of the thyroid from a patient with subacute thyroiditis (de Quervain), *Acta Pathol. Jpn.,* 25, 449, 1975.

156. **Satoh, M.,** Ultrastructure of the giant cell in de Quervain's subacute thyroiditis, *Acta Pathol. Jpn.,* 26, 133, 1976.
157. **Carney, J. A., Moore, S. B., Northcutt, R. C., Woolner, L. B., and Stillwell, G. K.,** Palpation thyroiditis (multifocal granulomatous folliculitis), *Am. J. Clin. Pathol.,* 64, 639, 1975.
158. **Volpe, R.,** Pathology of thyroiditis, *Hum. Pathol.,* 9, 429, 1978.
159. **Rosenbaum, H. and Reveno, W. S.,** Subacute thyroiditis. Difficulties in diagnosis and treatment, *Harper Hosp. Bull.,* 19, 1. 1961.
160. **Volpe, R.,** Acute suppurative thyroiditis, in *The Thyroid,* Werner, S. C. and Ingbar, S. H., Eds., Harper and Row, New York, 1971, 899.
161. **Jaffe, R. H.,** Tubercle-like structures in human goiters, *Arch. Surg.,* 21, 719, 1930.
162. **Klassen, K. P. and Curtis, G. M.,** Tuberculous abscess of the thyroid gland, *Surgery,* 17, 552, 1945.
163. **Goldfarb, H., Schifrin, D., and Graig, F. A.,** Thyroiditis cased by tuberculous abscess of the thyroid gland, *Am. J. Med.,* 38, 825, 1965.
164. **Thompson, W. D., McGrouther, D. A., and Stockdell, G.,** Thyrotoxicosis with sarcoid-like granulomata, *J. Pathol.,* 111, 289, 1973.
165. **Lender, M. and Dollberg, L.,** Coincidence of sarcoidosis and Hashimoto's thyroiditis, *Am. Rev. Respir. Dis.,* 112, 113, 1975.
166. **von Knorring, J. and Selroos, O.,** Sarcoidosis with thyroid involvement, polymyalgia rheumatica and breast carcinoma, *Scand. J. Rheumatol.,* 5, 77, 1976.
167. **Karlish, A. J. and MacGregor, G. A.,** Sarcoidosis, thyroiditis and Addison's disease, *Lancet,* 2, 330, 1970.
168. **Higgins, H. P., Bayley, T. A., and Diosy, A.,** Suppression of endogenous TSH: a treatment of subacute thyroiditis, *J. Clin. Endocrinol. Metab.,* 23, 235, 1963.
169. **Crile, G. and Schneider, R. W.,** Diagnosis and treatment of thyroiditis with special reference to the use of cortisone and ACTH, *Cleveland Clin. Q.,* 19, 219, 1952.
170. **Volpe, R.,** Treatment of thyroiditis, *Mod. Treatment.,* 6, 474, 1969.
171. **Wolfish, P. G. and Volpe, R.,** Irradiation related thyroid cancer, *Ann. Intern. Med.,* 88, 261, 1978.
172. **Torikai, T. and Kumaoka, S.,** Subacute thyroiditis treated with salicylate: report of 5 cases, *N. Engl. J. Med.,* 259, 1265, 1958.
173. **Ivy, H. K.,** Permanent myxedema: an unusual complication of granulomatous thyroiditis, *J. Clin. Endocrinol.,* 21, 1384, 1961.
174. **Sheets, R. F.,** The sequential occurrence of acute thyroiditis and thyrotoxicosis, *JAMA,* 157, 139, 1955.
175. **Werner, S. C.,** Graves' disease following acute (subacute) thyroiditis, *Arch. Intern. Med.,* 139, 1313, 1979.
176. **Bastenie, P.,** Etude anatomo-clinique et experimentale des inflammations chroniques et des scleroses du corps thyoide, *Arch. Int. Med. Exp.,* 12, 1, 1937.
177. **Lee, J. G.,** Chronic nonspecific thyroiditis, *Arch. Surg. Chicago,* 31, 982, 1936.
178. **Weyeneth, R.,** Die nicht spezifischen Entzundungen der Schilddruse mit besonderer Berucksichtigung der Riesenzellthyreoiditis Typus de Quervain, *Arch. Klin. Chir.,* 201, 457, 1941.

Chapter 5

PALPATION THYROIDITIS

Virginia A. LiVolsi

TABLE OF CONTENTS

I.	Introduction	44
II.	Description	44
III.	Histology of Palpation Thyroiditis	44
IV.	Differential Diagnosis	44
V.	Pathogenesis of Palpation Thyroiditis	50
VI.	Significance of Palpation Thyroiditis	50
VII.	Summary	50
References		51

I. INTRODUCTION

Two major forms of granulomatous thyroiditis have been described in earlier chapters of this volume: infectious types (including mycobacteria and fungal granulomata involving the thyroid) and subacute thyroiditis. In 1975, Carney et al.[1] described multifocal granulomatous folliculitis or palpation thyroiditis, an entity which may produce confusion in histopathologic examination of the thyroid.

II. DESCRIPTION

These authors[1] noted that this lesion was not related to specific microbiologic or chemical factors, but rather resulted from trauma. Evidence for this conclusion was based on several facts elucidated by their study. First, the incidence of palpation thyroiditis in surgically resected thyroids exceeded 90%, whereas only 39% of autopsied patients who died in the hospital, and 0% of patients dying at home, showed the lesion. This marked difference in incidence was explained by the greater likelihood of surgically resected glands to have been subjected to physical examination. Similarly, in-hospital patients would have been more likely to have undergone physical examination (including palpation of the thyroid) than individuals who died at home without recent examination by a physician.[1]

The second piece of evidence for a traumatic cause for this type of thyroiditis was obtained from animal experiments. A histologic lesion, identical to palpation thyroiditis, was produced in anesthetized dogs by vigorous squeezing of the thyroid gland. In these animals, one lobe was used as the test and the opposite lobe as the control. The thyroiditis was identified only in the test lobes.[1] This result indicates strongly that the lesion was not caused by microbiologic or chemical agents whose effect would be expected to involve the entire gland.

Finally, Carney[1] and his colleagues noted that the severity of the lesion (number and size of foci) increased with the vigor and intensity of the palpation.*

Since the original description of this lesion, the present author has evaluated surgically resected thyroid glands and has identified palpation thyroiditis in 85% of such glands. In my own experience, the lesion has been found most often in glands removed for adenomatous nodules and papillary carcinoma. Palpation thyroiditis has been noted only rarely in routine sections of the gland at autopsy on hospital patients (less than 10% of cases), and has never been encountered in forensic autopsies performed on individuals dying suddenly (by accidental, suicidal, or homicidal means).

III. HISTOLOGY OF PALPATION THYROIDITIS

The lesion involves scattered isolated follicles, ranging from one to three. Initially, the lining cells swell and are replaced by a semicircumferential or circumferential collection of histiocytes, occasionally giant cells, lymphocytes, plasma cells, and probably altered follicular epithelium (Figure 1). Often, evidence of hemorrhage with blood or siderophages is noted. These lesions may occur in or near the follicular well, within the follicle, or in a perifollicular location (Figures 2, 3).

IV. DIFFERENTIAL DIAGNOSIS

The histologic differential diagnosis of palpation thyroiditis includes granulomatous

---

* It must be recalled that this trauma represents minor, minimal injury and needs to be distinguished from gross traumatic disruption of the gland.[2-5] The latter may produce a portal of entry for microorganisms, leading to acute suppurative thyroiditis and may prove fatal.[5]

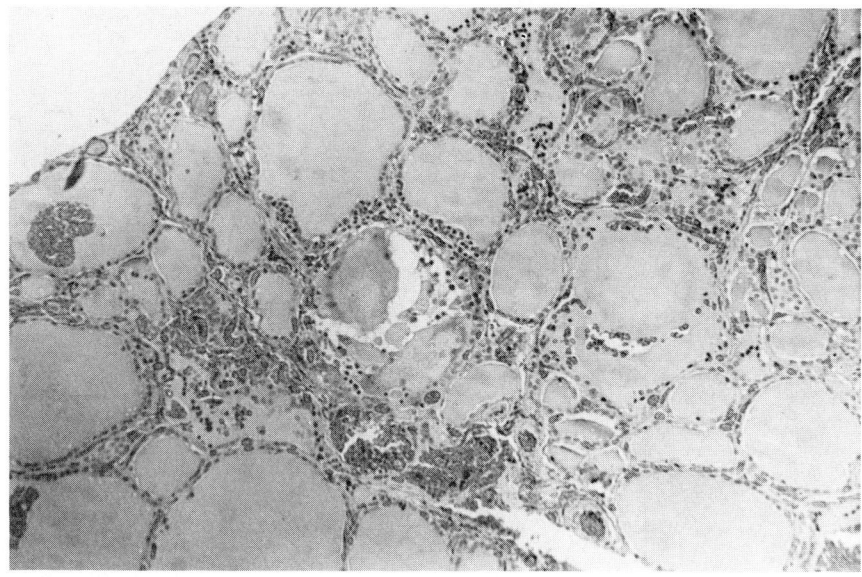

FIGURE 1. Low power view demonstrates relatively normal thyroid tissue in the center of which is one follicle affected by palpation thyroiditis. Note giant cell formation and follicular disruption. This gland was removed at the time of total laryngectomy for squamous carcinoma of the vocal cord. No thyroid pathology was found; no thyroid dysfunction had been identified clinically. (Hematoxylin-eosin; magnification × 125.)

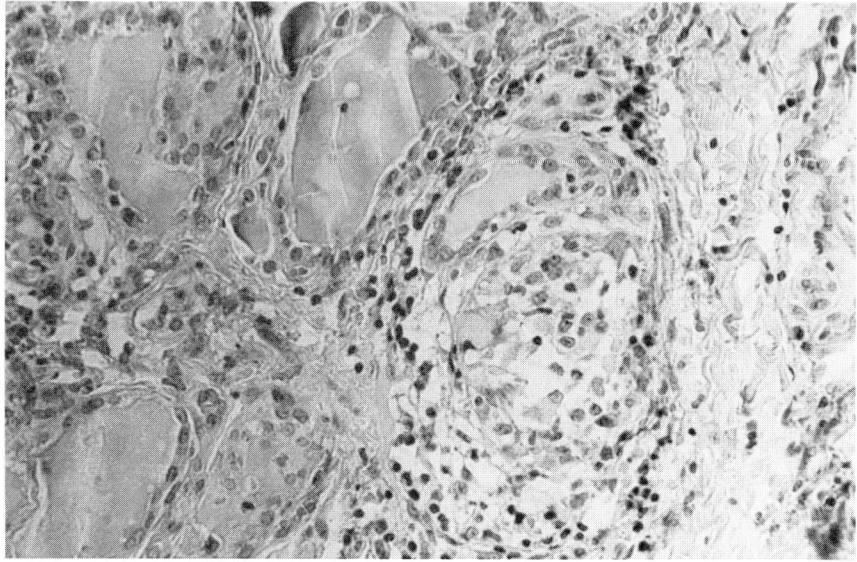

FIGURE 2. Higher power of another granulomatous focus in thyroid affected by nodular goiter. Note histiocytes, lymphocytes, and plasma cells in a focus pushing a follicle superiorly. Giant cells are absent in this area. (Hematoxylin-eosin; magnification × 200.)

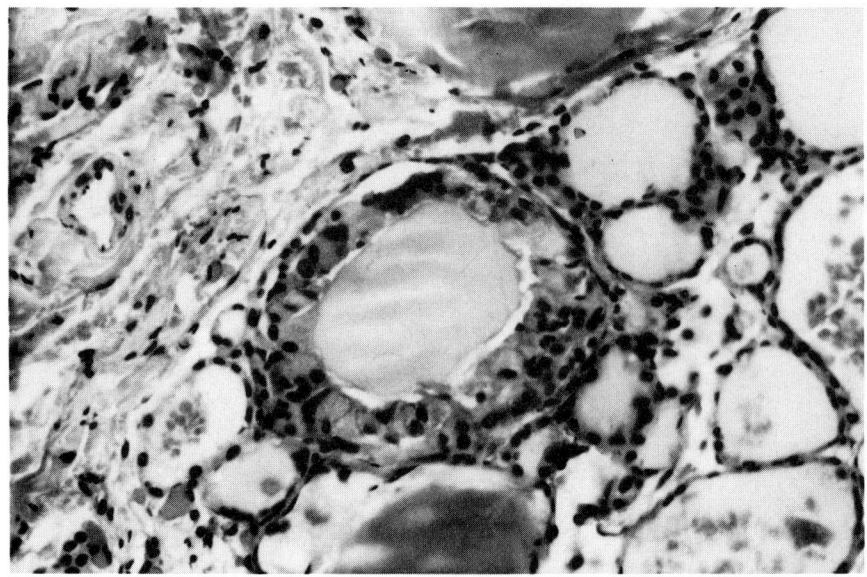

FIGURE 3. Circumferential follicular distribution of histiocytes is illustrated in this thyroid from a patient with papillary carcinoma elsewhere in the gland. (Hematoxylin-eosin; magnification × 250.)

Table 1
GRANULOMAS IN THE THYROID

Condition	Frequency
Palpation thyroiditis	Common
Histiocytic granulomatous inflammation around hemorrhage	Common
Subacute thyroiditis	Unusual
Tuberculosis	Very rare
Fungal thyroiditis	Rare
Sarcoidosis	Very rare
Granulomatous vasculitis	Very rare
Storage diseases	Very rare

thyroiditis of infectious etiology, necrotizing granulomatous vasculitides, subacute thyroiditis, Graves' disease, C-cell hyperplasia, desquamation of follicular cells (especially in autopsy specimens), tangential sectioning of follicular epithelium, colloidophagy, histiocytic reactions in areas of hemorrhage of adenomatous (nontoxic nodular) goiter, sarcoidosis, and storage diseases.[1] The distinction of these entities will be considered in Table 1.

Infectious granulomatous thyroiditis — This very rare condition should be easily distinguishable from palpation thyroiditis since, in the former, true granulomas are formed. These contain not only epithelioid histiocytes, but also lymphocytes and plasma cells; frequently, central necrosis is found. Special stains will disclose microorganisms (either tubercle bacilli or fungi) in these cases[6-8] (see Chapter 3).

Necrotizing granulomatous vasculitis — Necrotizing granulomatous vasculitis, such as that found in polyarteritis nodosa,[9] hypersensitivity states,[10] or Wegener's granulomatosis,[11] may rarely involve the thyroidal or perithyroidal vessels. The propensity

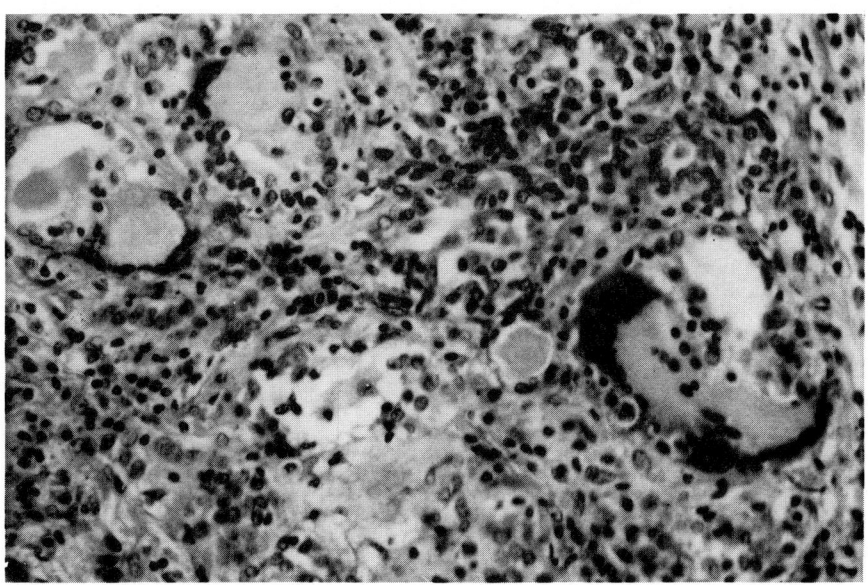

FIGURE 4. In subacute (? viral) thyroiditis numerous, multinucleated giant cells with more marked leukocytic and lymphoplasmacytic response is seen. Scant follicles are difficult to identify. The lesion of subacute thyroiditis is more extensive in size and intensity of the inflammatory component. (Hematoxylin-eosin; magnification × 250.)

for predominantly or exclusively vascular lesions, as well as the clinical recognition of a multisystem disorder, should easily differentiate this from palpation thyroiditis.

Subacute thyroiditis — This condition, discussed in Chapter 4, has certain clinical and laboratory findings which separate it from palpation thyroiditis. Whereas no symptoms or signs can be attributed to the latter and the thyroid function tests give normal results, clinical symptoms are often noted in subacute thyroiditis, including painful neck swelling and generalized malaise. Thyroid-function tests are abnormal often and, depending upon the stage of the illness, may reflect hyper- or hypothyroidism.[12-14] One crucial difference between the two is that subacute thyroiditis represents a disease, and palpation thyroiditis is merely a histological finding. Histologically, although giant cells can be identified in both conditions, they are noted more commonly in subacute thyroiditis. Indeed, many of the giant cells in the latter may represent not histiocytes, but virally-infected follicular epithelial cells[15,16] (see Chapter 4). In addition in subacute thyroiditis, there appears to be a spectrum of lesions ranging from granulomata to fibrosis; in palpation thyroiditis, the lesions tend to show a uniform pattern (Figure 4).

Graves' disease — Carney et al.[1] point out that in Graves' disease, hyperplastic follicular epithelial cells may plug follicles and this, associated with colloid depletion, may simulate palpation thyroiditis. However, the absence of lymphoplasmacytic infiltrate and epithelial hyperplasia with papillations in the latter are useful in differentiating the two entities.

C-cell hyperplasia — Although C-cells tend to occur in interfollicular areas, occasionally, when these elements are increased in number, they will form a small nodule protruding into a follicle.[17-19] However, a layer of follicular epithelium will always separate C-cells from the intrafollicular colloid. In addition, the clear cytoplasm of the C-cells differs from the foamy appearance of the histiocytes in palpation thyroiditis

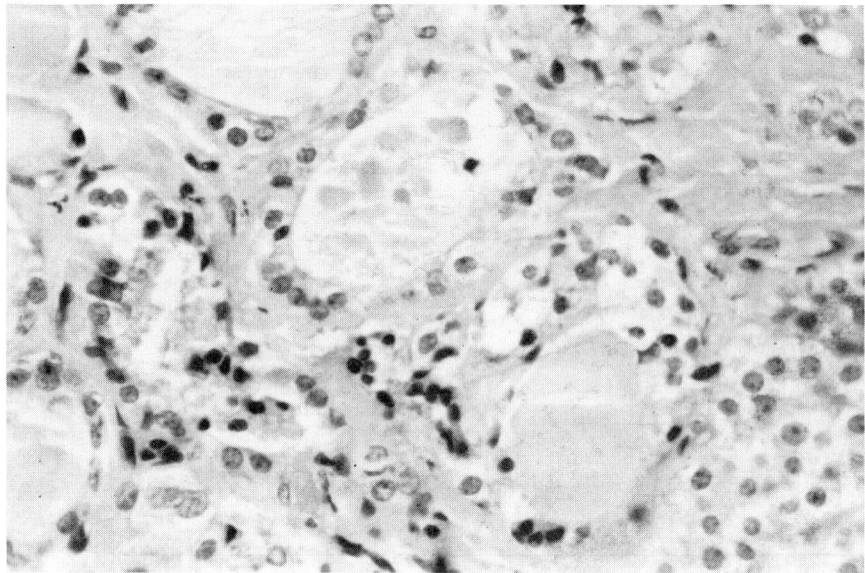

FIGURE 5. Foci of C-cells are seen: they are found in an interfollicular area. Lack of giant cells and inflammation and intact follicles distinguish this from palpation thyroiditis. (Hematoxylin-eosin; magnification × 300.)

(Figure 5). Intact follicles, absence of giant cells, and inflammation differentiate C-cell foci from palpation thyroiditis. Immunoperoxidase staining for localization of calcitonin in C-cells will resolve the issue.[19]

Desquamation of follicular cells — This problem, encountered in autopsy specimens, can be distinguished by the pyknotic nuclei of the desquamated cells[1] which differ from those of the histiocytes in palpation thyroiditis.

Tangential sectioning of follicular epithelium — This is readily identified by the obviously epithelial nature of the cells "filling" the lumen;[1] these cells resemble follicular elements and not histiocytes.

Colloidophagy — This phenomen, described by Hellwig,[20] consists of phagocytosis of colloid by macrophages. It is considered a normal mechanism for colloid resorption. When these colloid-laden macrophages do not reenter the circulation, they remain in the thyroid, may fuse to form syncytial masses, or may dislodge the colloid attracting a local lymphocytic reaction. Although histologically simulating palpation thyroiditis, in colloidophagy epithelial degeneration can be found more commonly than in palpation thyroiditis. However, the underlying mechanism is probably similar in that disruption of follicles with colloid leakage into the stroma elicits a macrophage response (see V. below).

Histiocytic reaction around hemorrhage in the thyroid — This is a frequently encountered change in adenomatous or colloid goiter.[21,22] Bleeding into or around cystic areas evokes the usual inflammatory response to hemorrhage, including histiocytes laden with hemosiderin. The focal nature of this reaction and its proximity to a cyst or scar (Figures 6, 7), serve to distinguish it from the multifocal palpation thyroiditis.

Sarcoidosis — Noncaseating granulomata have been described in patients with systemic sarcoidosis.[23-26] These tend to occur in the interfollicular regions and not to involve follicles per se. Occasionally, these lesions are associated with thyroid dysfunction (either hyper- or hypothyroidism). The mechanism is unknown.[27] The presence of nodal involvement (unknown in palpation thyroiditis, rare in subacute thyroiditis[27]),

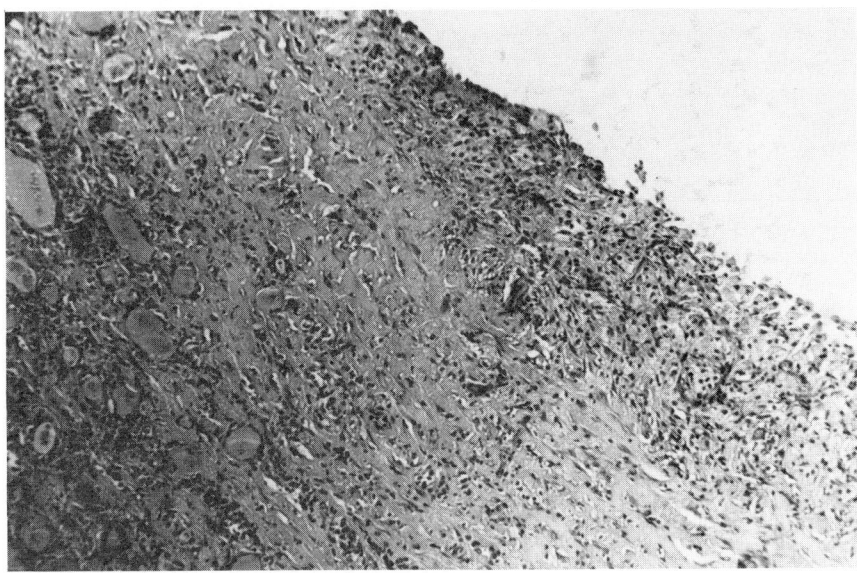

FIGURE 6. Hemorrhage into a cyst in nodular goiter will often invoke a macrophage response which not infrequently assumes the position of lining the cyst totally or partly. On the right of this photograph, such a row of histiocytes lines a cyst. Note pericyst fibrosis. (Hematoxylin-eosin; magnification × 125.)

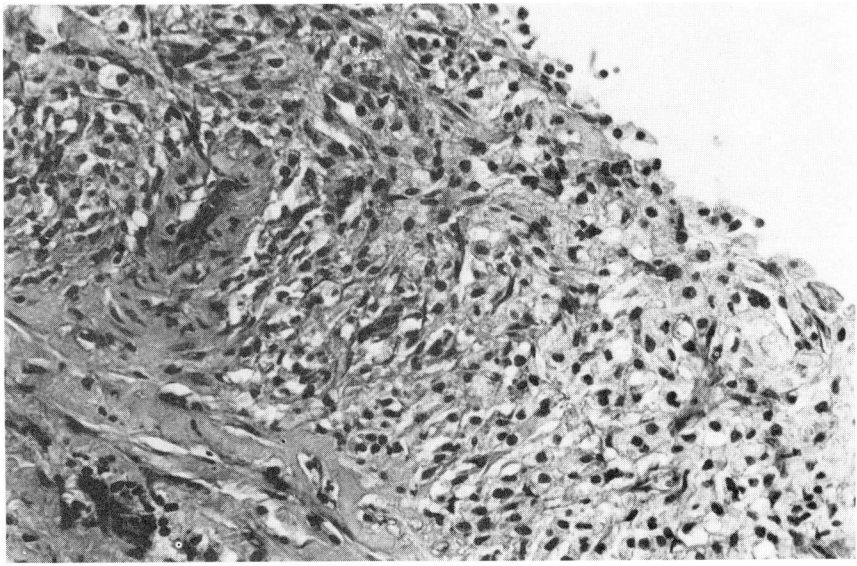

FIGURE 7. Higher power demonstrates the foamy cytoplasm and small, dark nuclei of the histiocytes. Note total absence of follicular epithelium and lack of giant cells. Iron stain would accentuate hemosiderin pigment phagocytized by these cells. (Hematoxylin-eosin; magnification × 250.)

the failure to demonstrate organisms, and the recognition of a systemic disease should be useful in distinguishing the rare case of sarcoidosis involving the thyroid.

Storage diseases — Dayan and Trickey[28] describe the finding of large amounts of lipofuscin-like material in thyroid follicular epithelial cells of patients with Batten's disease (juvenile amaurotic familial idiocy). The significance or chemical composition of this pigment is unknown. Its silvery-yellow color should serve to differentiate this follicular abnormality from palpation thyroiditis. Dayan and Trickey[28] noted no abnormalities in the thyroids of patients with other storage diseases. The present author has studied one patient with adult Gaucher's disease who underwent thyroid lobectomy for adenomatous goiter. Within the stroma of the gland, classical Gaucher's cells were found. These were identified only in an interfollicular location and would not be confused with palpation thyroiditis. Iron may localize in follicular epithelial cells in patients with hemochromatosis. The classic stain reactions, absence of inflammation, and diffuse involvement of follicles should distinguish this diagnosis for the histologist.[29,30]

V. PATHOGENESIS OF PALPATION THYROIDITIS

This lesion appears to represent a manifestation of the final, common pathway of the thyroid's response to noxious stimuli. Thus, Carney et al.[1] postulated that trauma produces injury to the follicular epithelium and possibly extrusion of colloid, both of which evoke an inflammatory reaction of predominantly histiocytic type. These cells undergo fusion and develop into giant cells of the foreign body type.[31] In this way, the resemblance at the pathogenetic, as well as histologic, level to subacute thyroiditis is apparent. In the latter, the stimulus is believed to be a virus (see Chapter 4).

VI. SIGNIFICANCE OF PALPATION THYROIDITIS

Palpation thyroiditis is a commonly found lesion if one is aware of it and looks for it. It has not been associated with any specific thyroid disease more commonly than another.[1]

Carney et al.[1] felt this lesion had little, if any, significance. The sequella of palpation thyroiditis appears to be microscopic focal scars which presumably do not affect thyroid function. These authors did caution, however, that such injury to the thyroid could lead to vascular disruption which, if a carcinoma is present in the gland, could induce dissemination.[32] This theoretical possibility remains to be substantiated.

VII. SUMMARY

Palpation thyroiditis represents a histiologic reaction commonly encountered in the thyroid. Its clinical significance is minimal, if any. The relevance of this lesion rests in the pathologist's recognition and distinction of this entity from other, more important, thyroid lesions.

REFERENCES

1. **Carney, J. A., Moore, S. B., Northcutt, R. C., Woolner, L. B., and Stillwell, G. K.**, Palpation thyroiditis (multifocal granulomatous folliculitis), *Am. J. Clin. Pathol.*, 64, 639, 1975.
2. **Hazard, J. B.**, Thyroiditis: a review, *Am. J. Clin. Pathol.*, 25, 289, 1955.
3. **Bishop, H. M. and Durman, D. C.**, Traumatic rupture of the thyroid gland, *Am. J. Surg.*, 75, 524, 1948.
4. **Burhans, E. C.**, Acute thyroiditis, *Surg. Gynecol. Obstet.*, 47, 478, 1928.
5. **Stein, O.**, Acute inflammation of the thyroid gland, *Laryngoscope*, 22, 1020, 1912.
6. **Jaffe, R. H.**, Tubercle-like structures in human goiters, *Arch. Surg.*, 21, 719, 1930.
7. **Klassen, K. P. and Curtis, G. M.**, Tuberculous abscess of the thyroid gland, *Surgery*, 17, 552, 1945.
8. **Goldfarb, H., Schifrin, D., and Graig, F. A.**, Thyroiditis caused by tuberculous abscess of the thyroid gland, *Am. J. Med.*, 38, 825, 1965.
9. **Moskowitz, R. W. and Baggenstoss, A. H.**, Histopathologic classification of periarteritis nodosa: a study of 56 cases confirmed at necropsy, *Mayo Clin. Proc.*, 38, 345, 1963.
10. **Zeek, P. M.**, Periarteritis nodosa and other forms of necrotizing angiitis, *N. Engl. J. Med.*, 248, 764, 1953.
11. **Godman, G. C. and Churg, J.**, Wegener's granulomatosis, *Arch. Pathol.*, 58, 533, 1954.
12. **Volpe, R.**, Etiology pathogenesis and clinical aspects of thyroiditis, II. *Pathol. Annu.*, 13, 399, 1978.
13. **Volpe, R.**, The pathology of thyroiditis, *Hum. Pathol.*, 9, 429, 1978.
14. **Hurley, J. R.**, Thyroiditis, *Disease-A-Month*, December, 1977.
15. **Stancekova, M., Stancek, D., Ciampor, F., Mucha, V., and Hnilica, P.**, Morphological, cytological and biological observations on viruses isolated from patients with subacute thyroiditis of de Quervain, *Acta Virol. Praha*, 20, 183, 1976.
16. **Satoh, M.**, Virus-like particles in the follicular epithelium of the thyroid from a patient with subacute thyroiditis (de Quervain), *Acta Pathol. Jpn.*, 25, 499, 1975.
17. **Wolfe, H. J., Melvin, K. E. W., Cervi-Skinner, S. J., Al-Saadi, A. A., Julian, J. F., Jackson, C. E., and Tashjian, A. H.**, C-cell hyperplasia preceding medullary thyroid carcinoma, *N. Engl. J. Med.*, 289, 437, 1973.
18. **DeLellis, R. A. and Balogh, K.**, Histochemical characteristics of parafollicular cells and medullary carcinoma, *Am. J. Pathol.*, 72, 119, 1973.
19. **LiVolsi, V. A., Feind, C. R., LoGerfo, P., and Tashjian, A. H.**, Demonstration by immunoperoxidase staining of hyperplasia of parafollicular cells in the thyroid gland in hyperparathyroidism, *J. Clin. Endocrinol. Metab.*, 37, 550, 1973.
20. **Hellwig, C. A.**, Colloidophagy in the human thyroid gland, *Science*, 113, 725, 1951.
21. **Meissner, W. A.**, Surgical pathology, in *Surgery of the Thyroid Gland*, Sedgwick, C. E., Ed., W. B. Saunders, Philadelphia, 1974, 24.
22. **Spjut, H. J., Warren, D. W., and Ackerman, L. V.**, Clinical-pathologic study of 76 cases of recurrent Graves' disease, toxic (non-exophthalmic) goiter, and nontoxic goiter, *Am. J. Clin. Pathol.*, 27, 367, 1957.
23. **Thompson, W. D., McGrouther, D. A., and Stockdill, G.**, Thyrotoxicosis with sarcoid-like granulomata, *J. Pathol.*, 111, 289, 1973.
24. **Lender, M. and Dollberg, L.**, Coincidence of sarcoidosis and Hashimoto's thyroiditis, *Am. Rev. Resp. Dis.*, 112, 113, 1975.
25. **vonKnorring, J. and Selroos, O.**, Sarcoidosis with thyroid involvement, polymyalgia rheumatica and breast carcinoma, *Scand. J. Rheumatol.*, 5, 77, 1976.
26. **Karlish, A. J. and MacGregor, G. A.**, Sarcoidosis, thyroiditis and Addison's disease, *Lancet*, 2, 339, 1970.
27. **Danyluk, J. M., Stirrat, J. H., and Laskin, M. M.**, Subacute (granulomatous) thyroiditis associated with granulomatous changes in adjacent lymph nodes, *Can. Med. Assoc. J.*, 100, 388, 1969.
28. **Dayan, A. D. and Trickey, R. J.**, Thyroid involvement in juvenile amaurotic familial idiocy (Batten's disease), *Lancet*, 2, 296, 1970.
29. **Sheldon, J. H.**, *Hemachromatosis*, Oxford University Press, London, 1935.
30. **Bloodworth, J. M. B., Ed.**, *Endocrine Pathology*, Williams and Wilkins, Baltimore, 1968.
31. **Mariano, M. and Spector, W. G.**, The formation and properties of macrophage polykaryons (inflammatory giant cells), *J. Pathol.*, 113, 1, 1974.
32. **Fisher, E. R. and Turnbull, R. B.**, The cytologic demonstration and significance of tumor cells in the mesenteric venous blood in patients with colorectal carcinoma, *Surg. Gynecol. Obstet.*, 100, 102, 1955.

Chapter 6

HASHIMOTO'S THYROIDITIS

Alan Seplowitz

TABLE OF CONTENTS

I.	Introduction	54
II.	Occurrence	54
III.	Incidence	54
IV.	HLA Frequencies in Patients with Hashimoto's Thyroiditis	55
V.	Pathogenesis	55
VI.	Animal Models	56
VII.	Clinical Features	57
VIII.	Laboratory Findings	57
IX.	Course	59
X.	Treatment	60
XI.	Summary	60
References		60

I. INTRODUCTION

In 1912, Hashimoto described a lymphocytic infiltration in four goitrous thyroid glands.[1] He referred to this condition as struma lymphomatosa and considered the disease to be quite rare (see Chapter 7). Other observers began to find similar pathology more frequently and it became apparent that Hashimoto's disease, or chronic lymphocytic thyroiditis, occurs much more commonly than originally believed. In addition, several variants have been described: asymptomatic thyroiditis, fibrosing thyroiditis, and adolescent lymphocytic goiter.

After the initial descriptive clinical and histological observations, about four decades lapsed before the autoimmune character of the disease was uncovered. The discovery of thyroid-specific autoantibodies in Hashimoto patients helped trigger a proliferation of research into immune mechanisms in this and other disorders. Some authors actually refer to Hashimoto's disease as autoimmune thyroiditis. Indeed, a wealth of circumstantial evidence implicates autoimmunity as the etiology of chronic lymphocytic thyroiditis. However, we will reserve the term autoimmune thyroiditis for experimental animal models, since the establishment of autoimmunity as the cause of human Hashimoto's thyroiditis, rather than as a response to injury by some other agent (e.g., a virus), awaits absolute proof.

II. OCCURRENCE

As in many other putative autoimmune diseases, females develop Hashimoto's thyroiditis much more frequently than do males. The female-to-male ratio probably exceeds 10:1.[2-14] Whether this phenomenon may be attributable to the X chromosome or to the female hormonal milieu remains a subject of speculation. The disease may affect people of all ages, with the peak incidence occurring among women 30 to 50 years old. Relatives of patients with Hashimoto's thyroiditis often have circulating autoantibodies, nonthyroidal as well as thyroidal.[6-20] Graves' disease and Hashimoto's disease are particularly likely to coexist in the same family and may even be found in the same individual.[16,21-29] Other disorders of autoimmune type (e.g., lupus, giant cell arteritis, chronic liver disease) may be found in a patient with chronic thyroiditis or in that subject's family.[15,30-33]

III. INCIDENCE

The distribution of Hashimoto's thyroiditis appears to be world-wide and the incidence may well be increasing. Observed incidence rates will tend to be underestimates, as many cases of Hashimoto's thyroiditis undoubtedly never come to medical attention. In Rochester, Minnesota, 246 cases of the disease were diagnosed between 1935 and 1967. Incidence rates in that city increased markedly during the period studied.[34] The average, annual incidence rates per 100,000 rose from 6.5 (1935-1944) to 21.4 (1945-1954) to 67.0 (1955-1964) to 69.0 (1965-1967). Over the same span of time, no change was observed in the incidence of Graves' disease in Rochester, and the authors contend that the change in incidence which they found for Hashimoto's thyroiditis is not merely an artifactual result of heightened awareness and improved diagnostic techniques. Indeed, other investigators[35] have reported an increasing prevalence of lymphocytic thyroiditis among autopsy cases, which they attribute to the greater availability of dietary iodine. A recent epidemiological study from Japan also links iodine ingestion to the development of chronic lymphocytic thyroiditis.[36] In this study, which encompasses over 10,000 children between the ages of 6 and 18, biopsy-proven lymphocytic thyroiditis occurred at a rate of 5.3/1000 in a seaside community (high iodine intake) versus 1.4/1000 in an urban community. Perhaps future studies will reveal the precise nature, if any, in which iodine interacts with genetic and immune factors in the development of this condition.

IV. HLA FREQUENCIES IN PATIENTS WITH HASHIMOTO'S THYROIDITIS

The search for an association between Hashimoto's thyroiditis and specific human histocompatibility antigens (HLA) represents an area of active research. Such investigations have been motivated by the ubiquitous nature of thyroid autoimmunity in Hashimoto's thyroiditis, by the increased frequency of thyroid antibodies in blood relatives of patients with Hashimoto's thyroiditis,[37] by findings suggestive of an association between histocompatibility genes and experimental or spontaneous autoimmune thyroiditis in animals,[38-41] and by an apparent association between Graves' disease and HLA-B8.[42] In addition, individuals with Turner's syndrome[43,44] and Down's syndrome[7,45] have an increased incidence of chronic thyroiditis. Each of these conditions is associated with major genetic abnormalities.

Until very recently, virtually all attempts have failed to demonstrate a significant association between Hashimoto's thyroiditis and HLA antigens.[13,42,46-51] This apparent lack of linkage may have reflected the investigation of an insufficient number of HLA antigens. Recently, two different teams of investigators have claimed an association between Hashimoto's thyroiditis and one of two different HLA antigens. The University of California (Los Angeles) group, which had previously reported a statistically insignificant association between Hashimoto's thyroiditis and HLA-B8,[42] now has found a highly significant increase in HLA-Aw30 among 41 patients (37 of whom were female) with Hashimoto's thyroiditis.[13] In their study, HLA-Aw30 had a frequency of 27% among all patients and 29% when analysis was restricted to the female patients. The Newfoundland team, which had also shown the absence of an association between Hashimoto's thyroiditis and HLA-B8,[14] now has studied 40 patients and 54 controls and has concluded that Hashimoto's thyroiditis is strongly linked to HLA-DRw3.[50] They found 55% of their patients to be positive for HLA-DRw3, as compared to 26% of controls. The findings of these two groups of investigators will require confirmation in larger studies as well as more precise dissection of the heterogeneous HLA-DRw3 locus.[51]

V. PATHOGENESIS

For more than two decades, evidence has been accumulating that strongly implicates the immune system in the pathogenesis of Hashimoto's thyroiditis.[2,9-11,52-60] If sufficiently sensitive assays are used (i.e., radioimmunoassay), virtually all patients with Hashimoto's thyroiditis can be shown to have circulating antithyroid antibodies. These autoantibodies may be directed against thyroglobulin (and/or a "second colloid antigen"), microsomal lipoproteins, certain cell-surface components, or a nuclear antigen. The thyroid-stimulating immunoglobulins, typical of Graves' disease, react with the thyrotropin receptor and sometimes occur in cases of Hashimoto's thyroiditis. Occasionally, antibodies against circulating thyroid hormones may be found. In clinical practice, only the thyroglobulin and microsomal antibodies are generally measured.

Though ubiquitous among cases of Hashimoto's thyroiditis, antithyroid antibodies apparently cannot, by themselves, initiate this disease. Transfusion of serum from Hashimoto's patients into Rhesus monkeys has failed to produce thyroid damage.[2]

Transplacental passage of thyroglobulin antibodies probably does not produce fetal thyroid damage.[52] On the other hand, experimental evidence does suggest a pathogenetic role for autoantibodies in conjunction with cell-mediated immune mechanisms. Some authors postulate an interaction between killer-lymphocytes and antigen-antibody complexes as the pathogenetic mechanism of Hashimoto's thyroiditis.[38,50-53] Volpe favors the theory that chronic lymphocytic thyroiditis results from a deficiency of suppressor T-lymphocytes, permitting proliferation of helper (activator) T-lymphocytes and B-lymphocytes which direct cell-mediated and humoral immune mechanisms, respectively, against the thyroid.[4-11] In vitro study of lymphocytes removed from Hashimoto's goiters shows that about 40% are B-cells and another 40% are T-cells.[54,55]

The killer (K) lymphocyte theory requires the presence of thyroid-specific, antigen-antibody complexes to facilitate lysis of thyroid acinar cells by these lymphocytes. Such complexes circulating in antibody excess could sensitize K cells to the antigen and enable the sensitized lymphocytes to destroy antigen-coated cells in the thyroid. Alternatively, immune complexes affixed to the target cells themselves could bind to K-lymphocytes at the acinar cell surface, with cell lysis then ensuing. This theory has several lines of experimental support. First, lymphocytes from patients with Hashimoto's thyroiditis can cause in vitro lysis of target cells (e.g., chicken erythrocytes) coated with thyroglobulin or thyroid microsomal antigen.[56] Second, incubation of control lymphocytes in Hashimoto's serum renders these lymphocytes capable of destroying thyroglobulin-coated target cells.[57] Finally, immune complex deposits have been described recently in Hashimoto's glands[58] and the existence of a thyroid cell-membrane-related cytotoxic antibody has been demonstrated.[57] Such an antibody could facilitate cytotoxicity by K cells.

The suppressor lymphocyte theory bypasses the need to postulate formation of thyroid-specific, antigen-antibody complexes as the event initiating thyroid damage. In the presence of a genetic defect in immune surveillance, a thyroid-directed clone of helper T-lymphocytes could emerge. The clone could produce a local cell-mediated immune reaction and could also facilitate thyroid-directed antibody production by B-lymphocytes. The argument for the pathogenicity of T-lymphocytes rests upon inconsistently substantiated reports about the presence in Hashimoto's serum of such substances as macrophage migration inhibiting factor. This is an area which requires further investigation.

The recent demonstration of antibodies to *Yersinia* sp. in patients with Graves' or Hashimoto's disease has raised the possibility of either an infectious etiology or, more likely, an abnormal immune response with cross-reacting antibodies to the organism and to thyroid components.[61,62] Some groups believe this finding does not reflect etiology, but is merely fortuitous.[63]

VI. ANIMAL MODELS

Research into animal models of autoimmune thyroiditis has contributed both to our knowledge and confusion about Hashimoto's thyroiditis. Spontaneous autoimmune thyroiditis occurs in beagles, in the Obese Strain of white Leghorn chickens, and in certain rats.[64-66] Experimental autoimmune thyroiditis has been induced in a variety of species, generally by such a procedure as inoculation with heterologous (e.g., bovine) thyroglobulin and killed tubercle bacilli in Freund's adjuvant.[67]

In Obese Strain Leghorns, neonatal bursectomy and neonatal thymectomy decrease and increase, respectively, the frequency of development of spontaneous thyroiditis.[8,64] In contrast, experimental autoimmune thyroiditis in other species is prevented by neonatal thymectomy, but not affected by bursectomy.[67] Thus, B-lymphocytes are likely to cause spontaneous thyroiditis, whereas T-cells probably mediate the experimental (induced) disease. Actually, the B-cell response in spontaneous autoimmune thyroiditis may occur because of a defect in immune surveillance by the suppressor T-lymphocytes. Indeed, thymectomized Obese Strain chickens often develop autoantibodies against nonthyroidal antigens as well.[40]

Experimental autoimmune thyroiditis may result from the action on thyroid cells of a soluble product (thyroid cytotoxic factor) of T-lymphocytes. Sensitized lymphocytes from guinea pigs with experimental autoimmune thyroiditis will lyse, in vitro and without direct cell-to-cell contact, thyroid cells from other guinea pigs.[68] The authors of this work failed to demonstrate cytolysis from incubation of guinea pig thyroid cells with hyperimmune antithyroglobulin serum. In contrast, others have induced experimental thyroiditis in vivo by passive transfer of immune serum.[69] Possible differences in end-organ sensitivity to cellular or humoral attack have not been investigated.

It should be emphasized that the various putative pathogenetic mechanisms for Hashimoto's and experimental autoimmune thyroiditis are not mutually exclusive. The full-blown disease may result from the interaction of B-, T-, and K-lymphocyte mechanisms. Thus, an inherited deficiency in suppressor T-lymphocytes might lead to thyroid autoantibody production in response to leakage of normal amounts of thyroid antigens into the circulation. If antigen-antibody complexes then formed, K-lymphocyte-mediated destruction of thyroid cells could occur.

In addition, as yet unidentified factors may influence the development and severity of Hashimoto's thyroiditis. As stated earlier, absolute proof is still lacking that the initiating event in the disease is autoimmune in nature, though all circumstantial evidence points strongly towards an autoimmune etiology. (See also Chapter 15.)

VII. CLINICAL FEATURES

Patients with chronic lymphocytic thyroiditis generally have firm, painless goiters. Occasionally, when goiterogenesis has been very rapid, neck discomfort may occur and mimic the presentation of subacute thyroiditis.[5,9,11,12,14,18,34] Estimates of thyroid size on physical examination will frequently fall between 40 and 60 g, though smaller or considerably larger glands may be encountered. The goiter, though generally diffuse and rubbery, is sometimes markedly asymmetrical and may feel quite hard and lobular to the point of suggesting nodularity. When large enough, the Hashimoto's goiter may encroach upon other structures in the neck and cause dyspnea, dysphagia, hoarseness, or a Horner's syndrome. Thus, the atypical Hashimoto's goiter might be mistaken for carcinoma of the thyroid.[3-5]

In addition to symptoms and signs referable to the size of the gland, one may find clinical evidence of hypothyroidism or, less often, of hyperthyroidism (as discussed below). Indeed, patients with Hashimoto's disease not infrequently first seek medical attention because of fatigability, constipation, or other symptoms of myxedema. Rarely, patients with histologically proven chronic lymphocytic thyroiditis have exhibited exophthalmos, even without concomitant thyrotoxicosis.[5]

VIII. LABORATORY FINDINGS

Thyroid function may cover the gamut from hypo- to hyperthyroidism.[5,9,11,14,18,34] The frequency of overt hypothyroidism increases with duration of disease, though the exact incidence remains doubtful since patients are often placed on suppressive therapy while functionally euthyroid. So-called subclinical hypothyroidism has been described in patients with Hashimoto's thyroiditis.[70,71] In such patients, (a) signs and symptoms of hypothyroidism are lacking or equivocal, (b) conventional thyroid function tests are normal (T_4, T_3 resin uptake, PBI), and (c) serum thyroid-stimulating hormone (TSH) is high and/or hyperresponds to exogenous thyrotropin-releasing hormone (TRH). Neither the frequency nor the time course of the progression from subclinical to symptomatic hypothyroidism is known.

Serum concentrations of T_4 and T_3 will generally reflect the patient's clinical thyroid status. Occasionally, antibodies directed against the thyroid hormones may increase the circulating reservoir of T_4 and/or T_3 without affecting free hormone levels.[72] Not infrequently, the Hashimoto's gland may release nonhormonal iodomolecules that bind to plasma proteins, especially albumin, and thereby increase the PBI-T_4 difference.[5]

Hashimoto's disease with hyperthyroidism, dubbed Hashitoxicosis, may occur with or without concomitant Graves' disease.[13,16,23,25-29,73-75] The incidence of hyperthyroidism among patients with Hashimoto's thyroiditis has been estimated at less than 10%. Fisher et al.[76] found 8 of 217 patients (3.7%) to be hyperthyroid, whereas Gharib et al.[77] diagnosed hyperthyroidism in 4 of 51 patients (8%). If untreated, Hashitoxicosis may persist for months or years.[18] Volpe[78] cautions that some cases of painless thyroiditis with toxicity represent variants of subacute disease and resolve completely.

This field remains confused however. Some patients with painless thyroiditis and hyperthyroidism spontaneously remit;[76] others may indeed progress to significant fibrosis and myxedema.[75] At present, distinction between these two prognostically different conditions is difficult, not only clinically, but also histologically (needle biopsy).[74]

Twenty-four hr radioiodine uptake may be low, normal, or high. An elevated ^{131}I uptake may reflect either Hashitoxicosis or dyshormonogenesis.[5] In the latter case, serum T_4 will be normal or low. The triad of low ^{131}I uptake, painless goiter, and hyperthyroidism has been labeled "painless subacute thyroiditis", and considered to be a variation of subacute, or granulomatous, thyroiditis.[78-80] Recent biopsy studies performed after[74,81] and during[82] the transient hyperthyroid phase have shown that such patients may have thyroid glands characterized by extensive lymphocytic infiltration rather than granulomatous involvement. As a result of these findings, some authors feel that such patients represent a form of Hashimoto's thyroiditis rather than a subacute thyroiditis.[83] Militating against a diagnosis of Hashimoto's thyroiditis were the normal or low titers of thyroglobulin and microsomal antibodies[74,82] in these patients. However, the conventional antibody assays using erythrocyte hemagglutination, complement fixation, or colloid and microsomal fluorescence may miss significant antibody titers detectable by more sensitive radioimmunoassay techniques. Using a radioimmunoassay for thyroglobulin antibodies, Dorfman and co-workers[84] demonstrated persistently elevated antibody levels in eight women with painless thyroiditis, transient thyrotoxicosis, and low radioactive iodine uptake (but without goiter). These studies raise provocative questions about possible early clinical manifestations of chronic lymphocytic thyroiditis and about the relationship of chronic lymphocytic to subacute thyroiditis. In particular, the possible pathogenetic role of viral damage in both entities merits investigation.

Radioactive iodine scans of thyroid glands affected by Hashimoto's disease may show either a normal pattern or diffusely patchy uptake. Fluorescent thyroid scanning, which indicates the stable iodine pool of the gland, generally shows a virtual absence of intrathyroidal iodine.[85] The iodine-perchlorate discharge test is frequently abnormal, implying a defect in iodine organification. The erythrocyte sedimentation rate is often elevated, though generally not so much as in subacute thyroiditis.

High titers of thyroglobulin and/or microsomal antibodies are frequently present, as previously discussed. The detection of antibodies is partly a function of the assay techniques employed. When radioimmunoassay is used, virtually all patients with Hashimoto's thyroiditis exhibit microsomal antibodies; the hemagglutination test will detect antibodies in only 90% of patients. Also, the presence of circulating thyroid antibodies, particularly in low titer, is not pathognomonic of Hashimoto's disease. For example, thyroglobulin antibodies may occur in patients with Graves' disease and various other autoimmune disorders, as well as in relatives of such patients.

IX. COURSE

True remission of Hashimoto's thyroiditis has been observed in young women or girls[86] with mild forms of the disease. The general rule, however, is progression to hypothyroidism. Goiters may or may not regress as hypothyroidism develops.

In some instances, hypothyroidism may occur (and recur) transiently. Patients with painless thyroiditis and transient hyperthyroidism may experience temporary hypothyroidism following their thyrotoxic episodes[87] and postpartum women with "autoimmune thyroiditis" may develop transient hypothyroidism.[46] Transient thyrotoxicosis has also been noted during the postpartum period[80] and such phenomena may reflect the influence of physiological postpartum immunological changes on preexistent thyroiditis.

Treatment, as discussed below, may alter the natural history of Hashimoto's thyroiditis by shrinking the goiter and by providing normal circulating thyroid hormone levels. Doniach and associates reported that about 10 to 20% of such goiters show no regression even after 10 to 15 yr of full levothyroxine replacement.[14] Within a 5-yr followup of treated goiters, this group found a 25% rate of nearly total disappearance of goiter and an additional 50% rate of regression to less than half the initial size.[14]

The clinical history of patients with chronic lymphocytic thyroiditis may also reflect the presence of associated diseases. Hashimoto's thyroiditis may coexist with a variety of disorders, at least some of which involve autoimmunity. Prominent among these are Graves' disease, Sjogren's syndrome (and other rheumatic conditions), pernicious anemia, and adrenal insufficiency.[10,14-16,30-32,45] Occasional case reports have also sought to link Hashimoto's disease to such entities as myasthenia gravis, idiopathic thrombocytopenic purpura, immunoblastic lymphadenopathy, and relapsing polychondritis.[14,15,31] Patients with Turner's or Down's syndromes have an increased likelihood of developing Hashimoto's thyroiditis.[43-45] In addition, it has been suggested that chronic thyroiditis may be associated with coronary heart disease,[5] possibly on the basis of mild or subclinical hypothyroidism with hyperlipidemia.[88,89] A recent study of hyperlipidemic survivors of myocardial infarction disclosed 12 elevated TSH levels among 122 subjects.[90] This investigation failed to demonstrate a significant correlation between TSH elevation and hypercholesterolemia, but did show a significantly increased prevalence of abnormal TSH values among women with sporadic hypertriglyceridemia. The biological importance of these findings will require further study, particularly of a prospective nature.

A possible association between Hashimoto's thyroiditis and cancer has also been examined. Hashimoto's disease may predispose slightly to development of lymphoma of the thyroid, but probably not to thyroid carcinoma[5] (see Chapter 10). Some investigators have shown an association between Hashimoto's thyroiditis[91] or elevated TSH (interpreted as an index of thyroid damage[92]) and breast cancer. Such associations will also require prospective study.

As has been noted above, other disorders considered autoimmune in nature have been found in patients with Hashimoto's disease.[14] These include pernicious anemia,[31]

Addison's disease,[31] lupus,[33] thymoma,[93] and chronic liver disease.[30] In some patients, these associated conditions will predominate and determine the patient's course.

X. TREATMENT

Treatment is indicated in cases of overt or subclinical (as defined above) hypothyroidism, or in instances where the size of the goiter is producing symptoms. Suppressive therapy, e.g., with levothyroxine 0.15 to 0.20 mg daily, will generally shrink the gland while ensuring a euthyroid state.[9,11,14,18] The suppression of small, asymptomatic goiters in euthyroid patients is more controversial. However, given that the natural course of Hashimoto's thyroiditis often leads to hypothyroidism, it would seem prudent to place such patients, as well, on life-long suppression. Spontaneous remissions have been reported; but, even disappearance of antibody titers during suppressive therapy does not guarantee against recrudescence of the disease if treatment is discontinued.

When hyperthyroidism coexists with Hashimoto's thyroiditis, the hyperthyroidism should be corrected and then levothyroxine instituted. Those hyperthyroid patients with low radioactive iodine uptakes may be presumed to have a self-limited phase of thyrotoxicosis, as discussed above. In such cases, symptomatic treatment with propranolol is preferable to more specific antithyroid therapy. Levothyroxine should be started when the thyrotoxic episode has passed.

In patients with painful goiters, temporary use of corticosteroids may be of some value, although suppressive therapy alone should generally prove adequate for reducing gland size and alleviating symptoms. Subtotal thyroidectomy should be reserved for goiters that fail to respond to levothyroxine treatment. Studies have suggested that resistance to suppressive therapy may correlate with increased cell-mediated immunity (either as a pathogenetic mechanism or as a response to injury) as measured by tests of leukocyte migration inhibition.[94]

XI. SUMMARY

Hashimoto's thyroiditis is the eponym applied to goiters characterized by lymphocytic infiltration. The disease occurs mainly in women. The precise etiology remains to be elucidated, but the pathogenesis clearly involves autoimmunity of both a cellular and humoral nature. The disease process classically culminates in permanent hypothyroidism, though variants exist with hyperthyroidism or transient hypothyroidism. For the classical presentation of the disease, a suppressive dose of levothyroxine is the treatment of choice, with the dual aim of minimizing goiter size and maintaining a euthyroid state.

REFERENCES

1. **Hashimoto, H.**, Zur Kenntnisse der Lymphomatosen Veranderungen der Schilddruse (Struma Lymphomatosa), *Langenbecks Arch. Chir.*, 9, 219, 1912.
2. **Roitt, I. M. and Doniach, D.**, Thyroid autoimmunity, *Br. Med. Bull.*, 16, 152, 1960.
3. **Buchanan, W. W. and Harden, R. M.**, Primary hypothyroidism and Hashimoto's thyroiditis, *Arch. Intern. Med.*, 115, 411, 1965.
4. **Al-Sarraf, M. and Waller, F. J.**, Hashimoto's disease: a ten year review at the Grace Hospital, *Grace Hosp. Bull.*, 45, 50, 1967.

5. Neve, P., Ermans, A. M., and Bastenie, P. A., Struma lymphomatosa (Hashimoto), in *Thyroiditis and Thyroid Function: Clinical, Morphological and Physiopathological Studies*, Pergamon Press, Oxford, 1972, 109.
6. Thier, S. O., Black, P., Williams, H. E., and Robbins, J., Chronic lymphocytic thyroiditis: report of a kindred with viral, immunological and chemical studies, *J. Clin. Endocrinol.*, 25, 65, 1965.
7. Vanhaelst, L., Hayez, F., Bonnyms, M., and Bastenie, P. A., Thyroid autoimmune disease and thyroid function in families of subjects with Down's syndrome, *J. Clin. Endocrinol.*, 30, 792, 1970.
8. Volpe, R., Ezrin, C., Johnston, M. W., and Steiner, J. W., Genetic factors in Hashimoto's struma, *Can. Med. Assoc. J.*, 88, 915, 1963.
9. Volpe, R., Thyroiditis: current views of pathogenesis, *Med. Clin. North Am.*, 59, 1163, 1975.
10. Volpe, R., The role of autoimmunity in hypoendocrine and hyperendocrine function, *Ann. Intern. Med.*, 87, 86, 1977.
11. Furszyfer, J., Kurland, L. T., Woolner, L. B., Elveback, L. R., and McConahey, W. M., Hashimoto's thyroiditis in Olmsted County, Minnesota 1935 through 1967, *Mayo Clin. Proc.*, 45, 586, 1970.
12. Volpe, R., Lymphocytic (Hashimoto's) thyroiditis, in *The Thyroid*, Werner, S. C. and Ingbar, S. H., Eds., Harper and Row, Baltimore, 1978, 996.
13. Brown, J., Solomon, D. H., Beall, G. N., Terasaki, P. I., Chopra, I. J., Van Herle, A. J., and Wu, S.-Y., Autoimmune thyroid disease — Graves' and Hashimoto's, *Ann. Intern. Med.*, 88, 379, 1978.
14. Doniach, D., Bottazzo, G. F., and Russell, R. C. G., Goitrous autoimmune thyroiditis (Hashimoto's disease), *Clin. Endocrinol. Metab.*, 8, 63, 1979.
15. Segal, B. M. and Weintraub, M. I., Hashimoto's thyroiditis, myasthenia gravis, idiopathic thrombocytopenic purpura, *Ann. Intern. Med.*, 85, 761, 1976.
16. Buchanan, W. W., Crooks, J., Alexander, W. D., Koutras, D. A., Wayne, E. J., Anderson, J. R., and Goudie, R. B., Association of thyrotoxicosis and autoimmune thyroiditis, *Br. Med. J.*, 1, 843, 1961.
17. Doniach, D. and Hudson, V., Lymphadenoid goiter: diagnostic and biochemical aspects, *Br. Med. J.*, 1, 672, 1957.
18. Doniach, D., Hudson, V., and Roitt, I. M., Human autoimmune thyroiditis: clinical studies, *Br. Med. J.*, 1, 365, 1960.
19. Share, L. L., Valensi, Q. J., Sorbevilla, L., and Gabrilove, N. Y., Chronic thyroiditis: a potentially confusing clinical picture, *Am. J. Med. Sci.*, 250, 532, 1965.
20. Hazard, J. B., Thyroiditis: a review, *Am. J. Clin. Pathol.*, 25, 399, 1955.
21. Joll, C. A., The pathology, diagnosis and treatment of Hashimoto's disease (struma lymphomatosa), *Br. J. Surg.*, 27, 351, 1939.
22. Farid, N. R., Munro, R. E., Row, V. V., and Volpe, R., Peripheral thymus-dependent (T) lymphocytes in Graves' disease and Hashimoto's thyroiditis, *N. Engl. J. Med.*, 228, 1313, 1973.
23. Wyse, E., McConahey, W. M., Woolner, L. B., Scholz, D. A., and Kearns, T. P., Ophthalmopathy without hyperthyroidism in patients with histologic Hashimoto's thyroiditis, *J. Clin. Endocrinol.*, 28, 1623, 1968.
24. Liddle, G. W., Heysell, R. M., and McKenzie, J. M., Graves' disease without hyperthyroidism, *Am. J. Med.*, 39, 845, 1965.
25. Anderson, S. R., Seedorff, H. H., and Halberg, P., Thyroiditis with myxoedema and orbital pseudotumor, *Acta Ophthal.*, 41, 120, 1963.
26. Mahaux, J., L'association exophthalmie ophthalmopleguque-thyroidite chronique avec reactions d'autoimmunite antithyroide, *Acta Clin. Belg.*, 16, 292, 1961.
27. Mason, R. E. and Walsh, F. B., Exophthalmos in hyperthyroidism due to Hashimoto's thyroiditis, *Bull. Johns Hopkins Hosp.*, 112, 323, 1963.
28. Eversman, J. J., Skillern, P. G., and Senhauser, D. A., Hashimoto's thyroiditis and Graves' disease with exophthalmos without hyperthyroidism, *Cleveland Clin. Q.*, 33, 179, 1966.
29. Jayson, M. I. V., Doniach, D., Benhamou-Glynn, N., Roitt, I. M., and El-Kabir, D. J., Thyrotoxicosis and Hashimoto goitre in a pair of monozygotic twins with long acting thyroid stimulator, *Lancet*, 2, 15, 1967.
30. Doniach, D., Autoimmunity in liver disease, in *Progress in Clinical Immunology*, Vol. 1, Schwartz, R. S., Ed., Grune & Stratton, New York, 1972, 45.
31. Dent, R. G. and Edwards, D. M., Autoimmune thyroid disease and the polymyalgia rheumatica-giant cell arteritis syndrome, *Clin. Endocrinol.*, 9, 215, 1978.
32. Doniach, D. and Bottazzo, G. F., Autoimmunity and the endocrine pancreas, *Pathobiol. Ann.*, 7, 327, 1977.
33. Doniach, D., Nilsson, L. R., and Roitt, I. M., Autoimmune thyroiditis in children and adolescents. II. Immunological correlations and parent study, *Acta Paediatr.*, 54, 260, 1965.

34. Furszyfer, J., Kurland, L. T., McConahey, W. M., Woolner, L. B., and Elveback, L. R., Epidemiologic aspects of Hashimoto's thyroiditis and Graves' disease in Rochester, Minnesota (1935-1967), with special reference to temporal trends, *Metabolism,* 21, 197, 1972.
35. Weaver, D. K., Batsakis, J. G., and Nishiyama, R. H., Relationship of iodine to "lymphocytic goiters", *Arch. Surg.,* 98, 183, 1969.
36. Inoue, M., Taketani, N., Sato, T., and Nakajima, H., High incidence of chronic lymphocytic thyroiditis in apparently healthy school children: epidemiological and clinical study, *Endocrinol. Jpn.,* 22, 483, 1975.
37. Hall, R. and Stanbury, J. B., Familial studies of autoimmune thyroiditis, *Clin. Exp. Immunol.,* 15, 467, 1973.
38. Valditiu, A. O. and Rose, N. R., Autoimmune murine thyroiditis-relation to histocompatibility (H-2) type, *Science,* 174, 1137, 1971.
39. Bacon, L. D., Kite, J. H., and Rose, N. R., Relation between the major histocompatibility (B) locus and autoimmune thyroiditis in obese chickens, *Science,* 186, 274, 1974.
40. Bigazzi, P. E. and Rose, N. R., Spontaneous autoimmune thyroiditis in animals as a model of human disease, *Prog. Allergy,* 19, 245, 1975.
41. Maron, R. and Cohen, I. R., Mutation at the H-2k locus influences susceptibility to autoimmune thyroiditis, *Nature (London),* 279, 715, 1979.
42. Chopra, I. J., Solomon, D. H., Chopra, U., Yoshihara, E., Terasaki, P. I., and Smith, I., Abnormalities in thyroid function in relatives of patients with Graves' disease and Hashimoto's thyroiditis: lack of correlation with inheritance of HLA-B8, *J. Clin. Endocrinol. Metab.,* 45, 45, 1977.
43. Hamilton, C. R., Moldawer, M., and Rosenberg, H. S., Hashimoto's thyroiditis and Turner's syndrome, *Arch. Intern. Med.,* 122, 69, 1968.
44. McHardy-Young, S., Doniach, D., and Polani, P. E., Thyroid function in Turner's syndrome and allied conditions, *Lancet,* 2, 1161, 1970.
45. Reid, A. H., Adamson, D. G., Browning, M. C., and Donald, J. M., A case of idiopathic Addison's disease and probable autoimmune thyroiditis in a Mongol, *J.Ment. Defic. Res.,* 19, 205, 1975.
46. Bode, H. H., Dorf, M. E., and Forbes, A. P., Familial lymphocytic thyroiditis: analysis of linkage with histocompatibility and blood group, *J. Clin. Endocrinol. Metab.,* 37, 692, 1973.
47. VanRood, J. J., VanHoof, J. P., and Keuning, J. J., Disease predisposition, immune responsiveness and the fine structure of the HL-A supergene: a need for reappraisal, *Transplant. Rev.,* 22, 75, 1975.
48. Svejgaard, A. and Ryder, L. P., HLA and disease, in *HLA Systems — New Aspects,* Ferrara, G. B., Ed., Elsevier, Amsterdam, 1977, 143.
49. Farid, N. R., Barnard, J. M., and Marshall, W. H., The association of HLA with autoimmune thyroid disease in Newfoundland: the influence of HLA homozygosity in Graves' disease, *Tissue Antigens,* 8, 181, 1976.
50. Moens, H. and Farid, N. R., Hashimoto's thyroiditis is associated with HLA-DRw3, *N. Engl. J. Med.,* 299, 133, 1978.
51. Van den Berg-Loonin, E. M., deBruin, T., and Schellekens, P. T. A., The complex nature of human D-locus determinants: heterogeneity within Dw3, *Immunogenetics,* 5, 261, 1977.
52. Goldsmith, R. E., McAdams, A. J., Larsen, P. R., MacKenzie, M., and Hess, E. V., Familial autoimmune thyroiditis: maternal-fetal relationship and the role of generalized autoimmunity, *J. Clin. Endocrinol. Metab.,* 37, 265, 1973.
53. Allison, A. C., Self-tolerance and autoimmunity in the thyroid, *N. Engl. J. Med.,* 295, 821, 1975.
54. Totterman, T. H., Maenpaa, J., Gordin, A., Makinen, T., Taskinen, E., Andersson, L. C., and Hayry, P., Blood and thyroid-infiltrating lymphocyte subclasses in juvenile autoimmune thyroiditis, *Clin. Exp. Immunol.,* 30, 193, 1977.
55. Totterman, T. H., Distribution of T-, B- and thyroglobulin-binding lymphocytes infiltrating the gland in Graves' disease, Hashimoto's thyroiditis and de Quervain's thyroiditis, *Clin. Immunol. Immunopathol.,* 10, 270, 1978.
56. Calder, E. A., McLeman, D., and Irvine, W. J., Lymphocyte cytotoxicity induced by pre-incubation with serum from patients with Hashimoto's thyroiditis, *Clin. Exp. Immunol.,* 15, 467, 1973.
57. Calder, E. A. and Irvine, W. J., Cell-mediated immunity and immune complexes in thyroid disease, *J. Clin. Endocrinol. Metab.,* 40, 287, 1975.
58. Kalderon, A. E. and Bogaars, H. A., Immune complex deposits in Graves' disease and Hashimoto's thyroiditis, *Am. J. Med.,* 63, 729, 1977.
59. DeGroot, L. J. and Stanbury, J. B., *The Thyroid and Its Diseases,* John Wiley and Sons, New York, 1975, 587.
60. Roberts, I. M., Whittingham, S., and MacKay, I. R., Tolerance to an autoantigen thyroglobulin, *Lancet,* 2, 936, 1973.
61. Editorial, Thyroid disease and antibodies to Yersinia, *Lancet,* 1, 734, 1977.

62. Beck, K., Clemmensen, O., Larsen, J. H., and Bendixen, G., Thyroid disease and Yersinia, *Lancet*, 1, 1060, 1977.
63. Keddie, N., Metcalf-Gibson, C., and Tooth, J. A., Yersinia and thyroid disease, *Lancet*, 2, 1368, 1977.
64. Wick, G., Sundick, R. S., and Albini, B. A., A review: the Obese Strain (OS) of chickens: an animal model with spontaneous autoimmune thyroiditis, *Clin. Immunol. Immunopathol.*, 3, 272, 1974.
65. Rose, N. R., Bigazzi, P. E., and Noble, B., Spontaneous autoimmune thyroiditis in the BUF rat, *Adv. Exp. Med. Biol.*, 73, 209, 1976.
66. Fritz, T. E., Zeman, R. C., and Zelle, M. R., Pathology and familial incidence of thyroiditis in a closed beagle colony, *Exp. Mol. Pathol.*, 12, 14, 1970.
67. Weigle, W. O., Experimental autoimmune thyroiditis, *Pathol. Annu.*, 8, 329, 1973.
68. Lin, M. S. and Salvin, S. B., In vitro and in vivo studies on the mechanism of experimental autoimmune thyroiditis in guinea pigs, *Cell Immunol.*, 27, 177, 1976.
69. Tomazic, V. and Rose, N. R., Autoimmune murine thyroiditis. VII. Induction of the thyroid lesions by passive transfer of immune serum, *Clin. Immunol. Immunopathol.*, 4, 511, 1975.
70. Gordin, A., Saarinen, P., Pelkonen, R., and Lamberg, B. A., Serum thyrotropin and the response to thyrotropin-releasing hormone in symptomless auto-immune thyroiditis, *Acta Endocrinol.*, 75, 274, 1974.
71. Takeda, R., Nakabayashi, H., Kawato, M., Ueda, M., and Matsubara, F., Clinical value of the thyrotropin releasing hormone stimulation test in predicting mild hypothyroid state in chronic thyroiditis, *Endokrinologie*, 65, 171, 1975.
72. Staeheli, V., Vollotton, M. B., and Burger, A., Detection of anti-thyroxine and anti-triiodothyronine antibodies in different thyroid conditions, *J. Clin. Endocrinol. Metab.*, 41, 669, 1975.
73. Fatourechi, V., McConahey, W. M., and Woolner, L. B., Hyperthyroidism associated with histologic Hashimoto's thyroiditis, *Mayo Clin. Proc.*, 46, 682, 1971.
74. Gluck, F. B., Nusynowitz, M. C., and Plymate, S., Chronic lymphocytic thyroiditis, thyrotoxicosis, and low radioactive iodine uptake, *N. Engl. J. Med.*, 293, 624, 1975.
75. Gordin, A. and Lamberg, B. A., Natural course of symptomless autoimmune thyroiditis, *Lancet*, 2, 1234, 1975.
76. Fisher, D. A., Oddie, T. H., Johnson, D. E., and Nelson, J. C., The diagnosis of Hashimoto's thyroiditis, *J. Clin. Endocrinol. Metab.*, 40, 795, 1975.
77. Gharib, H., Wahner, H. W., and McConahey, W. M., Serum levels of thyroid hormones in Hashimoto's thyroiditis, *Mayo Clin. Proc.*, 47, 175, 1972.
78. Volpe, R., Subacute (de Quervain's) thyroiditis, *Clin. Endocrinol. Metab.*, 8, 81, 1979.
79. Papapetrou, P. D. and Jackson, I. M. D., Thyrotoxicosis due to "silent" thyroiditis, *Lancet*, 1, 361, 1975.
80. Ginsberg, J. and Walfish, P. G., Postpartum transient thyrotoxicosis with painless thyroiditis, *Lancet*, 1, 1125, 1977.
81. Woolf, P. D. and Daly, R., Thyrotoxicosis with painless thyroiditis, *Am. J. Med.*, 60, 73, 1976.
82. Gorman, C. A., Duick, D. S., Woolner, L. B., and Wahner, H. W., Transient hyperthyroidism in patients with lymphocytic thyroiditis, *Mayo Clin. Proc.*, 53, 359, 1978.
83. Cooper, D. S., Ridgeway, E. C., and Maloof, F., Unusual types of hyperthyroidism, *Clin. Endocrinol. Metab.*, 7, 199, 1978.
84. Dorfman, S. G., Cooperman, M. T., Nelson, R. L., Depuy, H., Peake, R. L., and Young, R. L., Painless thyroiditis and transient hyperthyroidism without goiter, *Ann. Intern. Med.*, 86, 24, 1977.
85. Hoffer, P. B., Gottschalk, A., and Refetoff, S., Thyroid scanning techniques: the old and the new, *Curr. Probl. Radiol.*, 2, 5, 1972.
86. Rallison, M. L., Dobyns, B. M., Keating, F. R., Rall, J. E., and Tyler, F. H., Occurrence and natural history of chronic lymphocytic thyroiditis in childhood, *J. Pediat.*, 86, 675, 1975.
87. Amino, N., Miyai, K., Kuro, R., Tanizawa, O., Azukizawa, M., Takai, S., Tanaki, F., Nishi, K., Kawashima, M., and Kumahara, Y., Transient postpartum hypothyroidism: fourteen cases with autoimmune thyroiditis, *Ann. Intern. Med.*, 87, 155, 1977.
88. Vessby, B. and Wide, L., Serum levels of thyroid-stimulating hormone in hyperlipoproteinemia, *Clin. Chim. Acta*, 62, 293, 1975.
89. Fowler, P. B. S., Swale, J., and Andrews, H., Hypercholesterolemia in borderline hypothyroidism: stage of premyxoedema, *Lancet*, 2, 488, 1970.
90. Green, W. L., Hazzard, W. R., and Hershman, J. M., Thyrotropin levels in hyperlipidemic survivors of myocardial infarction, *Metabolism*, 25, 465, 1976.
91. Itoh, K. and Maruchi, N., Breast cancer in patients with Hashimoto's thyroiditis, *Lancet*, 2, 1119, 1975.
92. Mittra, I. and Hayward, J. L., Hypothalamic-pituitary-thyroid axis in breast cancer, *Lancet*, 1, 885, 1974.

93. **Dawson, M. A.**, Thymoma associated with pancytopenia and Hashimoto's thyroiditis, *Am. J. Med.*, 52, 406, 1972.
94. **Wartenberg, J., Doniach, D., Brostoff, J., and Roitt, I. M.**, Leucocyte migration inhibition in thyroid disease: effect of thyroid microsomes and thyroglobulin, *Int. Arch. Allergy Appl. Immunol.*, 44, 396, 1973.

Chapter 7

CHRONIC THYROIDITIS: PATHOLOGIC ASPECTS

Virginia A. LiVolsi

TABLE OF CONTENTS

I.	Introduction		66
II.	The Pathology of Hashimoto's Thyroiditis		67
	A.	Classic Form	67
		1. Gross Features	67
		2. Microscopic Features	68
		3. Ultrastructure	68
	B.	Hashitoxicosis	71
	C.	Juvenile Lymphocytic Thyroiditis	71
	D.	The Fibrosing Variant of Hashimoto's Thyroiditis	72
		1. Gross Features	73
		2. Microscopic Appearance	73
		3. Clinicopathologic Correlation	76
		4. Differential Diagnosis	77
		5. Squamous Cells in the Thyroid	77
	E.	Chronic Lymphocytic Thyroiditis Resembling Lymphoma	78
	F.	Hashimoto's Thyroditis Presenting as a Nodule	79
III.	The Hurthle Cell		80
	A.	Microscopic Appearance	80
	B.	Ultrastructure	80
	C.	Histochemistry	80
	D.	Hurthle Cells in the Thyroid	80
		1. Thyroiditis	80
		2. Tumors	81
IV.	So-Called Chronic Nonspecific Thyroiditis		81
V.	The Pathology of Hypothyroidism		82
	A.	Case Report	82
	B.	Myxedema — Primary	83
	C.	Myxedema — Secondary	83
	D.	The Pathology of Cretinism	84
VI.	Extrathyroid Pathology in Hypothyroidism		84
VII.	Associations in Hashimoto's Thyroiditis		84
VIII.	Differential Diagnosis: Fibrosis in the Thyroid		85

IX.	Hypothyroidism Due to Infiltrative Disorders of the Thyroid	86
	A. Amyloid	86
	B. Tumoral Replacement	86
	C. Other Infiltrations	86
X.	Lymphocytes in the Thyroid	86
	A. Hashimoto's Disease and Variants	86
	B. Graves' Disease	86
	C. Other Thyroiditides	87
	D. Nodular Goiter	87
	E. Tumors	87
	F. Lymphoma	87
	1. Systemic	87
	2. Primary	87
XI.	Summary	88
References		91

I. INTRODUCTION

Hashimoto, in 1912, described four patients with a thyroid disorder which bears his name.[1] The thyroids were symmetrically enlarged and firm grossly. Histologically, the epithelium ranged from hyperplastic to atrophic, follicles were focally dilated or atrophic, and the gland was infiltrated by lymphocytes, both in the lobules and the interstitium. Germinal centers were present and fibrosis ranged from mild to very prominent. In this initial description, two striking findings were emphasized: eosinophilic change in the follicular epithelium (now known as Hurthle cells) and a shrinkage of the colloid which exhibited altered staining characteristics described as "dirty eosinophilic lumps".* To his credit, Hashimoto[1] separated the disorder he reported from both granulomatous (de Quervain) and Riedel's thyroiditis.

As has been noted earlier in this monograph, confusion about the interrelationships among these diseases continued after the classical descriptions.[1-4] Indeed, even today, clinical features in certain cases suggest overlap.[5,6]

From the pathologic viewpoint, confusion has arisen also, especially in distinguishing fibrosing Hashimoto's disease from Riedel's struma.[7] In addition, the relationship between chronic nonspecific thyroiditis[8,9] and Hashimoto's disease is not clear. A further problem involves the distinction between tumor associated thyroiditis and Hashimoto's disease; the premalignant potential of the latter remains disputed[10-17] (see Chapter 10).

This chapter will (a) review the pathologic anatomy of chronic thyroiditis, including Hashimoto's disease and its variants, and of primary (idiopathic) and secondary myxedema, (b) discuss the differential diagnosis of the various features of chronic thyroidi-

---

* This is a loose translation as per Dr. Gary Pasternak from the original German.

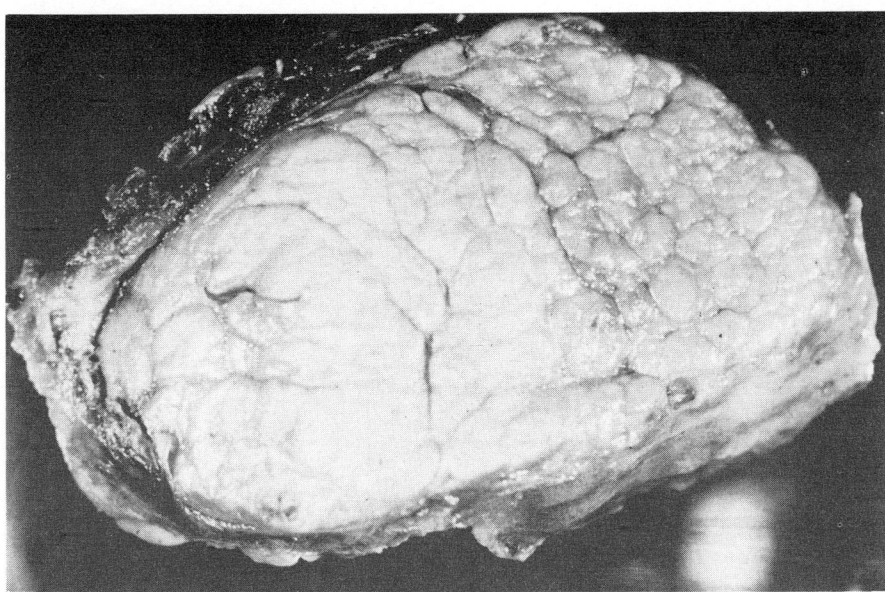

FIGURE 1. Gross photograph of classic Hashimoto's thyroiditis shows accentuation of lobular architecture of the gland.

tis, (c) summarize those pathologic features of systemic lesions in myxedema, (d) list unusual thyroid causes of hypothyroidism, and (e) evaluate the primary thyroid lymphoma and plasmacytoma and the relationship of these neoplasms to Hashimoto's thyroiditis. Chronic thyroiditis has been subdivided into three groups:[18,19]

1. Diffuse Hashimoto type with either hyperplastic, atrophic or predominantly oxyphilic epithelium
2. Lymphocytic with hyperplastic epithelium
3. Focal thyroiditis

II. THE PATHOLOGY OF HASHIMOTO'S THYROIDITIS

A. Classic Form
1. Gross Features

The gland is moderately enlarged from two to four times normal size although occasionally larger glands may be seen.[8,13,18-30] Gland weights range from 25 to 250 grams.[8,13,18,22,23] Typically, the enlargement is symmetrical with prominent involvement of the pyramidal lobe.[13,27] The capsule tends to be thin allowing the observer to view the lobulated appearance of the gland.[8,13,18-30] No adherence to periglandular tissues is noted.[8,13,27,28] The gland is described as firm, but not woody or hard;[8,13,18-30] Hurley[29] emphasizes that the degree of firmness correlates with the amount of collagen present.

On cut surface, the lobulation of the normal thyroid is accentuated and the individual lobules bulge to varying degrees depending upon the amount of septal fibrous tissue present.[8,13,27-29] The normal brown-red color of the thyroid is replaced by a pink-tan to yellow.[8,13,18-30] Bastenie et al.[13] stress the absence of shininess attributed to colloid depletion. These authors compare the gross appearance of the Hashimoto's gland to a hypertrophied thymus.[13] The diffuse nature of the process aids in differentiation from cancer of the thyroid. (Figure 1.)

Table 1
MAJOR VARIANTS OF HASTIMOTO'S THYROIDITIS

Features	Juvenile lymphocytic type	Oxyphil classic variant	Fibrosing variant
Sex (female:male) ratio	5:1	20:1	5:1
Incidence	Common	Common	Rare
Age	Childhood; Adolescence	Middle aged	Elderly
Thyroid function	Normal or hyperthyroid	Normal initially	Hypothyroid
Size of gland	Small or slightly enlarged	Moderate, (60-100 g)	Large
Consistency	Soft-firm	Firm	Hard
Prognosis	Remission; some recur	50% become hypothyroid	Myxedema
Antibodies (microsomal)	Low to moderate titer	Moderate to high titers	High titers
Thyroglobulin	Absent	Rarely present	High titers

Adapted from Doniach, D., Bottazzo, G. F., and Russell, R. C. G., *Clin. Endocrinol. Metab.*, 8, 63, 1979. With permission.

2. Microscopic Features

Histologically, at low power, the lobulation of the gland is recognized;[8,13,18-30] this distinguishes the lesion from carcinoma. Characteristically, the thyroid follicles are small and atrophic with sparse or absent colloid.[8,13,18-30] The colloid stains gray-pink and appears quite dense[1] and focal hyperplasia of follicular epithelium may be noted.[8,18-30] Oxyphilic metaplasia of much, or all, of the follicular epithelium is recognized.[8,13,18-30] These Hurthle or Askanazy cells appear larger than normal and contain large, sometimes bizarre and hyperchromatic nuclei and abundant eosinophilic cytoplasm.

Perhaps the most prominent histologic characteristic is the infiltration of lymphocytes with the formation of germinal centers; in the latter, plasma cells, immunoblasts, and macrophages are recognized.[8,13,18-30] Fibrosis, which varies in extent, is found predominantly in the interlobular stroma in the classic form of Hashimoto's disease (Table 1).

Occasionally, giant cells may be identified, but these never occur in large numbers nor are they associated with granulomatous inflammation as in subacute thyroiditis[8,13,27] (see Chapter 4). Although the gross changes appear diffuse in classic forms of the disease, microscopically, variations in extent of lymphoid infiltration, follicular atrophy, and fibrosis from one area of the gland to another are encountered commonly.[8,13,27,28] (Figures 2-5.)

3. Ultrastructure

Bastenie et al.[13] have reported on the electron microscopic appearance of the Hashimoto's thyroid. They divide the epithelial cells into three types:

1. Nonspecific — these correspond to hyperplastic cells, show normal mitochondria, dilated endoplasmic reticulum, well developed Golgi complexes, and colloid droplets. The authors believed these were stimulated cells with increased secretory activity; these elements are recognized more commonly in hyperplastic stages of the disease including juvenile thyroiditis.[13]

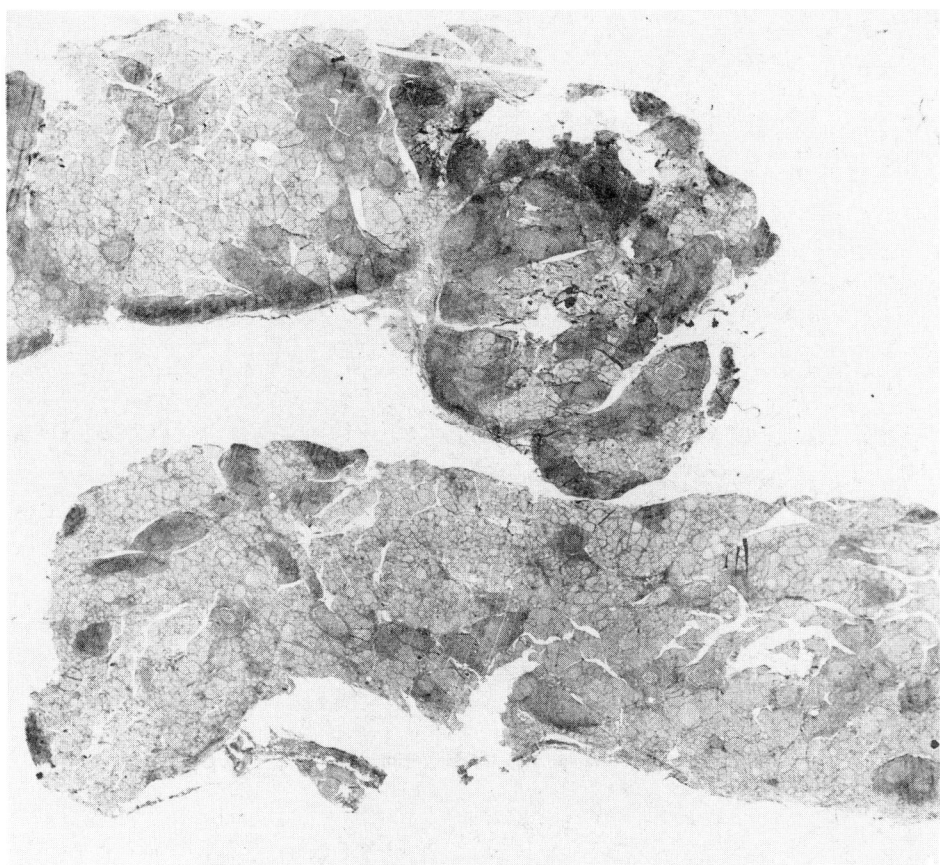

FIGURE 2. Low power view shows diffusely scattered lymphoid aggregates throughout the gland in classic thyroiditis (needle biopsy). (Hematoxylin-eosin; magnification × 4.)

2. Hurthle cells (Askanazy, oncocytes or oxyphilic cells) — these demonstrate poorly developed Golgi complexes, decreased endoplasmic reticulum, and characteristically increased numbers of large mitochondria.[13,31]
3. Colloid cells, which contain a large homogeneous area (? colloid) and appear to be end-stage cells.

Reidbord and Fisher[31] confirm the Hurthle cell appearance with characteristic numerous mitochondria.

Each of the studies documents the presence of lymphocytes in various sizes corresponding to the transformation sequence of B-cells,[13,31,32] i.e., transformed cells, immunoblasts, and plasma cells.[33] Immunologic studies have shown 40% T-cells and 40% B-cells in the infiltrate.[34] Stuart[35] described fuchsinophilic material within the lymphoid follicles and considered it an immunoglobulin. Bastenie et al.[13] and others[36] demonstrated lymphocytes penetrating epithelial cells in Hashimoto's disorder; this does not occur in normal thyroids. Kalderon et al.[37] noted follicular basement membrane deposits in eight cases of Hashimoto's which they examined ultrastructurally.[37] They compared these deposits to those identified in immune complex nephropathies.

Immunofluorescent studies have demonstrated immunoglobulins and complement in the basement membrane.[38] The meaning of this finding is not understood since both

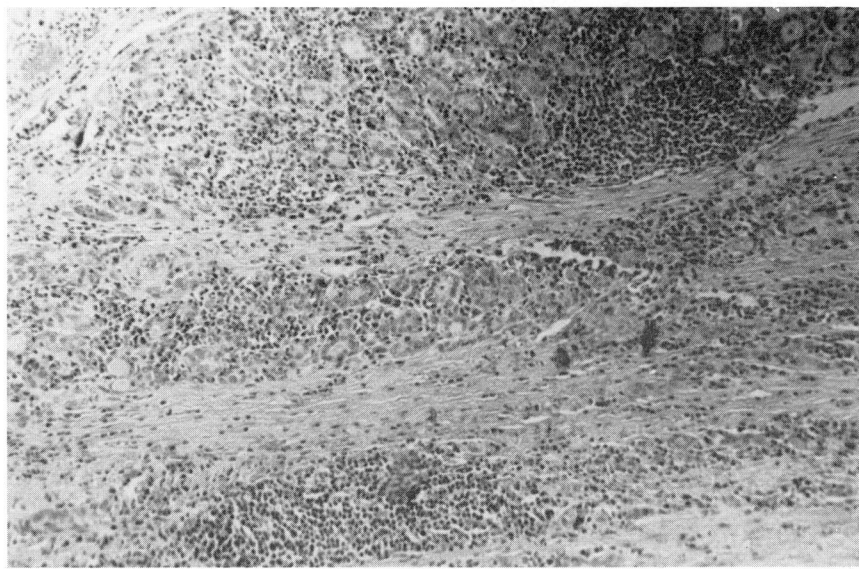

FIGURE 3. Fibrous band lymphocytic infiltrate and follicular atrophy are illustrated. (Hematoxylin-eosin; magnification × 100.)

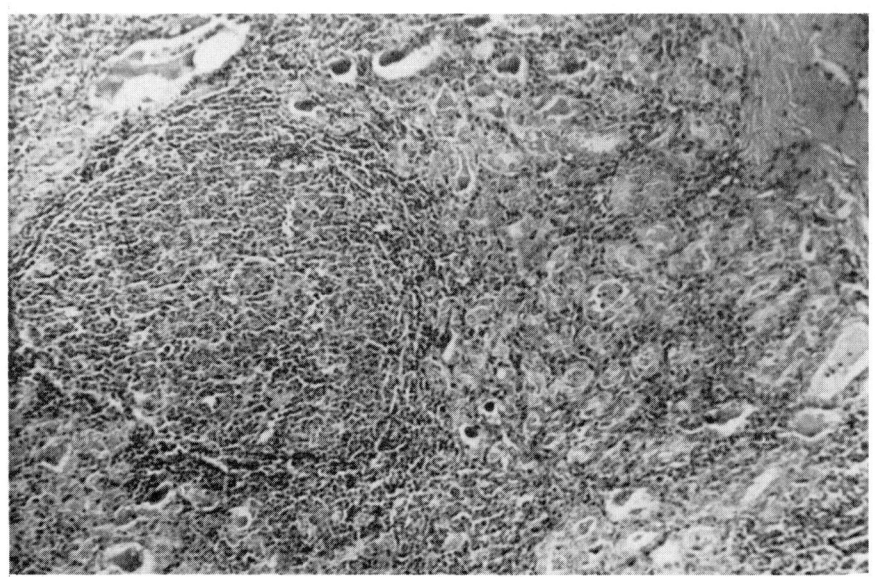

FIGURE 4. Germinal centers are surrounded by small colloid depleted follicles lined by Hurthle cells. (Hematoxylin-eosin; magnification × 125.)

Graves' disease and Hashimoto's disorder are lesions of uncertain etiology in which autoimmune phenomena of complex types (including cell-mediated and humoral factors) appear involved.[39] (Chapter 6). Hence, the mere demonstration of immunoglobulins in tissue must be interpreted cautiously. One report suggested the presence of "virus-like particles" in follicular epithelial cells in Hashimoto's disease;[40] the significance of these structures remains unclear.

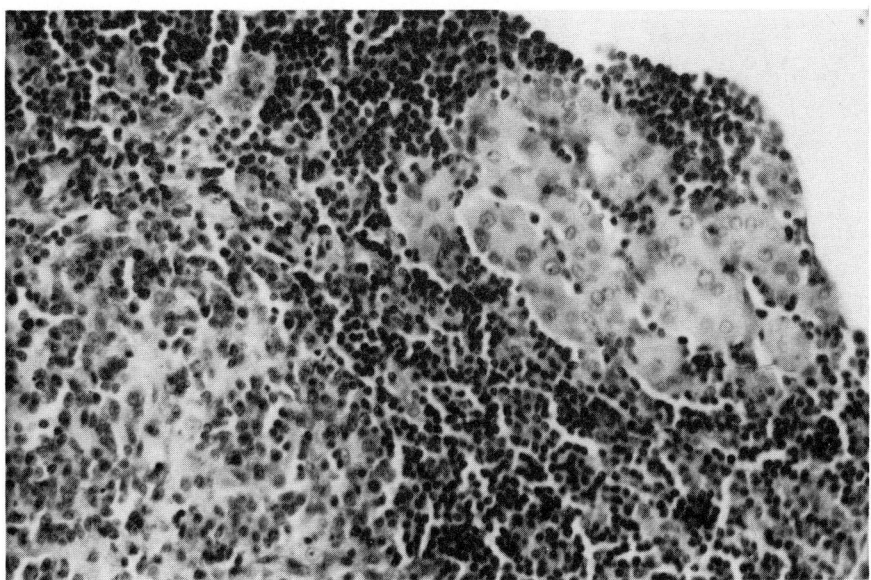

FIGURE 5. Hurthle cell cluster (upper right) is surrounded by lymphocytes. Germinal center is present in lower left. (Hematoxylin-eosin; magnification × 125.)

B. Hashitoxicosis

In 1971, the Mayo Clinic group described patients with hyperthyroidism and pathological features of Hashimoto's disease.[41] Since that time, the term Hashitoxicosis has been employed to refer to this disorder.[41,42] These authors[41] divided their subjects into three categories:

1. Group 1 included 9 individuals, ages 38 to 65 (male:female — 2:7) who had clinical and laboratory evidence of classical Graves' disease. On examination of their resected glands the histologic changes of Hashimoto's thyroiditis were recognized: lymphoid infiltration, oxyphilic epithelium, and follicular atrophy.
2. Group 2 was composed of five subjects (aged 14 to 54; malemale — 1:4) who showed clinical Graves' disease but whose thyroids demonstrated lymphocytic infiltration and focal epithelial hyperplasia. Hurthle cells were found rarely.
3. Group 3 included ten women (ages 15 to 63) with clinical Graves' disease and pathologic evidence of both epithelial hyperplasia and marked lymphoid infiltration.

These patients form a peculiar subgroup of autoimmune thyroid disease and lend support to Volpe's theory of a common pathogenesis for Graves' and Hashimoto's diseases.[39]

C. Juvenile Lymphocytic Thyroiditis

Lymphocytic thyroiditis tends to occur in children or adolescents[29,43] who have only slightly enlarged glands and may exhibit signs of hyperthyroidism. Pathologically lymphocytic infiltration predominates, but oxyphilic change and follicular destruction are absent or minimal.[6,18,26,29,43,44] Clinically, in lymphocytic thyroiditis, resolution may occur or the lesion may progress to myxedema.[6,29,43,44]

Painless thyroiditis[6,44-49] (see Chapter 4) with hyperthyroidism may represent this

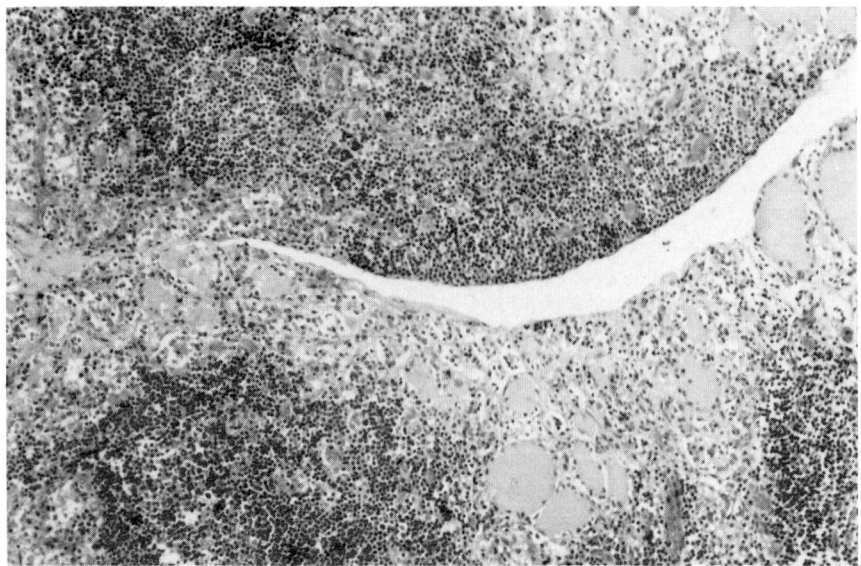

FIGURE 6. This case of juvenile lymphocytic thyroiditis illustrates lymphocytic infiltration, but no Hurthle cell change. Many thyroid follicles appear preserved. (Hematoxylin-eosin; magnification ×100.)

lymphocytic form or more commonly represents a variant of subacute thyroiditis[6,44-49] In this disorder, resolution with normal thyroid function is common, and recurrences are unusual. However, some patients with this disease do progress to myxedema.[6,43-50]

The thyroiditis cases associated with Graves' disease[41] (see above) partially overlap with juvenile lymphocytic thyroiditis[6,43,44] and painless subacute thyroiditis[6,42] (see Chapters 4 and 6) clinically and possible pathologically. Unfortunately, the Mayo Clinic series[41] was analyzed retrospectively, and adequate laboratory evaluation with modern techniques is lacking. These patients probably comprise a heterogeneous group[51-58] and the literature remains confused on this subject.

Some authors such as Doniach et al.[50] have divided Hashimoto's into three categories: juvenile lymphocytic, oxyphil (classic) variant, and fibrosing type (see Table 1). It is the first group which is not always easily delineated. Jackson[42] suggests that clinical distinction between Hashitoxicosis[41] and hyperthyroidism[6] may lie in the radioiodine uptake which is increased in the former and depressed in the latter.

In some cases dubbed juvenile lymphocytic thyroiditis, subacute onset is noted[55] or viral antigens are identified[58] leading to a confusing merging of various, probably distinct, entities. It must be recalled that antithyroid antibodies are measurable in subacute thyroiditis and that lymphocytes can be seen in that disorder.[49] Its prognosis and significance are so different that it would behoove all authorities to arrive at *definite* criteria (both clinical and pathologic) in order to define, modulate, and separate these entities. (Figure 6.)

D. The Fibrosing Variant of Hashimoto's Thyroiditis

In Hashimoto's original description,[1] one of his patients showed marked fibrosis and glandular destruction. He distinguished this case from Riedel's struma. Subsequent authors used cases of this type to support an interrelationship between Hashi-

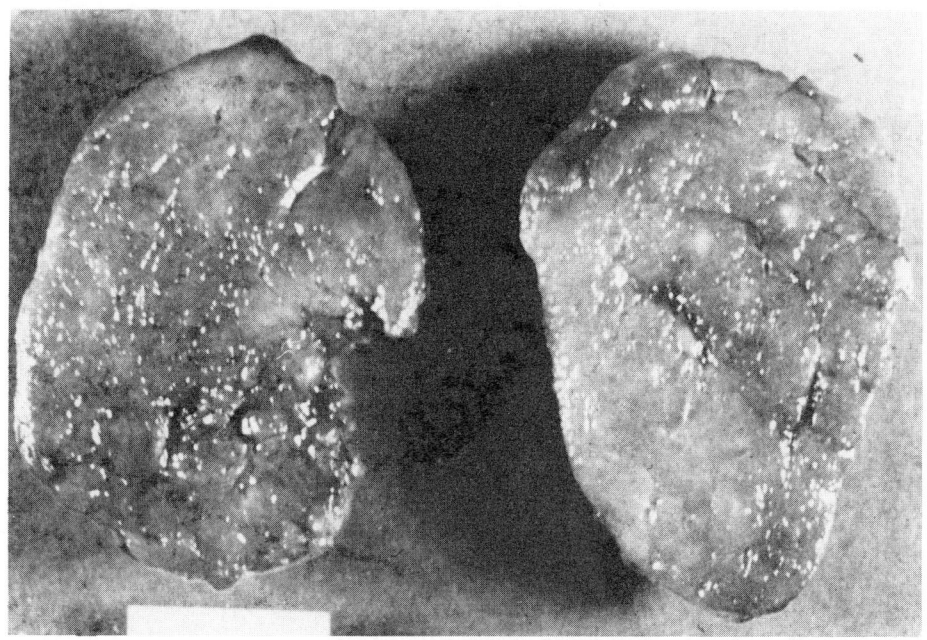

FIGURE 7. Gross appearance of fibrosing Hashimoto's thyroiditis initially diagnosed pathologically as Riedel's struma. Note containment within capsule of gland and suggestion of lobulation still present.

moto's and Riedel's disease, leading to great confusion in the literature. Katz and Vickery,[7] in 1974, elegantly redefined the fibrosing form of Hashimoto's thyroiditis. This disease comprises between 10 to 13% of all Hashimoto's lesion.[7,8,20]

1. Gross Features

The thyroid capsule is clearly demarcated from surrounding structures and few, if any adhesions are seen. This feature should reassure the surgeon and pathologist that they are not dealing with Riedel's disease.[7] Grossly, the thyroid is pale white to yellow, and very firm; on section a vaguely lobular pattern with extensive fibrosis is seen. The glands are often quite large (up to 200 g). (Figures 7 and 8.)

2. Microscopic Features

Histologically, at low power, the lobulation of the gland is retained (Figures 9 and 10); this finding serves in differentiating this lesion from cancer or Riedel's struma. Broad fibrous bands separate residual zones of degenerating thyroid (Figure 11). The latter shows changes reminiscent of classic Hashimoto's disease: follicular atrophy, oxyphil change, and lymphoid infiltrates with germinal centers. Inflammatory cells may also be identified within the fibrous bands. Although it may be found in other thyroid conditions (see below) and is not rare in the usual form of Hashimoto's disease,[8,18,20,29] squamous metaplasia is pronounced in the fibrous variant.[7] This change is considered a reaction of the damaged follicular epithelium from which the squamous or epidermoid cells arise.[7] Microscopically, distinction of this lesion from carcinoma may produce difficulty for the histopathologist.

Case Report — a 73-year-old man presented with weakness, fatiguability, and a large goiter. The patient had had a right parotidectomy 9 yr previously for "tumor".

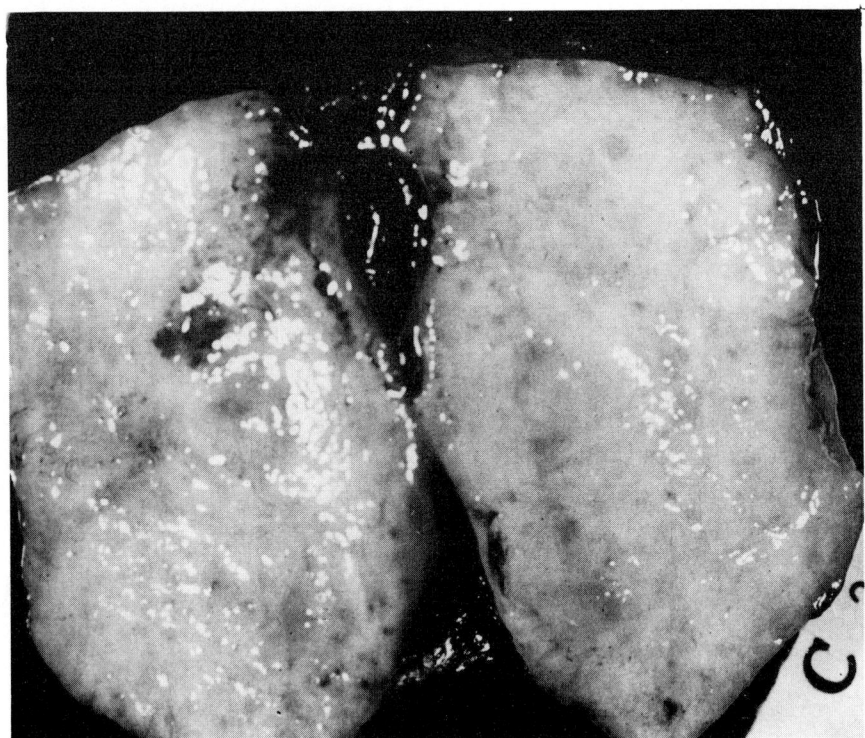

FIGURE 8. Another case of fibrosing variant shows intact capsule, pale, firm tissue, and slightly preserved lobulation (upper right).

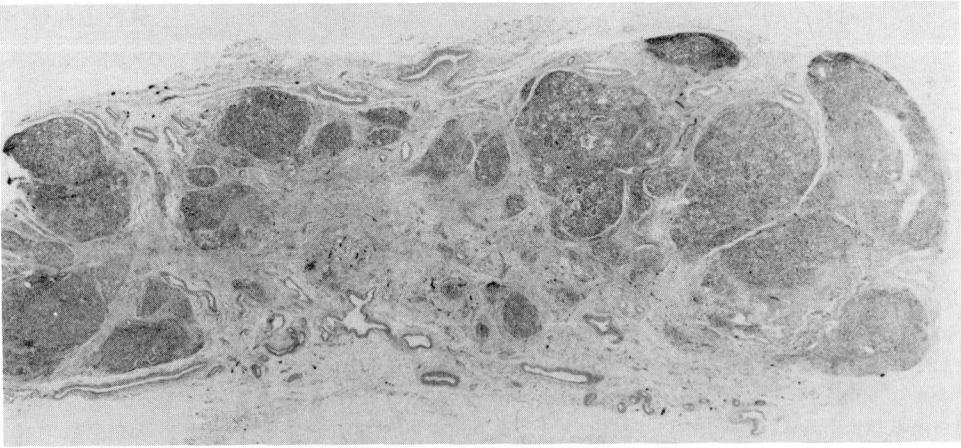

FIGURE 9. Low power view shows bridging fibrous bands separating preexisting lobules which contain lymphocytic infiltration and lobular atrophy. (Hematoxylin-eosin; magnification × 4.)

Because of the massive size of the goiter with extension to the lateral neck on the right, surgery was undertaken and a right cervical lymph node was excised. On frozen section, lymphoid tissue with germinal centers was seen in which scattered, rare epidermoid cell clusters were identified. The diagnosis of epidermoid carcinoma metastatic to lymph node was made and, prior to radical neck dissection, a portion of the goiter

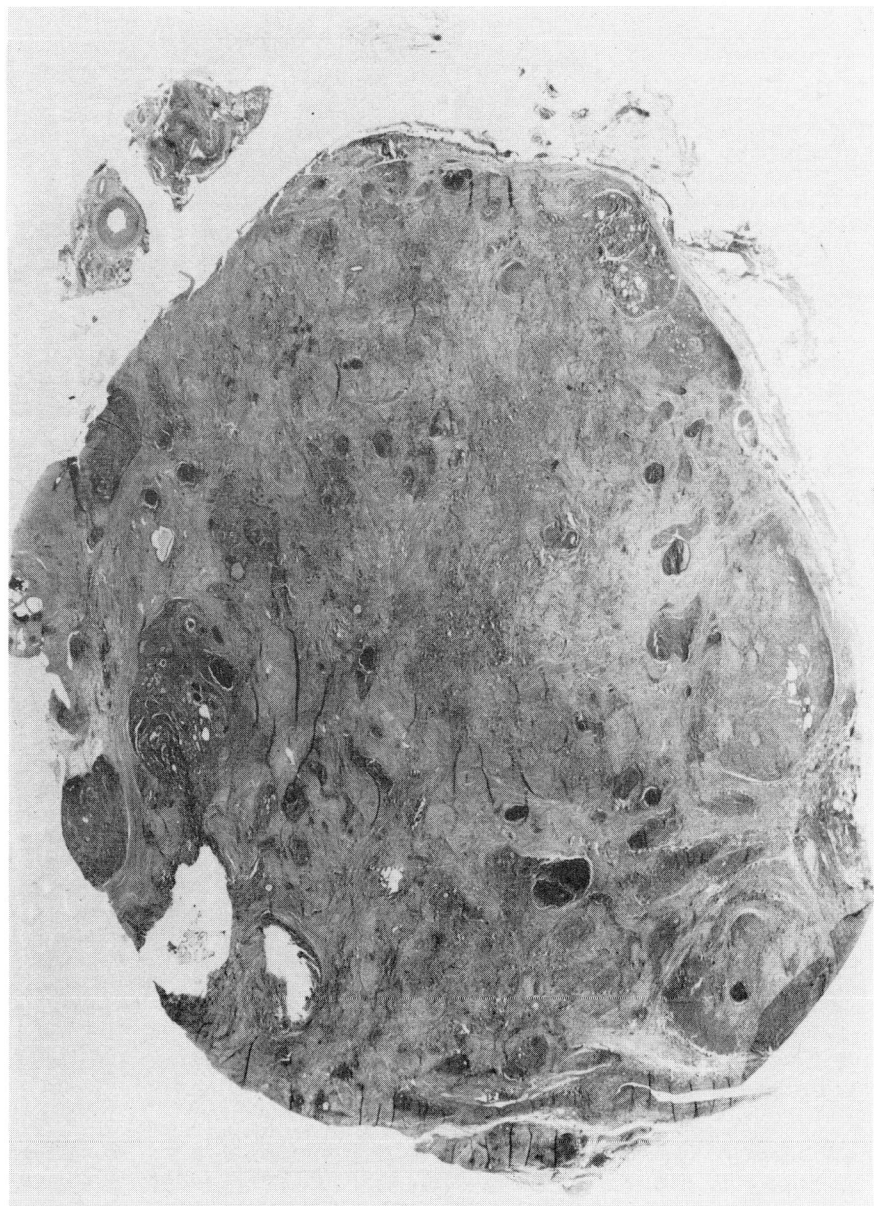

FIGURE 10. Same case as Figure 8 showing more obliterative fibrous pattern. (Hematoxylin-eosin; magnification × 4.)

was removed. This tissue showed extensive fibrosis and lobulation (Figure 10) and on frozen section, atrophic thyroid follicles were recognized, suggesting that the entire lesion represented thyroiditis (Figure 11). Reexamination of the initially removed node disclosed that it indeed did not represent lymph node (no sinuses present), but was merely a biopsy of the thyroid. Neck dissection was not performed. Postoperatively, thyroid function studies disclosed hypothyroidism; treatment with thyroid replacement elicited improvement in symptoms and shrinkage of the goiter. The slides of the paro-

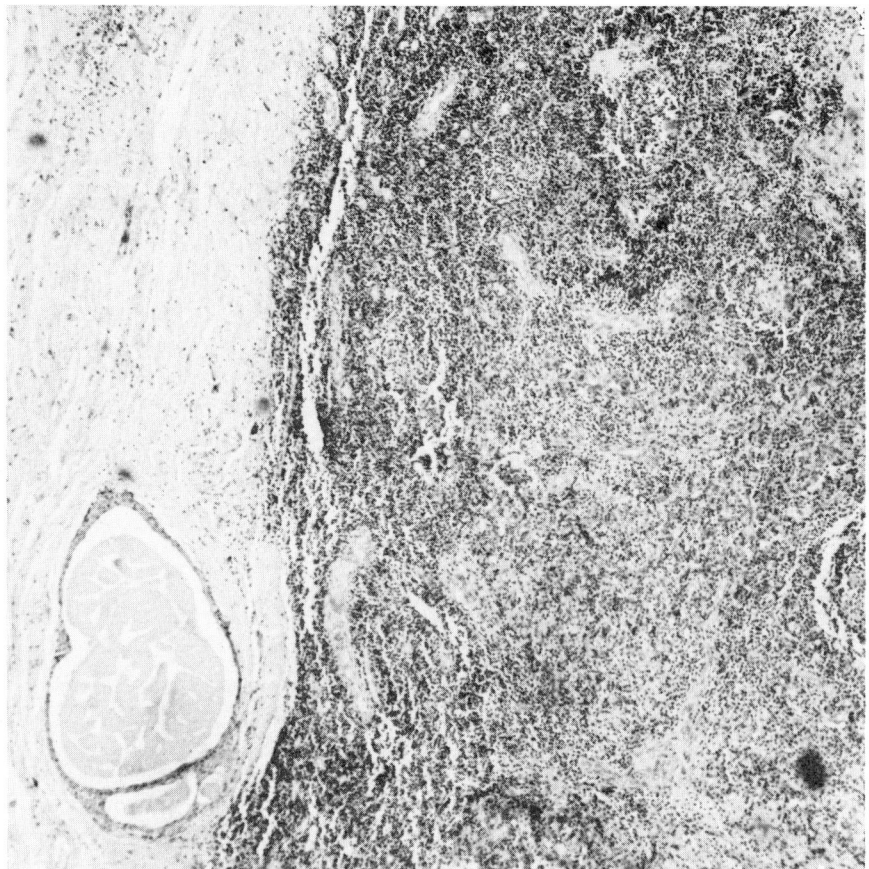

FIGURE 11. This photograph illustrates atrophic follicles obscured by lymphocytic infiltrate and fibrosis. Early squamous metaplasia of follicular epithelium is noted (lower left). (Hematoxylin-eosin; magnification × 125.)

tid tumor were obtained; review desclosed a Wasthin's tumor, considered unrelated to the patient's thyroiditis.

3. Clinicopathologic Correlation

As can be seen in Table 1, the fibrosing variant occurs in an older age group than ordinary Hashimoto's disease, often presents with large goiter and symptoms of hypothyroidism. Thyroglobulin antibodies are present in very high titers[7,50] more than any other subtype. This disorder often requires surgical treatment because of pressure symptoms due to goiter size.[7] Permanent hypothyroidism often results, whether surgical extirpation or needle biopsy only is used for diagnosis.[7]

The relationship of the fibrous variant to other subtypes of thyroiditis remains unclear. Katz and Vickery[7] suggest a progression from mild forms of Hashimoto's disease to fibrosis and older age at diagnosis supports this. Moreover, these authors report that three patients, in whom needle biopsy or surgical material from the thyroid was removed years before the diagnosis of fibrous Hashimoto's disease, demonstrated lymphocytic infiltration of the gland or a mild form of classic Hashimoto's thyroiditis.[7]

4. Differential Diagnosis

Three major diagnoses can be confused clinically and pathologically with fibrous Hashimoto's thyroiditis: Riedel's struma, carcinoma, and idiopathic myxedema.

Riedel's struma — Hashimoto[1] himself distinguished the disorder he described from Riedel's lesion.[4,8,13, 18-20,26,28,59-61] Grossly, the latter is woody or iron hard and the abnormal tissue is *adherent*[4,8,59,61] to surrounding structures; tissue planes are obliterated. As discussed in Chapter 11, Riedel's disease probably is not a disorder of the thyroid but a connective tissue proliferation involving the gland. No relationship between the Riedel's and Hashimoto's lesions (i.e., the former progresses to the latter) can be supported by present evidence.[59-61] Fibrosing Hashimoto's thyroiditis is characterized by nonviolation of thyroid capsule and intraglandular, not extraglandular, fibrosis. The thyroid demonstrates changes of classic Hashimoto's disease, and hypothyroidism is common.[7] In Riedel's struma, the noninvolved thyroid appears normal and euthyroidism is usually found.[8,59-61]

Carcinoma — most carcinomas of the thyroid present as discrete nodular lesions and should not cause confusion, clinically or pathologically. (The relationship between peritumor thyroiditis and Hashimoto's is discussed in Chapter 10; this would not produce confusion with the fibrosing variant, however.) Anaplastic carcinoma of the thyroid occurs in the same age group as fibrosing Hashimoto's and produces a large mass which is extremely hard to palpation. However, anaplastic cancer does not maintain the boundaries of the thyroid and often extends to surrounding tissues. Histological examination discloses a very cellular tumor different from the dense, relatively acellular collagen bands seen in Hashimoto's disease. In addition, lack of lobulation, mitoses, and cellular pleomorphism are found in the anaplastic carcinoma.[62-64]

Idiopathic myxedema — clinically presenting as hypothyroidism, often in elderly patients, idiopathic myxedema is distinguished from fibrosing Hashimoto's thyroiditis by small size of the gland. Histologic examination shows some similarity between the two disorders; each shows fibrosis, follicular destruction, lymphoid infiltration, oncocytes, and squamous metaplasia.[65]

Although these lesions may be related, i.e., both represent autoimmune thyroid destructive disorders, there is no evidence that fibrosing Hashimoto's disease is a transitional stage of idiopathic myxedema. Thus, patients with the latter rarely give a history of goiter.[7] Katz and Vickery postulate that the two lesions may represent different host responses to a common or related etiologic agent — one showing fibrous proliferation and the other fibrous atrophy.[7] (Figures 12 and 13.)

5. Squamous Cells in the Thyroid

A variety of cells have been called "squamous" in the thyroid.[66] These include (a) basaloid cells derived from ultimobranchial or thymic remnants, (b) clear cells (parafollicular of C-cells), and (c) epidermoid or true keratinizing squamous cells. The last group of these concerns us here. (Table 2.) Epidermoid cells may be derived from teratomas,[67-73] thyroglossal duct,[74-77] or from metaplasia of follicular epithelium.[78-80] In thyroiditis, the last mechanism is believed to be active.[78-80]

Klinck and Menk[78] and Harcourt-Webster[79] have studied the question of squamous metaplasia in the thyroid gland. Squamous cells may be encountered in the following conditions: adenomatous goiter, thyroiditis, primary or secondary myxedema, and carcinomas of various types, including pure squamous carcinoma.[81-86]

Evidence presented from histologic studies described above[78,79] supports the theory of metaplasia of follicular epithelial cells into squamous cells. Squamous elements are encountered commonly in inflammatory conditions in the thyroid. In these cases transitions between follicular and squamous cells can be recognized.[7,78,79,87] Gould et al.[88]

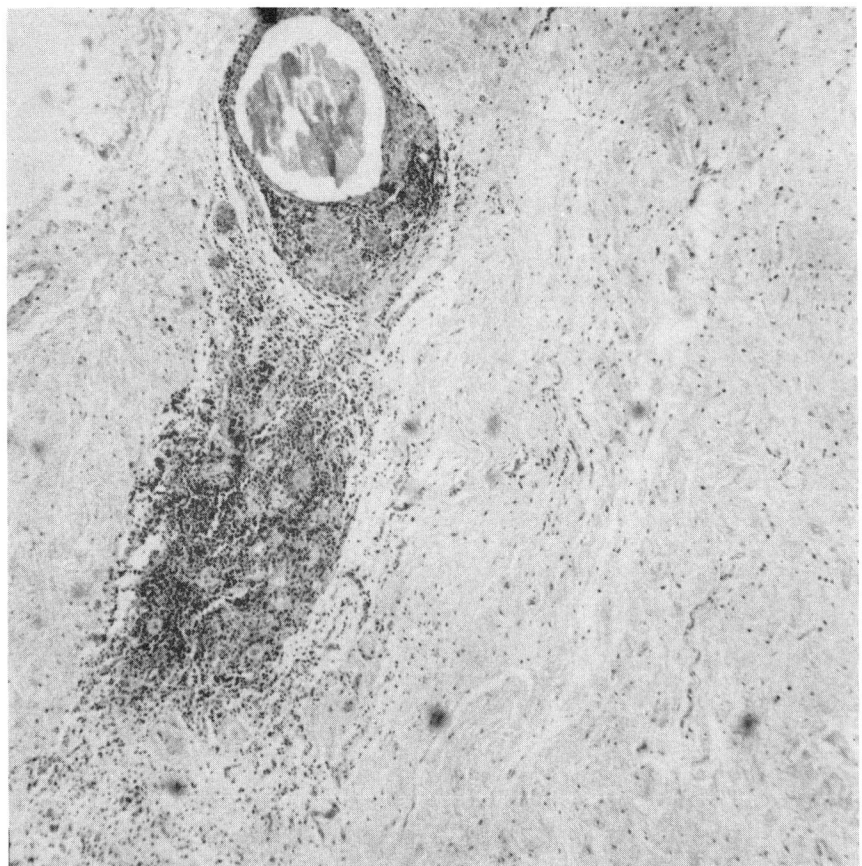

FIGURE 12. Tissue barely recognizable as thyroid shows fibrosis, lymphoid cells, and dilated follicle (upper mid portion) in case of idiopathic myxedema. (Hematoxylin-eosin; magnification × 100.)

examined squamous cells in papillary cancers of the thyroid by electron microscopy and concluded that these elements arose from altered follicular pithelium .

The squamous cells which may be epidermoid or truly squamous (with keratin), and which are derived from metaplasia of follicular epithelium, are identified only in association with other conditions. The clinical significance of this finding relates to the associated primary lesion. Adenomatous goiter[66] or thyroiditis[7,79] are the conditions which must be considered and treated. The most extreme examples of squamous metaplasia are encountered in chronic thyroiditis or myxedema.[7]

E. Chronic Lymphocytic Thyroiditis Resembling Lymphoma

Initially described by Woolner et al.,[18] this variant of Hashimoto's causes worries for the histopathologist since the lymphocytic infiltrate is so great as to mimic malignant lymphoma.[18] This variant occurs in less than 1% of cases and affects primarily elderly women.[18,29] The diffuse nature of the process, the presence of thyroid follicles,[18] and the reactive nature of the lymphoid nodules with a pleomorphic cell population, including macrophages, serves to distinguish this lesion from true malignant lymphoma.

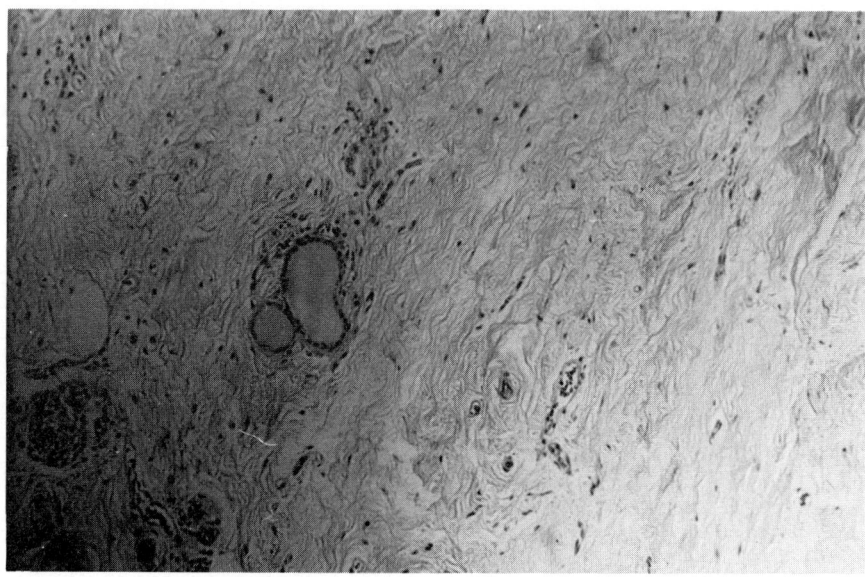

FIGURE 13. Focally a rare residual follicle enables one to identify the tissue as thyroid. (Hematoxylin-eosin; magnification × 100.)

Table 2
SQUAMOUS CELLS IN THE HUMAN THYROID

Basaloid
    Ultimobranchial body
    Thymic remnants
    Solid cell nests
Parafollicular cells
Epidermoid or true squamous cells
    Teratoma
    Thyroglossal duct remnants
    Metaplasia of normal, inflamed, or neoplastic follicular epithelium
    Squamous cell carcinoma, primary or metastatic

Adapted from LiVolsi, V. A. and Merino, M. J., *Am. J. Surg. Pathol.*, 2, 133, 1978. With permission.

F. Hashimoto's Thyroiditis Presenting as a Nodule

Occasionally, a cold or hypofunctioning nodule, clinically resembling a neoplasm, may represent the initial presentation of Hashimoto's thyroiditis.[7,8,13,89-91] In these cases, the diagnosis may be made only by the histologist. Bialas et al.[92] reported a patient with a functioning nodule who had Hashimoto's thyroiditis; they suggest that in patients with nodules, thyroid antibodies should be measured and the diagnosis might be confirmed by needle biopsy.[52] However, since histologic changes identical to Hashimoto's disease can be recognized in tissue surrounding thyroid tumors[10-13] (see Chapter 10), surgery might be undertaken to rule out a neoplasm.

The mechanism of nodule formation may include focal differences in severity of the lesion or the presence (preexistence) of nodular goiter (or adenomatous nodules). Such adenomatous foci are not unusual in classic Hashimoto's.[7,8,13]

III. THE HURTHLE CELL

A. Microscopic Appearance
Although not specific for Hashimoto's disease, the Hurthle cell is characteristic of that disease.[1,7,8,13,18,29] This cell is generally described as relatively large, contains finely granular eosinophilic cytoplasm, and large, sometimes bizarre, and even hyperchromatic nuclei. Often the hyperchromasia of the nuclei may be produced by a peculiar folding or crenation of this structure.[93,94]

The nature and significance of Hurthle cells in the thyroid (also called Askanazy cells, oxyphils, or oncocytes)[13,95,96] has elicited great interest. Biochemical studies on these elements have disclosed that, despite the presence of large amounts of various enzymes,[97,98] they are physiologically inert, do not produce thyroxine or thyroglobulin,[99] and probably represent a degenerative state of follicular epithelium.[13,93,94,99] Sometimes, in association with Hurthle cells or in the same gland, large cells with clear cytoplasm are found;[13,100,101] these are considered Hurthle-cell variants and hence related to follicular epithelium.

B. Ultrastructure
By electron microscopy,[13] Hurthle cells contain poorly developed endoplasmic reticulum which corresponds to a lack of protein synthesis,[99] but they possess many large mitochondria which fill the cytoplasm and are responsible for the cytoplasmic eosinophilia.[13] The significance of these mitochondria, which in biochemical terms would indicate tremendous physiologic activity, is unclear.[97-99] Similar cells are found in salivary glands and parathyroid, but here again, their meaning is unclear.

Heimann et al.[99] describe transitions between follicular epithelium and Hurthle cells and consider the evidence that Hurthle cells represent a degenerated state of follicular epithelium and not another cell line. Feidman et al.[102] also noted this resemblance to follicular cells in their ultrastructural examination of Hurthle cells.

C. Histochemistry
Tremblay and Pearse,[97] and Harcourt-Webster and Stott[98] have described the enzyme chemistry of Hurthle cells. These elements contain abundant Krebs cycle enzymes: succinate and beta-hydroxybutyrate dehydrogenase, glucose 6-phosphase dehydrogenase, glucose-6-phosphogluconate dehydrogenase, and lactate dehydrogenase. In addition, acid phosphatase and peroxidase are also recognized in large quantities. These findings suggest a hyperactive rather than a degenerative state; but no evidence for physiologic activity in these cells has been identified.

D. Hurthle Cells in the Thyroid
1. Thyroiditis
Hurthle cells are found in varying numbers in almost all cases of classic and fibrosing Hashimoto's[1,7,8,13,18,29] and less often in juvenile forms of the disease.[13,18,26,29] Such cells are rarely, if ever, identified in the other types of thyroiditis, or in Graves' disease. They may occur in isolated foci or as isolated cells in inflammatory conditions affecting the thyroid (such as in a nodular goiter), but this is rare.

The present author has identified Hurthle cells in large numbers, in otherwise normal thyroid glands, in 30 autopsied patients who died of malignancies, especially lymphoid and hematopoietic type. In each case, the patient had received chemotherapy in which one of the drugs was either cyclophosphamide or vinblastine. The significance of this finding warrants further investigation.(See Figure 5.)

2. Tumors

Pure Hurthle cell tumors — Hurthle cell tumors have presented difficulties for pathologists.[94,103] Some authors suggest that all Hurthle cell neoplasms be considered malignant;[103] others believe in the existence of a Hurthle cell adenoma which can be differentiated from a carcinoma by absence of anaplasia, high mitotic rate and capsule or vascular invasion. Hurthle cell carcinomas (and clear cell carcinomas) are regarded as variants of follicular carcinoma, which tumor they resemble in their biologic behavior (hematogenous metastases, unifocal lesion, sparing of regional nodes).[104-106]

Confusion with medullary carcinoma of the epithelial type — this may arise in Hurthle cell tumors. Amyloid, spindle cell areas, neurosecretory granules on electron microscopy, and localization of calcitonin by immunohistochemistry should distinguish the two.[107-108]

Other Tumors — Hurthle cells can comprise focal areas of otherwise characteristic follicular adenomas or carcinomas without altering prognosis. Indeed, several series report finding Hurthle cells in 20% of follicular thyroid carcinomas.[104-106] These authors argue that this represents further evidence for the origin of Hurthle cells from follicular epithelium.[104-106] Occasionally, a papillary carcinoma will be composed wholly or in part of Hurthle cells. Such tumors may behave somewhat more aggressively than ordinary papillary cancer, but this may be more related to larger size of these lesions at diagnosis.[109]

IV. SO-CALLED CHRONIC NONSPECIFIC THYROIDITIS

In Chapter 8, lymphocytic thyroiditis associated with ingestion of various drugs, including iodine (iodide), is discussed. It has been recognized that lymphocytic infiltration of the thyroid is found more frequently at autopsy and in surgical specimens since the addition of iodide to the water supplies in the U.S. some 40 to 50 years ago.[110-112] The possibility exists that iodide (iodine) acts as a hapten which combines with a protein, acts as an antigen, and evokes an immune response localized to the thyroid gland.[113]

Bastenie et al.[9] believe that these lymphocytic infiltrates share the meaning of autoimmune thyroiditis seen in other conditions such as around tumors.[9,13,18,114] They are distinguished clinically by older age of the patients, absence of symptoms, absent or low antithyroid antibodies,[9,114-116] and often the presence of nodules resembling nodular or adenomatous goiter.[9]

Pathologically, no gross lesions are seen except if nodules are present. Microscopically, focal aggregates of lymphocytes are seen, occasionally germinal center formation is noted, and (rarely) Hurthle cells are present.[26] The infiltrates tend to occupy only fibrous septa of the gland and spare adenomatous foci. Follicular atrophy is identified rarely.

Hurley[29] notes that the incidence of focal lymphoid thyroiditis parallels that of thyroidal antibodies in the general population,[117] and the finding increases with increasing age.[117,118] Thyroid function abnormalities also parallel increasing age.[119]

Sommers[26] postulates that nonspecific chronic thyroiditis represents a heterogeneous group of lesions which include residual inflammation following hemorrhage in nodular goiter, acute thyroiditis, trauma, chemical or radiation injury, and mild forms of Hashimoto's disease. This author[26] describes the entity of nonspecific thyroiditis, if it exists, as affecting women over 40 with slightly painful, minimally enlarged glands and with normal or low normal thyroid function.[24,120,121] It appears that again we are presented with a poorly defined, and confusing, entity, which awaits further evaluation.

V. THE PATHOLOGY OF HYPOTHYROIDISM

A. Case Report

A 79-yr-old white, unmarried, retired saleswoman was admitted to the hospital with complaints of lethargy (being "too weak to get out of bed"), cough, and chest pain. The patient was in good health until 12 years ago when she noted the onset of pressing substernal pain associated with exertion and relieved by rest. Three months later, she entered the hospital during one episode when this pain did not subside with rest, and subsequent studies demonstrated an anterolateral myocardial infarction. Serum cholesterol was 332 mg/dℓ. After an uncomplicated hospital course, she was discharged on phenobarbitol. Several months later, angina pectoris returned and was accompanied by leg edema. She was placed on a diuretic and digitalis. Two years later, leg edema, muscle weakness, thinning of the hair, and dry, pale skin were noted. Episodes of angina were treated with nitroglycerin.

Her condition remained relatively stable for 7 yr until approximately 6 weeks prior to this admission, when she began gaining weight, became pale, developed increased edema, and a cough. At this time she became confused, began to hallucinate, and complained of lethargy and coldness. Her private physician saw her 4 weeks prior to admission. Her temperature was 92°F and she was hyporeflexic. For a suspected diagnosis of hypothyroidism, increasing doses of dessicated thyroid were begun (0.25 grain, alternate days). She at first improved, but then developed symptoms of congestive heart failure.

Physical examination on admission revealed a confused, cyanotic female complaining of tiredness and difficulty breathing. Her pulse was 62, temperature 97°F, blood pressure 120/70, and respirations 18 per min. Her skin was dry and scaly with pallor and poor turgor. Alopecia and thin scalp hair were noted. Examination of the extremities showed pitting edema; facial and truncal edema were also present. The conjunctivae were pale and the pupils were round, equal, and reactive. The thyroid was not palpable, the trachea was in the midline, and no masses or enlarged lymph nodes were felt in the neck. Rales and expiratory wheezing were heard bilaterally over the entire lung field. Jugular veins were engorged. Auscultation of the heart revealed an irregular beat at the rate of 62 per min without murmurs or gallops. The abdomen was distended without organomegaly. Neurological exam disclosed obtundation, intact cranial nerves, and sensory system. Muscle strength was decreased. Reflexes were present and the relaxation period was increased after the knee and ankle jerks. Speech was slow and labored.

Admission lab values included hematocrit of 33.1, hemoglobin of 10.5, and a WBC count of 4700. There were 180,000 platelets. The ESR was 49. The red cell indices were: MCV = 105, MCH = 33.0, and MCHC = 31.9. A peripheral smear showed slight macrocytosis, slight aniso- and poikilocytosis, and few bizarre forms. Electrolytes, glucose, BUN, and creatinine were normal. Thyroxine (T_4) was 1.4 (normal = 4.2 to 9.2). The T_4 microsomal fraction complement fixation test was negative. Thyroglobulin-coated, sheep red cell antibody titer was positive at 1:2500.

The EKG demonstrated depressed ST segments, sinus rhythm with frequent, premature ventricular contractions, an old anterior myocardial infarction, and questionable left ventricular hypertrophy A chest X-ray demonstrated cardiomegaly and marked pulmonary congestive changes.

Treatment with digoxin and dessicated thyroid (0.75 grains per day) was given. However, the patient's dyspnea worsened and an X-ray on the third hospital day demonstrated increasing pulmonary edema. Furosemide was given. On the fourth day, the patient developed angina, and premature beats and confusion persisted. Her breathing

Table 3
PATHOLOGICAL FEATURES OF PRIMARY MYXEDEMA

Gross
    Gland small and atrophic (weights 10 to 15 g not uncommon)
    No adherence to neighboring structures
Microscopic
    Extensive fibrous replacement with loss of parenchyma; difficult to define lobules
    Follicular atrophy
    Lymphoplasmacytic infiltrate
    Hurthle cells present
    Squamous metaplasia is prominent

deteriorated and she required oxygen. However, respiratory arrest, followed by a cardiac arrest, ensued and despite attempts at cardiac massage and defibrillation, the patient died on the sixth hospital day.

Pathology — Autopsy disclosed severe generalized arteriosclerosis, myocardial fibrosis, cardiomegaly with anasarca, and pleural and pericardial effusions all reflecting heart failure. The thyroid weighed 12.5 g and was pale and firm. Microscopically, extensive fibrosis replaced 90% of the parenchyma (Figures 12 and 13); focally, lymphocytic infiltrates were noted in which markedly atrophic follicles lined by Hurthle cells were seen. Squamous metaplasia was prominent.

B. Myxedema — Primary

This case illustrates the classic findings in idiopathic myxedema. Although any of the Hashimoto's variants described above can produce hypothyroidism, the situation with primary myxedema differs in clinical and pathologic features. Thus, clinical symptoms tend to be of greater degree and duration, the gland tends to be small and, histologically, is almost totally replaced by fibrosis.[7,26,65] Since the etiology of none of these disorders is known, interrelationships among them can only be guessed at. Katz and Vickery suggest that fibrous Hashimoto's thyroiditis and idiopathic myxedema may represent two paths with similar beginnings but pathologically divergent ends.[7]

The classic paper by Sclare[65] outlines the various histologic changes in myxedematous glands: his group I corresponds to primary myxedema as in the case above. The findings include extensive fibrous replacement (making recognition of the gland as thyroid difficult), lymphoplasmacitic infiltrate, Hurthle cells, and squamous metaplasia with follicular atrophy (see Table 3).

Ultrastructural studies of myxedematous glands have disclosed alterations of follicular epithelial cells to Hurthle cells, and lymphoplasmacytic infiltration with penetration of the epithelial cells by lymphocytes;[122,123] this resembles the changes noted in the usual form of Hashimoto's disease.[13]

C. Myxedema — Secondary

Available evidence of thyroid pathology in secondary (pituitary, hypothalmic) myxedema[26,124-126] is scant. The present author has had the opportunity to examine the thyroid of an elderly man with an undiagnosed and untreated pituitary adenoma which replaced that organ. The thyroid in this case resembled that seen in primary myxedema with extensive lobular fibrosis and lymphoid infiltration. However, Hurthle cells were sparse and, focally, groups of follicles appeared intact.

D. The Pathology of Cretinism

It is not in the scope of a book on thyroiditis to discuss cretinism in detail, since this disorder does not entail inflammatory changes in the thyroid. Indeed, the pathologic features of hyperplastic goiter reflect enzymatic defects in thyroid hormone synthesis, such that thyrotropin continuously stimulates the gland without effect. Grossly, huge goiters with secondary degenerative changes, including hemorrhage, fibrosis, and calcification can be seen. Microscopically, extensive hyperplasia of follicular epithelial cells, papillary infoldings, and absent colloid are seen.[26,127-134]

VI. EXTRATHYROID PATHOLOGY IN HYPOTHYROIDISM

The major effects of hypothyroidism on the system appear to reflect on the cardiovascular system. Thus, accelerated atherosclerosis has been noted[135,136] as well as hypercholesterolemia,[26,137-139] premature myocardial infarcts,[140,141] and congestive heart failure.[142,143] Impaired myocardial contractility, bradycardia, and decreased cardiac output result from low-circulating thyroid hormone.[140,141] Impaired fluid excretion and renal tubular defects have also been reported.[144-149]

The gastrointestinal tract also malfunctions and constipation is a common complaint.[150,151] These changes are believed to be predominantly functional ones reversible by therapy. Nervous system and psychiatric disturbances have been described,[26,152-154] reflecting the overall low metabolic state and poor oxygenation.[155] Defects in the senses of taste and smell may occur.[156]

Alterations of the hepatocyte organelles[157] have been reported. Anemia,[158-161] deafness,[162] joint effusions and arthritis,[163-166] hypoinsulinism,[167] and sexual abnormalities[126,168-171] may occur. The skin characteristically is thickened because of mucopolysaccharide deposits in it.[172]

The pituitary changes in myxedema have been studied by several groups.[173-178] In both animal studies and in human myxedema, increased numbers of thyrotropes are found; at times these are so numerous as to cause gross pituitary enlargement.[173] The presumed mechanism is lack of feedback by absence of thyroxin from the thyroid gland. Cohen and Felig[168] suggest that the patient with primary hypothyroidism may seek medical attention because of amenorrhea-galactorrhea syndromes, presumably from excess prolactin secretion. The interrelationships to explain this phenomenon remain unknown, but the possibility exists that if one cell line (thyrotrophs) undergoes hyperplasia, neighboring ones (lactotrophs) may too. Alternatively, the same cell may be capable of secreting both hormones. More work is needed in this area.

VII. ASSOCIATIONS IN HASHIMOTO'S THYROIDITIS

In Chapter 6, Seplowitz has discussed the association of disorders of "autoimmune" nature with Hashimoto's disease. The common denominator in many of these conditions appears to be a specific genotype present in patients and their families.

Conditions commonly found in patients with Hashimoto's thyroiditis, or their close relatives, include lupus,[179,180] rheumatoid arthritis,[164] scleroderma,[180] liver disease,[182] Graves' disease,[50] purpura,[183] myasthenia gravis,[183] and giant cell arteritis.[184]

Two interesting associations are adrenal failure and ovarian failure. The combination of adrenal insufficiency and hypothyroidism without pituitary cause has been called Schmidt's syndrome.[185-188] Antibodies to both organs have been identified in these patients. Pathologically, the thyroid shows changes of classic Hashimoto's disease; in the adrenal, lymphocytic infiltration with cortical destruction is present. Antiovarian antibodies have been described in a patient with Hashimoto's thyroiditis and hypoparathyroidism.[189]

Table 4
FIBROSIS IN THE THYROID

Diffuse
    Thyroiditis
    Hashimoto's
      Classic variant
      Fibrosing variant
    Riedel's struma
    Subacute thyroiditis, sometimes
    Healed acute thyroiditis, sometimes
    Healed palpation thyroiditis
    Radiation
    Myxedema, primary and secondary
Focal
    Thyroiditis
      Healed acute thyroiditis
      Riedel's struma, sometimes
    Trauma
    Desmoplasia around tumors
    Nodular goiter

These unusual clinical situations shed light on the systemic disease which is dubbed Hashimoto's thyroiditis. The role of autoimmunity in these situations remains tempting as a pathogenetic mechanism, but is not adequately proven. Thymic dysfunction pathology[190] in these patients awaits evaluation by modern immunologic methods.

As has been noted elsewhere in this monograph, surgical series have implied an association between Hashimoto's thyroiditis and cancer of the thyroid[191-198] with estimates ranging from 8 to 22.5% coincidence. Other studies have not confirmed this view;[192,197] recent evidence suggests that the Hashimoto picture found around a thyroid carcinoma represents an immunologic response to the tumor (? abnormal anitgens), not evidence of preexisting Hashimoto's disease[28] (see Chapter 10).

Rarely, a neoplasm of, or in, the thyroid may clinically suggest thyroiditis. Rosen et al.[198] coined the term malignant pseudothyroiditis for this entity; the report by Rosen et al.[199] also emphasizes this phenomenon. These cases present clinical problems, not pathologic confusion as does the peritumor thyroiditis considered above.

VIII. DIFFERENTIAL DIAGNOSIS: FIBROSIS IN THE THYROID

Table 4 lists those conditions associated with fibrosis of the thyroid. As has been discussed earlier, fibrosis in the thyroid may be seen in Hashimoto's thyroiditis and its variants, in Riedel's disease, and in idiopathic myxedema. In these conditions, the degree of fibrosis varies as does the severity of thyroid destruction. Distinguishing Hashimoto's fibrosing thyroiditis from Riedel's disease and myxedema has been outlined above.

Focal scarring may occur in nodular goiter, especially in areas of colloid cysts, with collapse, hemorrhage and subsequent healing.[200] Similarly, healing following trauma (accident, surgical) or infection may leave focal areas of fibrosis.[201-203]

In subacute thyroiditis, minute perilobular scars may be noted after recovery. These apparently do not interfere with function.[203-206] Similar lesions are believed to occur after resolution of the granulomatous foci in palpation thyroiditis.[207]

Radiation to the thyroid, either external or internal produces fibrosis with concomitant atrophy and epithelial atypia;[208-211] the latter are noted more commonly with radioiodine.[210,211] Finally, desmoplastic responses around tumors, either primary or metastatic, produce focal zones of fibrosis.[104-107]

IX. HYPOTHYROIDISM DUE TO INFILTRATIVE DISORDERS OF THE THYROID

A. Amyloid

Glenner and Page[212] define amyloid as a proteinaceous substance deposited extracellularly in tissues, and composed of a homogeneous eosinophilic material. By electron microscopy, amyloid consists of nonbranching fibrils 80 to 100 Å wide. These fibrils produce the characteristic Congo red staining, toluidine blue metachromasia, and birefringence by polarized light. Chemical analyses indicate that amyloid consists of a protein composed of polypeptide chains arranged in a beta-pleated sheet configuration. This latter feature is shared by amyloids of various origins

Pearse[213] differentiated immunoamyloid from APUD-amyloid associated with neuroendocrine tumors. Thus, immunoamyloid is composed of immunoglobulin light chains[213] and APUD-amyloid contains prohormones secreted by neuroendocrine tumor cells.[213-215]

Amyloid may be found in the thyrid in several conditions. Medullary carcinoma is the most common. However, patients with systemic amyloidosis (as in multiple myeloma) can have amyloid in the thyroid; usually this substance which is by definition immunoamyloid, is deposited perivascularly.[212,216]

Amyloid goiter is a rare lesion of the thyroid in which a mass of amyloid material, unassociated with neoplasm or systemic disorder, replaces a portion of the thyroid.[216,217] Fat is commonly found associated with the amyloid.[216,218] Its nature is unclear; however, if large amounts of thyroid are replaced, hypofunction might occur.

B. Tumoral Replacement

It is unusual for a primary or metastatic cancer in the thyroid to replace such large amounts of the gland as to interfere with function. Occasionally, large masses such as primary anaplastic carcinoma or multifocal lesions (such as medullary cancer in familial cases[62-64,84,214]) might destroy much of the thyroid. Rarely, direct extension from a laryngeal or pharyngeal tumor may replace large areas of the gland and cause hypothyroidism.[219]

Metastases to the thyroid from patients with cancer of various sites have been identified at autopsy in up to 24% of cases.[84,219,220] Only rarely however, are these evident clinically because they interfere so infrequently with thyroid function.[219]

C. Other Infiltrations

Iron in hemochromatosis[221] and certain storage diseases, especially Batten's disease,[222] lipofusion in cystic fibrosis,[223] and cystinosis, affect the thyroid and may lead to hypofunction.[224]

X. LYMPHOCYTES IN THE THYROID

A. Hashimoto's Disease and Variants

Lymphocytic infiltration of the thyroid occurs most often in Hashimoto's thyroiditis, its variants, and in idiopathic myxedema. As noted above, many of these cells are B-cells and germinal center formation is common.[1,8,18]

B. Graves' Disease

Lymphocytes, including germinal center formation, can be identified in many cases of classic Graves' disease.[39,41,84,200] In distinguishing Graves' from Hashimoto's disease, histological clues which are helpful include lack of fibrosis, lack of Hurthle cells,

TABLE 5
LYMPHOCYTES IN THE THYROID

Hashimoto's disease and variants
Idiopathic myxedema
Graves' disease
Nontoxic goiter
Nonspecific lymphocytic thyroiditis
Drugs, especially lithium and iodide
Around tumors, especially papillary carcinoma
Lymphoma
   Primary
   Secondary
Ectopic thymic tissue

and presence of epithelial hyperplasia in the former. Obviously, the distinction may not always be possible as lesions of Hashitoxicosis and hyperthyroiditis, which overlap the two disorders, can and do occur.[39,41,42]

C. Other Thyroiditides

Other thyroiditides can show lymphoid infiltration, usually without the presence of germinal centers.[8,19,28,49,204-206] Thus, in subacute thyroiditis, especially in the later stages,[49,204-206] lymphocytes are common. Lack of Hurthle cells, presence of giant cells, and absence of germinal centers help the pathologist differentiate subacute from Hashimoto's thyroiditis. Clinical distinctions include painful gland, low antibody titers, low radioiodine uptake out of proportion to PBI, and generally complete recovery in the subacute form of the disease.[49,204-206]

D. Nodular Goiter

Nodular goiter may show changes of nonspecific thyroiditis as discussed above. The meaning of this change is not clear at present.[9]

E. Tumors

As discussed in Chapter 10, lymphocytic thyroiditis resembling Hashimoto's disease can be seen surrounding thyroid tumors, especially papillary carcinoma.[10,13,18,21,29] Most modern workers believe that this peritumor thyroiditis represents a host response to the tumor and does not impart a precancerous significance to the Hashimoto's lesion.[13,28,29]

F. Lymphoma of the Thyroid Gland

1. Systemic

About 20% of patients dying of malignant lymphoma will show thyroid involvement at autopsy,[84,200] although clinical dysfunction occurs rarely.[17] Occasionally, malignant lymphoma will arise primarily in the thyroid gland. Meissner and Warren[84] state that the incidence of this occurrence is unknown since histologic distinction between lymphoma and diffuse, small cell undifferentiated carcinoma may be impossible.[225-227]

2. Primary

Woolner et al.[17] reviewed 46 cases of primary thyroid lymphoma and found a 3:1 female:male ratio. Other authors[228-239] have reported a similar sex distribution. The disease affects individuals in the sixth to eighth decades of life.[228-238]

Grossly, the gland is enlarged and bulky (up to 300 g); it may show asymmetrical

Table 6
LYMPHOMA OF THE THYROID

Twenty percent of patients dying of systemic lymphoma will show thyroid involvement at autopsy; functional impairment is rare
Primary thyroid lymphoma occurs, probably always superimposed upon Hashimoto's disease
Most are follicular center cells (B-cell), transformed cells or immunoblastic sarcomas (histiocytic lymphoma of Rappaport)
If remain localized to gland, prognosis excellent
If regional nodes involved initially, course tends to follow that of nodal disease of similar stage
Pathologic distinction between lymphoma and small cell undifferentiated carcinoma may be facilitated by electron microscopy or immunohistochemical studies

or diffuse involvement.[228-238] The gland is whitish-tan in color and often the tumoral tissue will extend beyond the thyroid capsule and involve cervical soft tissues and nodes.[228-238]

Histologically, all varieties of lymphoma have been recorded, including Hodgkin's disease.[228-238] Most cases represent histiocytic lymphoma of Rappaport or reticulum cell sarcoma of the older literature.[229,230] According to present immunologic classifications,[32,240,241] these tumors are follicular center cell lesions, often immunoblastic sarcomas of B-cells (Figures 14 to 16). Plasmacytoid characteristics may be seen in some of the tumor cells.

The prognosis of lymphoma confined to the thyroid appears good; Woolner et al.[17,237] recorded generalized disease in only 1 of 16 individuals with initially localized tumor. If cervical nodes are involved at diagnosis, however, the course follows that of nodal disease with prognosis depending upon histologic subtype and clinical stage.[17,231-238] When the tumor disseminates, a peculiar proclivity to involve the gastrointestinal tract has been noted.[242]

Hashimoto's thyroiditis has been documented histologically in 25 to 100% of patients with primary thyroid lymphoma.[17,231,232,237,238] Most series are retrospective ones; adequate serologic documentation of Hashimoto's disease is often lacking.[17] Woolner et al. recorded twelve cases of malignant lymphoma occurring in 605 patients, followed with documented Hashimoto's thyroiditis.[18] These authors question the association. Goudie and Angouridakis[238] documented Hashimoto's disease by serologic testing in four of their six cases of primary thyroid lymphoma.

Immunologic reasoning strongly supports the development of extranodal malignant lymphoma in a previously immunologically abnormal tissue. Prospective studies of large numbers of patients with modern serologic techniques may resolve the debate. Immunohistochemical techniques[243-244] applied to such tumors have disclosed intracellular immunoglobulin (IgA and IgG).[245]

Such methods, as well as ultrastructural studies,[227] may prove useful in distinguishing lymphoma from anaplastic epithelial tumors. This confusion in histologic diagnosis is compounded when one recognizes that primary extranodal lymphomas can involve regional nodes partially when they spread, simulating metastatic carcinoma.

XI. SUMMARY

This chapter has reviewed the pathologic features of chronic thyroiditis and hypothyroidism. Several problems arise in classification of certain types of chronic thyroid disease. Crossovers, both clinical and pathological, have led to diagnoses of Hashitoxicosis and hyperthyroiditis. The pathology of primary myxedema and the extrathyroid effects are also discussed. Differential diagnostic pointers for fibrosis in the thyroid

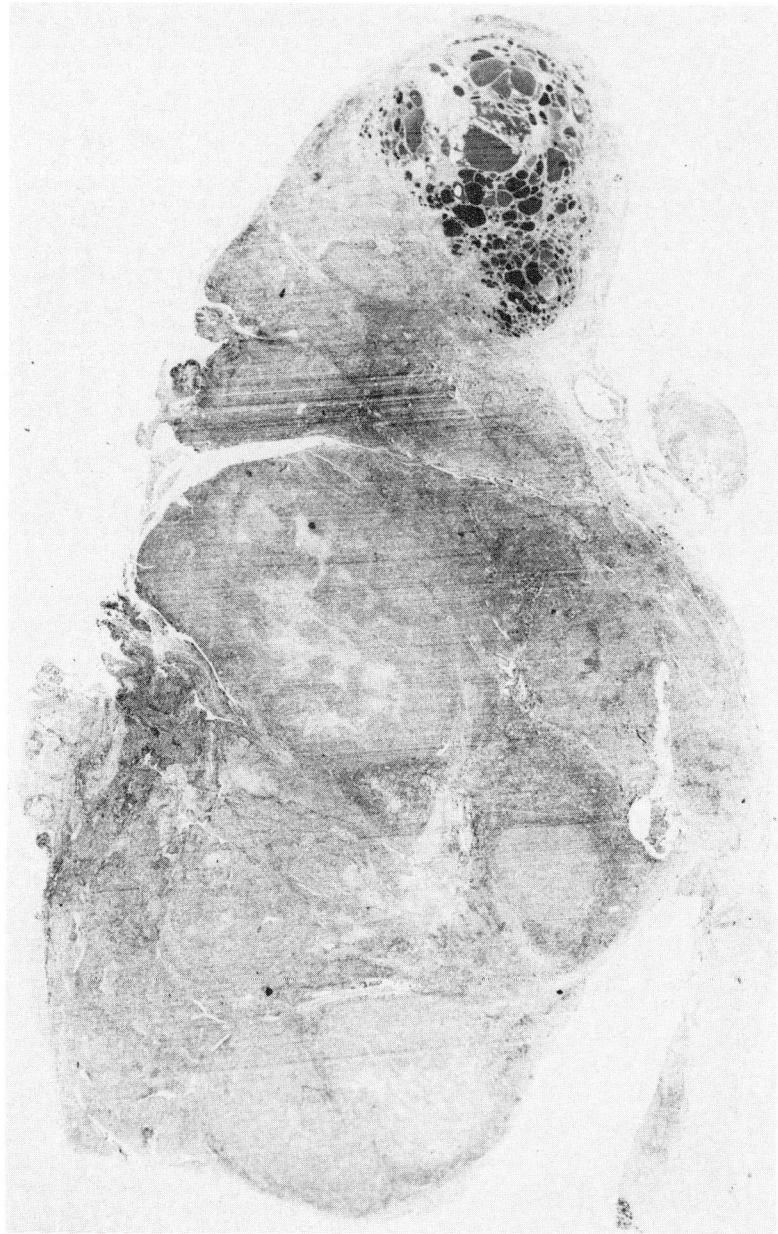

FIGURE 14. Low power view shows nodular tumor masses replacing large areas of the thyroid. (Hematoxylin-eosin; magnification × 4.)

and lymphocytic infiltration of the gland are outlined, and, finally, a discussion of malignant lymphoma of the thyroid is included.

In closing, it appears obvious that just as Evered et al.[246] define clinical grades of hypothyroidism, pathologic shadings and gradings can be found which lead to confusion and complexity. It is hoped that further study including the application of modern immunologic armamentaria may solve some of the problems .

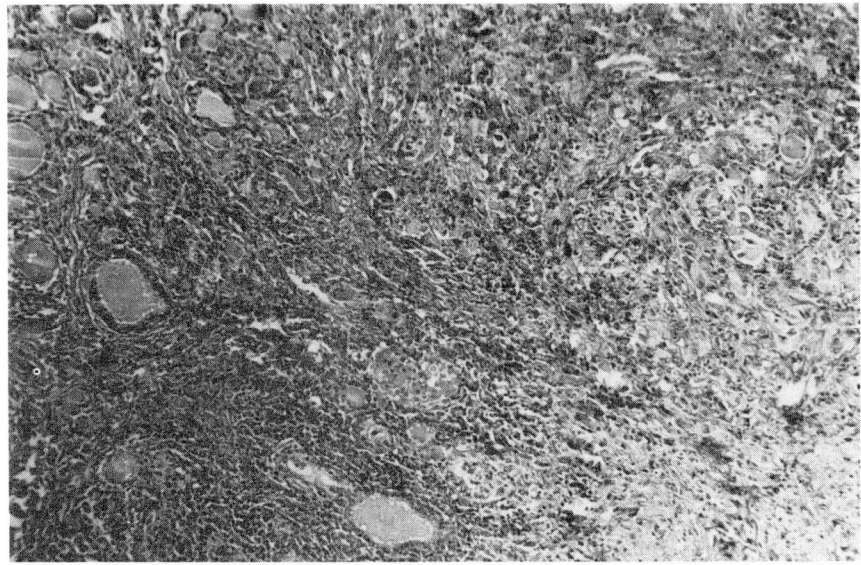

FIGURE 15. Markedly abnormal cells (right half of photograph) grow in sheets and solid masses from still recognizable gland affected by lymphocytic thyroiditis. (Hematoxylin-eosin; magnification × 125.)

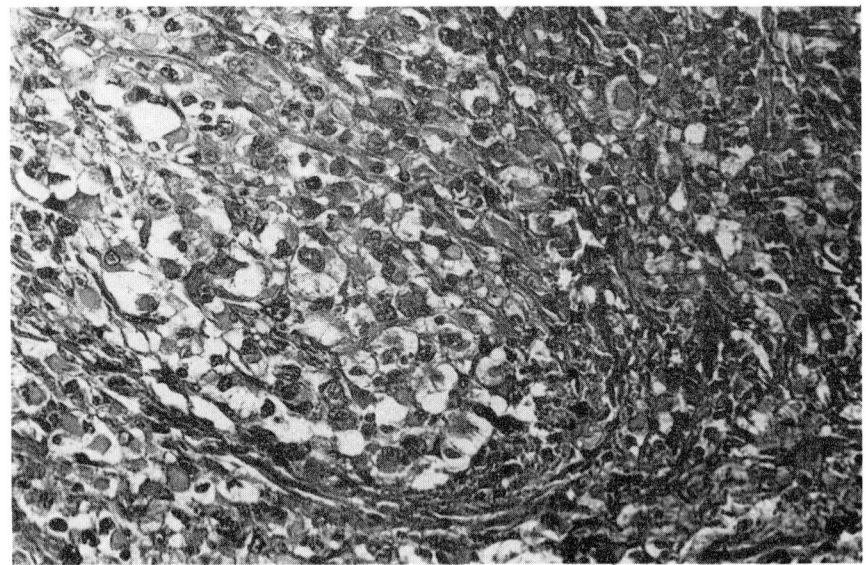

FIGURE 16. Higher power of same case as Figures 14 and 15 illustrates large immunoblastic tumor (immunoblastic sarcoma of B-cells). (Hematoxylin-eosin; magnification × 300.)

REFERENCES

1. **Hashimoto, H.**, Zur Kenntniss der lymphomatosen Veranderung der Schilddruse (Struma lymphomatosa), *Arch. Klin. Chir.*, 97, 219, 1912.
2. **de Quervain, F.**, Die akute, nicht eiterige Thyreoiditis und die Beteilung der Schilddruse an akuten Intoxikationem und Infektionen uberhaupt, *Mitt. Grenzgeb. Med. Chir. Jena,* 2, (Suppl.) 1, 1904.
3. **de Quervain F. and Giordanengo, G.**, Die akute und subakute nichteitrige Thyreoditis, *Mitt. Grenzgeb. Med. Chir.*, 44, 538, 1935-1937.
4. **Riedel, B. H. C. L.**, Ueber Verlauf und Ausgang der Strumitis chronica, *Muench. Med. Wochenschr.*, 57, 1946, 1910.
5. **Chopra, D., Wool, M. S., Crosson, A., and Sawin, C. T.**, Riedel's struma associated with subacute thyroiditis, hypothyroidism and hypoparathyroidism, *J. Clin. Endocrinol. Metab.*, 46, 869, 1978.
6. **Gluck, F. B., Nusynowitz, M. L., and Plymate, S.**, Chronic lymphocytic thyroiditis, thyrotoxicosis, and low radioactive iodine uptake, *N. Engl. J. Med.*, 293, 624, 1975.
7. **Katz, S. M. and Vickery, A. L.**, The fibrosing variant of Hashimoto's thyroiditis, *Hum. Pathol.*, 5, 161, 1974.
8. **Hazard, J. B.**, Thyroiditis: a review, *Am. J. Clin. Pathol.*, 25, 399, 1955.
9. **Bastenie, P. A., Ermans, A. M., and Neve, P.**, Focal lymphocytic thyroiditis in simple goiter, in *Thyroiditis and Thyroid Function: Clinical, Morphological and Physiopathological Studies,* Bastenie, P. A. and Ermans, A. M., Eds., Pergamon Press, Oxford, 1972, 143.
10. **Hirabayashi, R. N. and Lindsay, S.**, Thyroid carcinoma and chronic thyroiditis of the Hashimoto type: a statistical study of their relationship, in *Int. Coll. Tum. Thyroid Gland, Marseille,* S. Karger, Basel, 1966, 272.
11. **Meier, D. W., Woolner, L. B., Beahrs, O. H., and McConahey, W. M.**, Parenchymal findings in thyroidal carcinoma; pathologic study of 256 cases, *J. Clin. Endocrinol. Metab.*, 19, 162, 1959.
12. **Prior, J. T. and Fairchild, R. D.**, Thyroid neoplasms and coexistent thyroiditis: observations in 15 cases, *Am. J. Surg.*, 106, 57, 1963.
13. **Bastenie, P. A., Ermans, A. M., and Delaspesse, G.**, Chronic lymphocytic thyroiditis and cancer of the thyroid, in *Thyroiditis and Thyroid Function: Clinical, Morphological and Physiopathological Studies,* Bastenie, P. A. and Ermans, A. M., Eds., Pergamon Press, Oxford, 1972, 159.
14. **Perzik, S. L.**, *Surgery in Thyroid Disease,* Stratton Medical Book Corp., New York, 1976.
15. **Catz, B., Perzik, S. L., Friedman, N. B., and Sacks, H.**, Association of lymphocytic thyroiditis with other lesions of the thyroid, *Surg. Gynecol. Obstet.*, 136, 47, 1973.
16. **Holmes, H. B., Kreutner, A., and O'Brien, P. H.**, Hashimoto's thyroiditis and its relationship to other thyroid diseases, *Surg. Gynecol. Obstet.*, 144, 887, 1977.
17. **Woolner, L. B., McConahey, W. M., Beahrs, O. H., and Black, B. M.**, Primary malignant lymphoma of the thyroid, *Am. J. Surg.*, 111, 502, 1966.
18. **Woolner, L. B., McConahey, W. M., and Beahrs, O. H.**, Struma lymphomatosa (Hashimoto's thyroiditis) and related thyroidal disorders, *J. Clin. Endocrinol. Metab.*, 19, 53, 1959.
19. **Woolner, L. B.** Thyroiditis: classification and clinicopathologic correlation, in *The Thyroid,* Hazard, J. B. and Smith, D. E., Eds., Williams & Wilkins Co., Baltimore, 1964, 123.
20. **Lindsay, S., Dailey, M. E., Friedlander, J., Yee, G., and Soley, M. H.**, Chronic thyroiditis: a clinical and pathological study of 354 patients, *J. Clin. Endocrinol. Metab.*, 12, 1578, 1952.
21. **Harland, W. A. and Frantz, V. K.**, Clinicopathologic study of 261 surgical cases of so-called "thyroiditis", *J. Clin. Endocrinol.*, 11, 1433, 1956.
22. **Parmley, C. C. and Hellwig C. A.**, Lymphadenoid goiter: its differentiation from chronic thyroiditis, *Arch. Surg.*, 53, 190, 1946.
23. **Statland, H., Wasserman, M. M., and Vickery, A. L.**, Struma lymphomatosa (Hashimoto's struma): review of 51 cases with discussion of endocrinologic aspects, *Arch. Intern. Med.*, 88, 659, 1951.
24. **Marshall, S. F., Meissner, W. A., and Smith, D. C.**, Chronic thyroiditis, *N. Engl. J. Med.*, 238, 758, 1948.
25. **Schilling, J. A.**, Struma lymphomatosa, struma fibrosa and thyroiditis, *Surg. Gynecol. Obstet.*, 81, 533, 1945.
26. **Sommers, S. C.**, Thyroid gland, in *Endocrine Pathology,* Bloodworth, J. M. B., Ed., Williams & Wilkins Co., Baltimore, 1968, 133.
27. **DeGroot, L. J. and Stanbury, J. B.**, *The Thyroid and Its Diseases,* John Wiley and Sons, New York, 1975, 587.
28. **Volpe, R.**, The pathology of thyroiditis, *Hum. Pathol.*, 9, 429, 1978.
29. **Hurley, J. R.**, Thyroiditis, *Disease-a-Month,* December 1977.

30. Tasea, C. and Stefaneanu, L., A pathomorphic study of chronic thyroiditis, *Endocrinologie*, 14, 265, 1976.
31. Reidbord, H. E. and Fisher, E. R., Ultrastructural features of subacute granulomatous thyroiditis and Hashimoto's disease, *Am. J. Clin. Pathol.*, 59, 327, 1973.
32. Lukes, R. J. and Collins, R. D., New observations on follicular lymphoma, in *Gann Monograph on Cancer Research, No. 15: Malignant Diseases of the Hematopoietic System*, Akazaki, K., Rappaport, H., Berard, C. W., Bennett, J. M., and Ishikawa, E., Eds., University Park Press, Baltimore, 1973, 209.
33. Harris, M., The cellular infiltrate in Hashimoto's disease and focal lymphocytic thyroiditis, *J. Clin. Pathol.*, 22, 326, 1969.
34. Totterman, T. H., Distribution of T, B and thyroglobulin binding lymphocytes infiltrating the gland in Graves' disease, Hashimoto's thyroiditis and de Quervain's thyroiditis, *Clin. Immunol. Immunopathol.*, 10, 270, 1978.
35. Stuart, A. E., Fuchsinophilic material in the lymphoid follicles of Hashimoto's thyroiditis, *J. Pathol. Bacteriol.*, 86, 249, 1963.
36. Lupulescu, A. and Petrovici, A., *Ultrastructure of the Thyroid Gland*, Williams & Wilkins Co., Baltimore, 1968.
37. Kalderon, A. E., Bogaars, H. A., and Diamond, I., Ultrastructural alterations of the follicular basement membrane in Hashimoto's thyroiditis, *Am. J. Med.*, 55, 485, 1973.
38. Buckingham, B. A., Costin, G., Kogut, M. D., Isaacs, H., and Landing, B. H., Pathologic and immune factors in thyroid disease, *J. Pediatr.*, 91, 728, 1977.
39. Volpe, R., Farid, N. R., von Westrap, C., and Row, V. V., The pathogenesis of Graves' disease and Hashimoto's thyroiditis, *Clin. Endocrinol.*, 3, 239, 1974.
40. Kahn, L. B. and Dale, J., Virus-like particles in Hashimoto's disease and a variety of other tissues, *Lab. Invest.*, 29, 350, 1973.
41. Fatourechi, V., McConahey, W. M., and Woolner, L. B., Hyperthyroidism associated with histologic Hashimoto's thyroiditis, *Mayo Clin. Proc.*, 46, 682, 1971.
42. Jackson, I. "Hyperthyroiditis". A diagnostic pitfall, *N. Engl. J. Med.*, 293, 661, 1975.
43. Rallison, M. L., Dobyns, B. M., Keating, F. R., Rall, J. E., and Tyler, F. H., Occurrence and natural history of chronic lymphocytic thyroiditis in childhood, *J. Pediatr.*, 86, 675, 1975.
44. Gordin, A. and Lamberg, B. A., Natural course of symptomless autoimmune thyroiditis, *Lancet*, 2, 123, 1975.
45. Hamburger, J. I., Occult subacute thyroiditis — Diagnostic challenge, *Mich. Med.*, 70, 1125, 1971.
46. Blonde, L., Witkin, M., and Harris, R., Painless subacute thyroiditis simulating Graves' disease, *West. J. Med.*, 125, 75, 1976.
47. Dorfman, S. G., Cooperman, M. T., Nelson, R. L., Depuy, H., Peake, R. L., and Yonge, R. L., Painless thyroiditis and transient hyperthyroidism without goiter, *Ann. Intern. Med.*, 86, 24, 1977.
48. Ginsberg, J. and Walfish, P., Postpartum transient thyrotoxicosis with painless thyroiditis, *Lancet*, 1, 1125, 1977.
49. Volpe, R., Subacute (de Quervain's) thyroiditis, *Clin. Endocrinol. Metab.*, 8, 81, 1979.
50. Doniach, D., Bottazzo, G. F., and Russell, R. C. G., Goitrous autoimmune thyroiditis, *Clin. Endocrinol. Metab.*, 8, 63, 1979.
51. DeGroot, L. J., Hall, R., McDermott, W. V., and Davis, A. M., Hashimoto's thyroiditis: a genetically conditioned disease, *N. Engl. J. Med.*, 267, 267, 1962.
52. Vickery, A. L. and Hamlin, E., Struma lymphomatosa (Hashimoto's thyroiditis): Observation in repeated biopsies in 16 patients, *N. Engl. J. Med.*, 264, 226, 1961.
53. Greenberg, A. H., Czernichow, P., Hung, W., Shelley, W., Winship, T., and Blizzard, R. M., Juvenile chronic lymphocytic thyroiditis: Clinical, laboratory and histological correlations, *J. Clin. Endocrinol. Metab.*, 30, 293, 1970.
54. Joll, C. A., The pathology, diagnosis and treatment of Hashimoto's disease (struma lymphomatosa), *Br. J. Surg.*, 27, 351, 1939.
55. Humbert, J. R., Gotlin, R. W., Hostetter, G., Sherrill, J. G. and Silver, H. K. Lymphocytic (autoimmune Hashimoto's) thyroiditis: Presentation of an unusual case with subacute onset in a 14-year-old girl, *Arch. Dis. Child.*, 43, 80, 1968.
56. Shane, L. L., Valensi, Q. J., Sobrevilla, L., and Gabulove, J. L., Chronic thyroiditis: A potentially confusing clinical picture, *Am. J. Med. Sci.*, 250, 532, 1965.
57. Tung, K. S. K., Ramos, C. V., and Deodhar, S. D., Antithyroid antibodies in juvenile lymphocytic thyroiditis, *Am. J. Clin. Pathol.*, 61, 549, 1974.
58. Ziring, P. R., Gallo, G., Finegold, M., Biumovici-Klein, E., and Ogra, P., Chronic lymphocytic thyroiditis: Identification of rubella virus antigen in the thyroid of a child with congenital rubella, *J. Pediatr.*, 90, 419, 1977.

59. **Woolner, L. B., McConahey, W. M., and Beahrs, O. H.**, Invasive fibrous thyroiditis (Riedel's struma), *J. Clin. Endocrinol. Metab.*, 17, 201, 1957.
60. **Bastenie, P. A.**, Invasive fibrous thyroiditis (Riedel), in *Thyroiditis and Thyroid Function: Clinical, Morphological and Physiopathological Studies*, Bastenie, P. A. and Ermans, A. M., Eds., Pergamon Press, Oxford, 1972, 99.
61. **Volpe, R.**, Riedel's struma (struma fibrosa), in *The Thyroid*, Werner, S. C. and Ingbar, S. H., Eds., Harper and Row, New York, 1978, 1009.
62. **Hutter, R. V. P., Tollefsen, H. R., DeCosse, J. J., Foote, F. W., and Frazell, E. L.**, Spindle and giant cell metaplasia in papillary carcinomata of the thyroid, *Am. J. Surg.*, 110, 660, 1965.
63. **Nishiyama, R. H., Dunn, E. L., and Thompson, N. W.**, Anaplastic spindle cell and giant cell tumors of the thyroid gland, *Cancer*, 30, 113, 1972.
64. **Kyriakides, G. and Sosin, H.**, Anaplastic carcinoma of the thyroid, *Ann. Surg.*, 179, 295, 1974.
65. **Sclare, G.**, The thyroid in myxedema, *J. Pathol. Bacteriol.*, 85, 263, 1963.
66. **LiVolsi, V. A. and Merino, M. J.**, Squamous cells in the human thyroid gland, *Am. J. Surg. Pathol.*, 2, 133, 1978.
67. **Bale, G. F.**, Teratoma of the neck in the region of the thyroid gland, *Am. J. Pathol.*, 26, 565, 1950.
68. **Buckwalter, J. A. and Layton, J. W.**, Malignant teratoma in the thyroid gland of an adult, *Ann. Surg.*, 139, 218, 1954.
69. **Hajdu, S. I., Faruque, A. A., Hajdu, E. O., and Morgan, W. S.**, Teratoma of the neck in infants, *Am. J. Dis. Child.*, 111, 412, 1966.
70. **Keynes, W. M. M.**, Teratoma of the neck in relation to the thyroid gland, *Br. J. Surg.*, 46, 466, 1959.
71. **Newstedt, J. R. and Shirkey, H. C.**, Teratoma of the thyroid region, *Am. J. Dis. Child.*, 107, 88, 1964.
72. **Silberman, R. and Mendelson, I. R.**, Teratoma of the neck, *Arch. Dis. Child*, 35, 159, 1960.
73. **Weitzner, S.**, Benign teratoma of the neck in an infant, *Am. J. Dis. Child.*, 107, 84, 1964.
74. **Heuser, C. H.**, A human embryo with 14 pairs of somites, *Contrib. Embryol.*, 22, 135, 1930.
75. **Johnson, F. P.**, A human embryo with 24 pairs of somites, *Contrib. Embryol.*, 5, 125, 1917.
76. **LiVolsi, V. A., Perzin, K. H., and Savetsky, L.**, Carcinoma arising in median ectopic thyroid, *Cancer*, 34, 1303, 1974.
77. **Sugiyama, S.**, The embryology of the human thyroid gland including ultimobranchial body and others related, *Adv. Anat. Embryol. Cell Biol.*, 44, 6, 1971.
78. **Klinck, G. H. and Menk, K. F.**, Squamous cells in the human thyroid, *Mil. Surg.*, 109, 406, 1951.
79. **Harcourt-Webster, J. N.**, Squamous epithelium in the human thyroid gland, *J. Clin. Pathol.*, 19, 384, 1966.
80. **Jaffe, R. H.**, Epithelial metaplasia of the thyroid gland, *Arch. Pathol.*, 23, 821, 1937.
81. **Bahuleyan, C. K. and Ramachandran, P.**, Primary squamous cell carcinoma of the thyroid, *Indian J. Cancer*, 9, 89, 1972.
82. **Cocke, W. M. and Carrera, G. M.**, Mixed squamous cell carcinoma and papillary adenocarcinoma (adenoacantahoma) of the thyroid gland, *Am. J. Surg.*, 108, 432, 1964.
83. **Huang, T.-Y. and Assor, D.**, Primary squamous cell carcinoma of the thyroid gland, *Am. J. Clin. Pathol.*, 55, 93, 1971.
84. **Meissner, W. A. and Warren, S.**, *Tumors of the Thyroid*, AFIP fascicle IV, 2nd series, Washington, D. C., 1969.
85. **Prakash, A., Kukreti, B. C., and Sharma, M. P.**, Primary squamous cell carcinoma of the thyroid gland, *Intern. Surg.*, 50, 538, 1968.
86. **Rhatigan, R. M., Roque, J. L., and Bucher, R. L.**, Mucoepidermoid carcinoma of the thyroid gland, *Cancer*, 39, 210, 1977.
87. **Dube, V. E. and Joyce, G. T.**, Extreme squamous metaplasia in Hashimoto's thyroiditis, *Cancer*, 27, 434, 1971.
88. **Gould, V. E., Gould, N. S., and Benditt, E. P.**, Ultrastructural aspects of papillary and sclerosing carcinomas of the thyroid, *Cancer*, 29, 1613, 1972.
89. **Block, M. A., Horn, R. C., and Miller, J. M.**, Unilateral thyroid nodules with lymphocytic thyroiditis, *Arch. Surg.*, 86, 280, 1963.
90. **Paull, B. R., Alderson, P. O., Siegel, B. A., Bauer, W. C., and Evens, R. G.**, Thyroid imaging in lymphocytic thyroiditis, *Radiology*, 115, 139, 1975.
91. **Boyle, J. A., Thompson, J. A., Grieg, W. R., Jackson, I. M. D., and Boyle, I. T.**, The thyroid scan in patients with Hashimoto's disease, *Arch. Endocrinol.*, 51, 337, 1966.
92. **Bialas, P., Marks, S., Dekker, A., and Field, J. B.**, Hashimoto's thyroiditis presenting as a solitary functioning thyroid nodule, *J. Clin. Endocrinol. Metab.*, 43, 1365, 1976.

93. **Friedman, N. B.,** Cellular involution in the thyroid gland: Significance of Hurthle cells in myxedema, exhaustion atrophy, Hashimoto's disease and the reactions to irradiation, thiouracil therapy and subtotal resection, *J. Clin. Endocrinol.,* 9, 874, 1949.
94. **Horn, R. C.,** Hurthle cell tumors of the thyroid, *Cancer,* 7, 234, 1954.
95. **Askanazy, M.,** Pathologisch-anatomische Beitrage zur Kenntriss des Morbus Basedowii, insbesondere uber die dabei auftretende Muskelkrankung, *Dtsch. Arch. Klin. Med.,* 61, 118, 1898.
96. **Hurthle, K.,** Beitrage zur Kennthiss, des Secretions vargangs in der Schilddruse, *Pflugers Arch. Gesamte Physiol.,* 56, 1, 1894.
97. **Tremblay, G. and Pearse, A. G. E.,** Histochemistry of oxidative enzyme systems in the human thyroid, with special reference to Askanazy cells, *J. Pathol. Bacteriol.,* 80, 353, 1960.
98. **Harcourt-Webster, J. N. and Stott, N. C. H.,** Histochemical study of oxidative and hydrolytic enzymes in the human thyroid, *J. Pathol. Bacteriol.,* 92, 291, 1966.
99. **Heimann, P., Ljungren, J. G., Lowhagen, T., and Hjern, B.,** Oxyphilic adenoma of the human thyroid, *Cancer,* 31, 246, 1973.
100. **Kniseley, R. M. and Andrews, G. A.,** Transformation of thyroid carcinoma to clear cell type, *Am. J. Clin. Pathol.,* 26, 1427, 1956.
101. **Variakojis, D., Getz, M. L., Paloyan, E., and Strauss, F. H.,** Papillary clear cell carcinoma of the thyroid, *Hum. Pathol.,* 6, 384, 1975.
102. **Feldman, P. S. Horvath, E., and Kovacs, K.,** Ultrastructure of three Hurthle cell tumors of the thyroid, *Cancer,* 30, 1279, 1972.
103. **Thompson, N. W., Dunn, E. I., Batsakis, J. G., and Nishiyama, R. H.,** Hurthle cell lesions of the thyroid gland, *Surg. Gynecol. Obstet.,* 139, 55, 1974.
104. **Woolner, L. B.,** Thyroid carcinoma: Pathologic classification with data on prognosis, *Semin. Nucl. Med.,* 1, 481, 1971.
105. **Franssila K.,** Value of histologic classification of thyroid cancer, *Acta Pathol. Microbiol. Scand. Suppl.,* 225, 5, 1971.
106. **Woolner, L. B., Beahrs, O. H., Block, B. M., McConahey, W. M., and Keating F. R.,** Classification and prognosis of thyroid carcinoma, *Am. J. Surg.,* 102, 354, 1961.
107. **LiVolsi, V. A.,** Pathology of thyroid cancer, in *Thyroid Cancer,* Greenfield, L., Ed., CRC Press, Boca Raton, Fla., 1978, 85.
108. **LiVolsi, V. A., Feind C. R., LoGerfo, P., and Tashjian, A. H.,** Demonstration of immunoperoxidase staining by hyperplasia of parafollicular cells in the thyroid gland in hyperparathyroidism, *J. Clin. Endocrinol. Metab.,* 37, 550, 1973.
109. **Hawk, W. A. and Hazard, J. B.,** The many appearances of papillary carcinoma of the thyroid, *Cleveland Clin. Q.,* 43, 207, 1976.
110. **Beierwaltes, W. H.,** Iodine and lymphocytic thyroiditis, *Bull. All India Inst. Med. Sci.,* 3, 145, 1969.
111. **Weaver, D. K., Batsakis, J. G., and Nishiyama, R. H.,** Relationship of iodine to "lymphocytic goiter", *Arch. Surg.,* 98, 183, 1969.
112. **Inoue, M., Taketani, N., Sato, T., and Nakajima, H.,** High incidence of chronic lymphocytic thyroiditis in apparently healthy school children: Epidemiological and clinical study, *Endocrinol. Jpn.,* 22, 483, 1975.
113. **Volpe, R.,** Lymphocytic thyroiditis, in *The Thyroid,* Werner, S. C. and Ingbar, S. H., Eds., Harper & Row, New York, 1978, 996.
114. **Senhauser, D. A.,** Immune pathologic correlations in thyroid disease, in *The Thyroid,* Hazard J. B. and Smith, D. E., Eds., Williams & Wilkins Co., Baltimore, 1964, 167.
115. **Soto, R. J., Imas, B., Brunengo, A. M., and Goldberg, D.,** Endemic goiter in Misiones, Argentina: Pathophysiology related in immunological phenomena, *J. Clin. Endocrinol. Metab.,* 27, 1581, 1967.
116. **Buchanan, W. W., Harden, R. M., and Clark, D. H.,** Hashimoto's thyroiditis: A differentiation from simple goiter, thyroid neoplasm, drug-induced goiter and dyshormonogenesis, *Br. J. Surg.,* 52, 430, 1965.
117. **Williams, E. D. and Doniach, I.,** The postmortem incidence of focal thyroiditis, *J. Pathol. Bacteriol.,* 83, 255, 1962.
118. **Goudie, R. B., Anderson, J. R., and Gray, K. G.,** Complement-fixing antithyroid antibodies in hospital patients with asymptomatic thyroid lesions, *J. Pathol. Bacteriol.,* 77, 389, 1959.
119. **Sawin, C. T., Chopra, D., Azizi, F., Mannix, J. E., and Bacharach, P.,** The aging thyroid, *JAMA,* 242, 247, 1979.
120. **Thomas, W. C., Anderson, R. M., Jurkiewicz, M. J., Araujo, J. D., and Blizzard, R. M.,** Clinical studies in thyroiditis, *Ann. Intern. Med.,* 63, 808, 1965.
121. **Bullock, W. K., Hummer, G. J., and Kahler, J. E.,** Squamous metaplasia of thyroid gland, *Cancer,* 5, 966, 1952.
122. **Neve, P.,** The ultrastructure of thyroid in chronic autoimmune thyroiditis, *Virchows Arch. A,* 346, 302, 1969.

123. **Ketebant-Balasse, P. and Neve, P.,** Ultrastructural study of the thyroid in adult hypothyroidism, *Virchows Arch. A,* 362, 195, 1974.
124. **Hurxthal, L.,** Myxedema and its various causes, *Surg. Clin. North Am.,* 25, 657, 1945.
125. **Pittman, J. A.,** Hypothyroidism: Hypopituitarism, in *The Thyroid,* Werner, S. C. and Ingbar, S. H., Eds., Harper & Row, New York, 1978, 797.
126. **Kramer, M. S., Kauschamsky, A., and Genel, M.,** Adolescent secondary amenorrhea: Association with hypothalamic hypothyroidism, *J. Pediatr.,* 94, 300, 1977.
127. **Fisher, D. A.,** Hypothyroidism: Pediatric aspects, in *The Thyroid,* Werner, S. C. and Ingbar, S. H., Eds., Harper & Row, New York, 1978, 807.
128. **Fierro-Benitez, R., Penafiel, W., DeGroot, L. J., and Ramirez, I.,** Endemic goiter and endemic cretinism in the Andean region, *N. Engl. J. Med.,* 280, 296, 1969.
129. **Homoki, J., Birk, J., Loos, U., Rothenbucher, G., Fazekas, A. T. A., and Teller, W. M.,** Thyroid function in term newborn infants with congenital goiter, *J. Pediatr.,* 86, 753, 1975.
130. Editorial, New light in endemic cretinism, *Lancet,* 2, 365, 1972.
131. **Nusynowitz, M. L., Clark, R. F., Strader, W. J., Estrin, H. M., and Seal, U. S.,** Thyroxine-binding globulin deficiency in three families, and total deficiency in a normal woman, *Am. J. Med.,* 50, 458, 1971.
132. **Dussault, J. H., Letarte, J., Guyda, H., and Laberge, C.,** Serum thyroid hormone and TSH concentrations in newborn infants with congenital absence of thyroxine-binding globulin, *J. Pediatr.,* 90, 264, 1977.
133. **Ibbertson, H. K.,** Endemic goitre and cretinism, *Clin. Endocrinol. Metab.,* 8, 97, 1979.
134. **Barsano, C. P. and DeGroot, L. J.,** Dyshormonogenetic goitre, *Clin. Endocrinol. Metab.,* 8, 145, 1979.
135. **Weller, C. V., Wanstrom, R. C., Gordon, H., and Bugher, J. C.,** Cardiac histopathology in thyroid disease, *Am. Heart J.,* 8, 2, 1932.
136. Editorial, Thyroid heart disease, *Lancet,* 2, 232, 1977.
137. **Redgrave, T. G. and Snibson, D. A.,** Clearance of chylomicron triacylglycerol and cholesterol ester from the plasma of streptozotocin-induced diabetic and hypercholesterolemic hypothyroid rats, *Metabolism,* 26, 493, 1977.
138. **Tulloch, B. R., Lewis, B., and Fraser, T. R.,** Triglyceride metabolism in thyroid disease, *Lancet,* 1, 391, 1973.
139. **Fuller, C. H. and Sommers, C. L.,** The thyroid status in relation to atherosclerotic disease, *Boston Med. Q.,* 10, 1, 1959.
140. **Kurtzman, R. S., Otto, D. L., and Chepey, J. J.,** Myxedema heart disease, *Radiology,* 84, 624, 1965.
141. **Steinberg, A. D.,** Myxedema and coronary artery disease, a comparative autopsy study, *Ann. Intern. Med.,* 68, 338, 1968.
142. **Macaron, C. and Famuyima, O.,** Hyponatremia of hypothyroidism, *Arch. Intern. Med.,* 138, 820, 1978.
143. **Derubertis, F. R., Michelis, M. F., Bloom, M. E., Mintz, D. H., Field, J. B., and Davis, B. B.,** Impaired water excretion in myxedema, *Am. J. Med.,* 51, 41, 1971.
144. **Marsh, H. E.,** Myxedematous ascites removed by thyroid extract, *Am. J. Med. Sci.,* 172, 585, 1926.
145. **Papper, S. and Lancestremere, R. G.,** Certain aspects of renal function in myxedema, *J. Chronic Dis.,* 14, 495, 1961.
146. **Mason, A. M. S. and Golding, R. L.,** Renal tubular acidosis and autoimmune thyroid disease, *Lancet,* 2, 1104, 1970.
147. **Discala, V. A. and Kinney, M. J.,** Effects of myxedema on the renal diluting and concentrating mechanism, *Am. J. Med.,* 50, 325, 1971.
148. **Pettinger, W. A., Talner, L., and Ferris T. F.,** Inappropriate secretion of antidiuretic hormone due to myxedema, *N. Engl. J. Med.,* 272, 362, 1965.
149. **Kocen, R. S. and Atkinson, M.,** Ascites in hypothyroidism, *Lancet,* 1, 527 1963.
150. **Hohl, R. D. and Nixon, R. K.,** Myxedema ileus, *Arch. Intern. Med.,* 115, 145, 1965.
151. **Liechty, R. D., Miller, R. F., and Cohen, W. N.,** Myxedema causing adynamic ileus, serous effusions and inappropriate secretion of antidiuretic hormone, *Surg. Clin. North Am.,* 50, 1087, 1970.
152. **Davidoff, F. and Gill, J.,** Myxedema madness, *Conn. Med.,* 41, 618, 1977.
153. **Sanders, V.,** Neurologic manifestations of myxedema, *N. Engl. J. Med.,* 266, 547, 1962.
154. **Jellinek, E. H.,** Fits, faints, coma and dementia in myxoedema, *Lancet,* 2, 1010, 1962.
155. **Wilson, W. R. and Bedell G. N.,** The pulmonary abnormalities in myxedema, *J. Clin. Invest.,* 39, 42, 1960.
156. **McConnell, R. J., Menendez, C. E., Smith, F. R., Henkin R. I., and Rivlin, R. S.,** Defects of taste and smell in patients with hypothyroidism, *Am. J. Med.,* 59, 354, 1975.
157. **Klion F. M., Segal, R., and Schaffner, F.,** The effect of altered thyroid function on the ultrastructure of the human liver, *Am. J. Med.,* 50, 317, 1971.

158. **Tudhope, G. R. and Wilson, G. M.,** Anemia in hypothyroidism: Incidence, pathogenesis and response to treatment, *Q. J. Med.*, 29, 513, 1960.
159. **Kiely, J. M., Purnell, D. C., and Owen, C. A.,** Erythrokinetics in myxedema, *Ann. Intern. Med.*, 67, 533, 1967.
160. **Horton, L., Coburn R. J., England, J. M., and Himsworth, R. L.,** The haematology of hypothyroidism, *Q. J. Med.*, 45, 101, 1976.
161. **Wardrop, C. and Hutchison, H. E.,** Red cell shape in hypothyroidism, *Lancet*, 1, 1243, 1969.
162. **Thieme, E. T.,** Goiter and deaf mutism, *Ann. Surg.*, 182, 173, 1975.
163. Case Records of the Massachusetts General Hospital (Case 2-1975), *N. Engl. J. Med.*, 292, 95, 1975.
164. **Dorwart, B. and Schumacher, H. R.,** Joint effusions, chondrocalcinosis and other rheumatic manifestations in hypothyroidism, *Am. J. Med.*, 59, 780, 1975.
165. **Kabadi U., Levine, L. H., and Krishnamurthy, P. S.,** Familial hypothyroidism, manifested by painful swollen joints, *N.Y. State J. Med.*, 77, 1489, 1977.
166. **Bland, J. H. and Frymoyer, J. W.,** Rheumatic syndromes myxedema, *N. Engl. J. Med.*, 282, 1171, 1970.
167. **Shah, J. H. and Cerchio, G. M.,** Hypoinsulinemia of hypothyroidism, *Arch. Intern. Med.*, 132, 657, 1973.
168. **Cohen K. and Felig, P.,** Primary hypothyroidism and the pituitary, *Arch. Intern. Med.*, 139, 855, 1979.
169. **Barnes, N. D., Hayles, A. B., and Ryan, R. J.,** Sexual maturation in juvenile hypothyroidism, *Mayo Clin. Proc.*, 48, 849, 1973.
170. **Goldsmith, R. E., Sturgis, S. H., Lerman, J., and Stanbury, J. B.,** The menstrual pattern in thyroid disease, *J. Clin. Endocrinol. Metab.*, 12, 846, 1952.
171. **Ross, F. and Nusynowitz, M. L.,** A syndrome of primary hypothyrodism, amenorrhea and galactorrhea, *J. Clin. Endocrinol. Metab.*, 28, 591, 1968.
172. **Watanakunakorn, C., Hodges, R. E., and Evans, T. C.,** Myxedema: A study of 400 cases, *Arch. Intern. Med.*, 116, 183, 1965.
173. **Herlant M. and Pasteels, J. L.,** Pituitary changes in myxoedema and chronic thyroiditis, in *Thyroiditis and Thyroid Function: Clinical, Morphological and Physiopathological Studies*, Bastenie, P. A. and Ermans, A. M., Eds., Pergamon Press, Oxford, 1972, 251.
174. **Burt, A. S. and Cohen, R. B.,** Pituitary changes in thyroid aplasia: Possible significance, *Lab. Invest.*, 2, 357, 1953.
175. **Purves, H. D. and Griesbach, W. E.,** Pituitary cytology in relation to thyrotropic hormone secretion, *Ciba Found. Colloq. Endocrinol.*, 10, 51, 1957.
176. **Jawadi, M. H., Ballonoff, L. B., Stears, J. C., and Katz, F. H.,** Primary hypothyroidism and pituitary enlargement, *Arch. Intern. Med.*, 138, 1555, 1978.
177. **Russfield, A. B.,** Histology of the human hypophysis in thyroid disease — Hypothyroidism, hyperthyroidism and cancer, *J. Clin. Endocrinol. Metab.*, 15, 1393, 1955.
178. **Russfield, A. B.,** Combined bioassay and histological study of 73 human hypophyses, *Cancer*, 13, 790, 1960.
179. **Doniach, D., Nilsson, L. R., and Riott, I. M.,** Autoimmune thyroiditis in children and adolescents. II. Immunological correlations and parent study, *Acta Paediatrica* 54, 260, 1965.
180. **Garber, J. J., Randall, R. V., Worthington, J. W., and Kierland, R. R.,** Lupus erythematosus and Hashimoto's thyroiditis, *Postgrad. Med.*, 69, 100, 1969.
181. **Shoaleh, M., Momtaz, A. H., and Jamshidi, C.,** Scleroderma and hypothyroidism, *JAMA*, 235, 752, 1976.
182. **Doniach, D.,** Autoimmunity in liver disease, in *Progress in Clinical Immunology*, Vol. 1, Schwartz, R. S., Ed., Grune & Stratton, New York, 1972, 45.
183. **Segal, B. M. and Weintraub, M. I.,** Hashimoto's thyroiditis, myasthenia gravis, idiopathic thrombocytopenic purpura, *Ann. Intern. Med.*, 85, 761, 1976.
184. **Dent, R. G. and Edwards, D. M.,** Autoimmune thyroid disease and the polymyalgia rheumatica-giant cell arteritis syndrome, *Clin. Endocrinol.*, 9, 215, 1978.
185. **Schmidt, M. B.,** Eine biglandulare Erkrankung (Nebennieren und Schilddruse) bei morbus Addisonii, Verh. Dtsch *Ges. Pathol.*, 21, 212, 1926.
186. **Carpenter, C. C. J., Solomon, N., Silverberg, S. G., Bledsoe, T., Northcutt, R. C., Klinenberg, J. R., Bennett, I. L., and Harvey, A. M.,** Schmidt's syndrome (thyroid and adrenal insufficiency): A review of the literature and a report of 15 new cases including ten instances of coexistent diabetes mellitus, *Medicine*, 43, 153, 1964.
187. **Genant, H. K., Hoagland, H. C., and Randall, R. V.,** Addison's disease and hypothyroidism (Schmidt's syndrome), *Metabolism*, 16, 189, 1967.
188. **Gharit, H., Hodgson, S. F., Gastrineau, C. F., Scholz, D. A., and Smith, L. A.,** Reversible hypothyroidism in Addison's disease, *Lancet*, 2, 734, 1972.

189. Vazquez, A. M. and Kenny, F. M., Ovarian failure and antiovarian antibodies in association with hypoparathyroidism, moniliasis, and Addison's and Hashimoto's disease, *Obstet. Gynecol.,* 41, 414, 1973.
190. Hong, R., Gatti, R., Rathbun, J. C., and Good, R. A., Thymic hypoplasia and thyroid dysfunction, *N. Engl. J. Med.,* 282, 470, 1970.
191. Chesky, V. E., Hellwig, C. A., and Welch, J. W., Cancer of the thyroid associated with Hashimoto's disease: An analysis of forty-eight cases, *Am. Surg.,* 28, 678, 1962.
192. Schlicke, C. P., Hill, J. E., and Schultz, G. F., Carcinoma in chronic thyroiditis, *Surg. Gynecol. Obstet.,* 111, 552, 1960.
193. Dailey, W. E., Lindsay, S., and Skahen, R., Relation of the thyroid neoplasms to Hashimoto disease of the thyroid gland, *Arch. Surg.,* 70, 291, 1954.
194. Hirabayashi, R. N. and Lindsay, S., The relation of thyroid carcinoma and chronic thyroiditis, *Surg. Gynecol. Obstet.,* 121, 243, 1965.
195. Pollock, W. F. and Sprong, D. H., The rationale of thyroidectomy for Hashimoto's thyroiditis: A premalignant lesion, *West. J. Surg.,* 66, 17, 1958.
196. Shands, W. C., Carcinoma of the thyroid in association with struma lymphomatosa (Hashimoto's disease), *Ann. Surg.,* 151, 675, 1960.
197. Crile, G. and Hazard, J. B., Incidence of cancer in struma lymphomatosa, *Surg. Gynecol. Obstet.,* 115, 101, 1962.
198. Rosen, I. B., Strawbridge, H. G., Walfish, P. G., and Bain, J., Malignant pseudothyroiditis: A new clinical entity, *Am. J. Surg.,* 136, 445, 1978.
199. Rosen, F., Rowe, V. V., Volpe, R., and Ezrin, C., Anaplastic carcinoma of the thyroid with abnormal circulating iodoprotein, *Can. Med. Assoc. J.,* 95, 1039, 1966.
200. Meissner, W. A., Surgical pathology, in *Surgery of the Thyroid Gland,* Sedgwick, C. E., Ed., W. B. Saunders, Philadelphia, 1974, 24.
201. Volpe, R., Acute suppurative thyroiditis, in *The Thyroid,* Werner, S. C., Ingbar, S. H., Eds., Harper & Row, Inc. New York, 1971, 849.
202. Bishop, H. M. and Durman, D. C., Traumatic rupture of the thyroid gland, *Am. J. Surg.,* 75, 524, 1948.
203. Hazard, J. B., Thyroiditis: A review, *Am. J. Clin. Pathol.,* 25, 289, 1955.
204. Lindsay, S. and Dailey M. E., Granulomatous or giant cell thyroiditis: Clinical and pathologic study of 37 patients, *Surg. Gynecol. Obstet.,* 98, 197, 1954.
205. Woolner, L. B., McConahey, W. M., and Beahrs, O. H., Granulomatous thyroiditis (de Quervain's thyroiditis), *J. Clin. Endocrinol. Metab.,* 17, 1202, 1957.
206. Bastenie, P. A., Bonnyms, M., and Neve, P., Subacute and chronic granulomatous thyroiditis, in *Thyroiditis and Thyroid Function: Clinical, Morphological and Physiopathological Studies,* Bastenie, P. A. and Ermans, A. M., Eds., Pergamon Press, Oxford, 1972, 69.
207. Carney, J. A., Moore, S. B., Northcutt, R. C., Woolner, L. B., and Stillwell, G. K., Palpation thyroiditis (multifocal granulomatous folliculitis), *Am. J. Clin. Pathol.,* 64, 639, 1975.
208. Wagner, D. H., Recant, W. M., and Evans, R. H., A review of one hundred and fifty thyroidectomies following prior irradiation to the head, neck and upper part of the chest, *Surg. Gynecol. Obstet.,* 147, 903, 1978.
209. Komorowski, R. A. and Hanson, G. A., Morphologic changes in the thyroid following low-dose childhood radiation, *Arch. Pathol.,* 1019, 36, 1977.
210. Kennedy, J. S. and Thomas, J. A., The changes in the thyroid gland after irradiation with 131-I or partial thyroidectomy for thyrotoxicosis, *J. Pathol.,* 112, 65, 1974.
211. Curran, R. C., Eckert, H., and Wilson, G. M., The thyroid gland after treatment of hyperthyroidism by partial thyroidectomy or iodine-131, *J. Pathol. Bacteriol.,* 76, 541, 1958.
212. Glenner, G. G. and Page, D. L., Amyloid, amyloidosis and amyloidogenesis, *Intern. Rev. Exp. Pathol.,* 15, 1, 1976.
213. Pearse, A. G. E., Ewen, S. W. B., and Pollack, J. M., The genesis of apudamyloid in endocrine polypeptide tumors: Histochemical distinction from immunoamyloid, *Virchows Arch. B.,* 10, 93, 1972.
214. Ibanez, M. L., Medullary carcinoma of the thyroid, *Pathobiol. Annu.,* 9, 263, 1974.
215. Tashjian, A. H., Wolfe, M. J., and Voelkel, E. F., Human calcitonin: Immunologic assays, cytologic localization and studies on medullary thyroid carcinoma, *Am. J. Med.,* 56, 840, 1974.
216. Kennedy, J. S., Thomson, J. A., and Buchanan, W. M., Amyloid in the thyroid, *Q. J. Med.,* 43, 127, 1974.
217. James, P. D., Amyloid goitre, *J. Clin. Pathol.,* 25, 683, 1972.
218. Harcourt-Webster, N. and Stuart, A. E., Fat in thyroiditis, *J. Pathol. Bacteriol.,* 86, 240, 1963.
219. Gowing, N. F. C., The pathology and natural history of thyroid tumours, in *Tumours of the Thyroid Gland,* Smithers, D., Ed., E. & S. Livingstone, Edinburgh, 1970, 103.

220. Silverberg, S. and Vidone, R., Metastatic tumors in the thyroid, *Pac. Med. Surg.*, 74, 175, 1966.
221. Sheldon, J. H., *Hemachromatosis*, Oxford University Press, London, 1935.
222. Dayan, A. D. and Trickey, R. J., Thyroid involvement in juvenile amaurotic familial idiocy (Batten's disease), *Lancet*, 2, 296, 1970.
223. Chan, A. M., Lynch, M. J. G., Bailey, J. D., Ezrin, C., and Fraser, D., Hypothyroidism in cystinosis, *Am. J. Med.*, 48, 678, 1970.
224. Bovel, D. M. and Reddy, J. K., Excessive lipofuscin accumulation in the thyroid gland in mucoviscidosis, *Arch. Pathol.*, 96, 269, 1973.
225. Meissner, W. A. and Phillips, M. L., Diffuse small cell carcinoma of the thyroid, *Arch. Pathol.*, 74, 291, 1962.
226. Rayfield, E. J., Nishiyama, R. N., and Sisson, J. C., Small cell tumors of the thyroid, *Cancer*, 28, 1023, 1971.
227. Cameron, R. G., Seemayer, T. A., Wang, N. S., Ahmed, M. N., and Tabeth, E. J., Small cell malignant tumors of the thyroid, *Hum. Pathol.*, 6, 731, 1975.
228. Dinsmore, R. S., Dempsey, W. S., and Hazard, J. B., Lymphosarcoma of the thyroid, *J. Clin Endocrinol. Metab.*, 9, 1043, 1949.
229. Brewer, D. B. and Orr, J. W., Struma reticulosa: A reconsideration of the undifferentiated tumors of the thyroid, *J. Pathol. Bacteriol.*, 65, 193, 1953.
230. Winship, T. and Greene, R., Reticulum cell sarcoma of the thyroid gland, *Br. J. Cancer*, 9, 401, 1955.
231. Kenyon, R. and Ackerman, L. V., Malignant lymphoma of the thyroid apparently arising in struma lymphomatosa, *Cancer*, 8, 964, 1955.
232. Lindsay, S. and Dailey, M. E., Malignant lymphoma of the thyroid gland and its relation to Hashimoto disease: A clinical and pathologic study of 8 patients, *J. Clin. Endocrinol. Metab.*, 15, 1332, 1955.
233. Walt, A. J., Woolner, L. B., and Black, B. M., Small cell malignant lesions of the thyroid gland, *J. Clin. Endocrinol. Metab.*, 17, 45, 1957.
234. Walt, A. J., Woolner, L. B., and Black, B. M., Primary malignant lymphoma of of the thyroid, *Cancer*, 10, 663, 1957.
235. Cox, M. T., Malignant lymphoma of the thyroid, *J. Clin. Pathol.*, 17, 591, 1964.
236. Mikal, S., Primary lymphoma of the thyroid gland, *Surgery*, 55, 233, 1964.
237. Burke, J. S., Butler, J. J., and Fuller, L. M., Malignant lymphomas of the thyroid, *Cancer*, 39, 1587, 1977.
238. Goudie, R. B. and Angouridakis, C. E., Autoimmune thyroiditis associated with malignant lymphoma of the thyroid, *J. Clin. Pathol.*, 23, 377, 1970.
239. Fujimoto, Y., Suzuki, H., Abe, K., and Brooks, J. R., Autoantibodies in malignant lymphoma of the thyroid gland, *N. Engl. J. Med.*, 276, 380, 1967.
240. Lukes, R. J. and Collins, R. D., Immunologic characterization of human malignant lymphomas, *Cancer*, 34, 1488, 1975.
241. Nathwani, B. N., A critical analysis of the classifications of non-Hodgkins lymphomas, *Cancer*, 44, 347, 1979.
242. Smithers, D. W., Malignant lymphoma of the thyroid gland, in *Tumours of the Thyroid Gland*, Smithers, D., Ed., E. & S. Livingstone, Edinburgh, 1970, 141.
243. Mesa-Tejarda, R., Pascal, R. R., and Fenoglio, C. M., Immunoperoxidase immunohistochemical technique as a "special stain" in the diagnostic pathology laboratory, *Hum. Pathol.*, 8, 313, 1977.
244. Taylor, C. R., Immunoperoxidase techniques, *Arch. Pathol. Lab. Med.*, 102, 113, 1978.
245. LiVolsi, V. A. and Waldron, J. A., Unpublished observations.
246. Evered, D. C., Ormston, B. J., Smith, P. A., Hall, R., and Bud, T., Grades of hypothyroidism, *Br. Med. J.*, 1, 657, 1973.

Chapter 8

DRUG-ASSOCIATED THYROIDITIS

Virginia A. LiVolsi

TABLE OF CONTENTS

I. Introduction 100

II. Drugs Implicated in Thyroiditis 100
    A. Lithium 100
    B. Diphenylhydantoin 101
    C. Iodide 103
    D. Minocycline 104

III. Summary 105

References 105

I. INTRODUCTION

Although many prescription drugs may alter thyroid function or, at least, interfere with laboratory thyroid function tests, few have been implicated in the production of thyroiditis. Hence, hypothyroidism (or at least chemical hypothyroidism) has been associated with long term use of such common drugs as thiazides,[1] sulfonamides, and sulfonylureas.[2,3] Drugs which may interfere with thyroid function tests include oral contraceptive pills, salicylates, coumadin, anabolic steroids, prednisone, and iodine-containing compounds such as radiographic dyes, expectorants, and nasal sprays.[4] Thus, patients taking such agents may be euthyroid but give abnormal results in the laboratory tests.

The histopathologic changes that occur in the thyroids of these patients would be expected to be minimal or nonexistent since, in test situations, normal thyroid function is restored following discontinuance of the drug.[3] No studies of the histological evaluation of these patients have been reported.

The purpose of this chapter is to focus on those major prescription drugs in common use which have been associated not only with changes in thyroid function, but with documented histologic alterations of the gland. The drugs to be discussed are lithium compounds, dilantin (diphenylhydantoin), iodide, and minocycline.

II. DRUGS IMPLICATED IN THYROIDITIS

A. Lithium

Lithium salts (chiefly lithium carbonate) have been utilized for over a decade in the therapy of certain psychiatric disorders, chiefly manic and hypomanic states.[5] Prior to the discovery of the efficacy of this drug for psychiatric problems in 1949,[4] lithium was employed as a treatment for gout and as a sedative.[6]

The mode of action of lithium is as yet unclear,[7] but most hypotheses have suggested an effect of the lithium ion on cell membranes, including neurons.[8] Lithium ion may interfere with, or completely replace, the sodium ion at the cell membrane level and lead to failure of stimulated neuron membranes to conduct action potentials.[9,10] There exists some evidence that lithium may exert its effect through interference with neuronal synaptic transmission.[11] However, further evidence awaits to be accumulated to support or modify this hypothesis.

The benefits of any therapeutic agent must be weighed against the risks and side effects[12,13] Central nervous system effects, including confusion, lethargy, and visual and auditory disturbances, have been reported.[5,14] Renal effects including tubular damage have been noted;[15] since lithium is excreted solely by the kidney, local accumulation of this substance, especially after prolonged use, may be responsible for this effect. Pathologically, the kidney in prolonged lithium use shows fibrosis, tubular atrophy, and glomerular sclerosis.[16]

Goiter develops commonly in patients treated for prolonged periods with lithium salts,[5] and thyroid hypofunction can occur in 3 to 12% of such cases.[5,17] Perrild et al.[17] described two patients without goiter who became irreversibly myxedematous following prolonged lithium carbonate intake. Without histologic evidence, but by extrapolation of the kidney data,[16] Perrild et al. postulated that fibrosis of the thyroid may occur, accounting for the hypothyroidism.[17] These authors suggested that this complication may develop more commonly than is currently appreciated.

The present author has had the opportunity to study a case of a nodular goiter removed from a 54-yr old woman who had developed thyroidomegaly after taking lithium carbonate for 18 months. Thyroid function tests showed mild hypothyroidism;

thyroid autoantibodies were absent. Surgery and left lobectomy was performed for a palpable nodule which was "cold" on radioiodine scan. The gland proved to show several nodules, with the clinically evident one being the largest. The intervening thyroid gland showed interlobular fibrosis, follicular atrophy with colloid depletion, and infiltration by lymphocytes without the formation of follicular centers (Figures 1 and 2).

The relationship of the thyroid histology and function to the lithium ion intake remains unexplained. As Baldessarini and Lipinski[5] have noted most patients, when initially exposed to lithium ion, develop transient depression of serum protein-bound iodine and free thyroxine; these return to normal within a few weeks. However, a minority of patients develop goiter, a smaller number develop hypothyroidism, and rarely both occur.[5] Those individuals who will develop these problems cannot be predicted although studies have demonstrated that women are more frequently affected than men.[5]

Why are certain individuals affected? Is it a genetic tendency perhaps related to HLA subtype? Does the reaction occur on an allergic basis? Is there a direct toxic effect of lithium on the thyroid of some patients, who perhaps have abnormal enzymatic makeup? Do some individuals have an underlying subclinical thyroid abnormality? Answers to these questions await further study.

Experimental data on the effects of lithium on thyroid metabolism have been accumulated. Thus, lithium can interfere with accumulation of iodine, iodination and release of iodinated tyrosine, and possibly with the actions of thyroid-stimulating hormone.[18-21] However, the mechanism of lithium's thyroid effect in man remains to be elucidated.[22,23]

B. Diphenylhydantoin

Diphenylhydantoin (Dilantin®) has found wide clinical usefulness in the treatment of epileptic disorders for over 40 yr. The side effects associated with the use of this agent include true side effects on metabolic and endocrine functions and idiosyncratic reactions.[24]

Euthyroid patients (whether normal or on replacement therapy) receiving Dilantin® will experience a decrease in serum protein-bound iodine.[25] Diphenylhydantoin has been shown to compete with thyroxine for thyroxine-binding globulin binding sites.[26-28] Larsen et al.[29] have demonstrated that although thyroxine secretion rates remain normal, diphenylhydantoin increases urinary and fecal thyroxine excretion; this decrease in serum thyroxine may be enhanced by an apparent direct effect of Dilantin® on hepatic metabolism of thyroxine.[30,31]

Recently, Kuiper[32] described a young woman who developed lymphocytic thyroiditis while taking Dilantin® for epilepsy. This patient developed a rash and fever 3 weeks after beginning therapy; the drug was stopped but reinstated 2 weeks later. After another 3 weeks of treatment, she developed fever, a maculopapular rash, lymphadenopathy, and thyroidomegaly. The disease was accompanied by lymphocytosis, neutropenia, and eosinophilia. Cultures, lupus cell preparations, and a variety of serologic tests gave negative results. Thyroid function tests included elevated protein-bound iodine and thyroxine resin uptake but antibodies to thyroid cells and thyroglobulin were negative. Biopsy demonstrated lymphocytic infiltration, follicular atrophy, and slight fibrosis suggestive of Hashimoto's thyroiditis. Following cessation of Dilantin® therapy, the patient recovered and thyroid size and function tests reverted to normal. However, 2 yr later the patient's serum demonstrated cytotoxic antibodies to thyroid epithelial cell fractions.

Kuiper[32] indicated that he considered the Dilantin® to be etiologically related to the

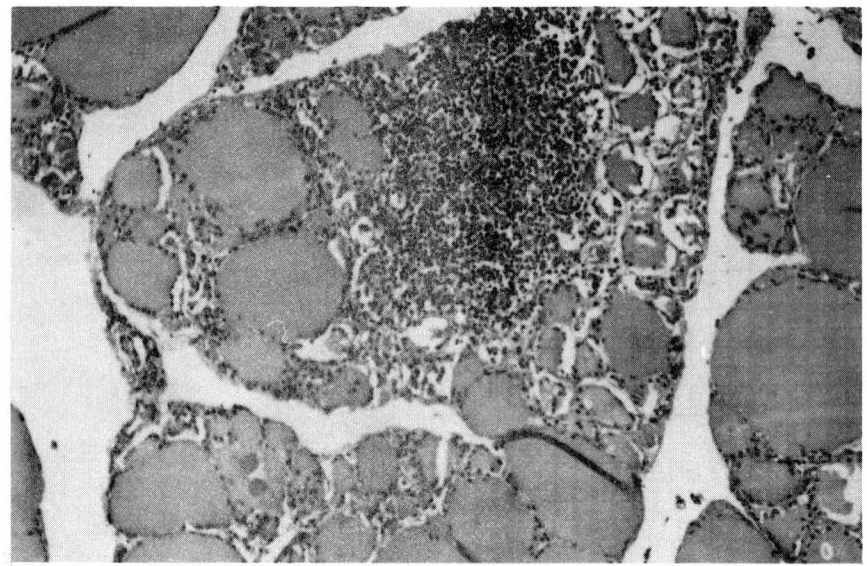

FIGURE 1. This thyroid was removed from a 54-yr old woman with multinodular goiter which had developed while she was taking lithium carbonate for manic-depressive illness. Note focal lymphocytic infiltration. (Hematoxylin-eosin; magnification × 100.)

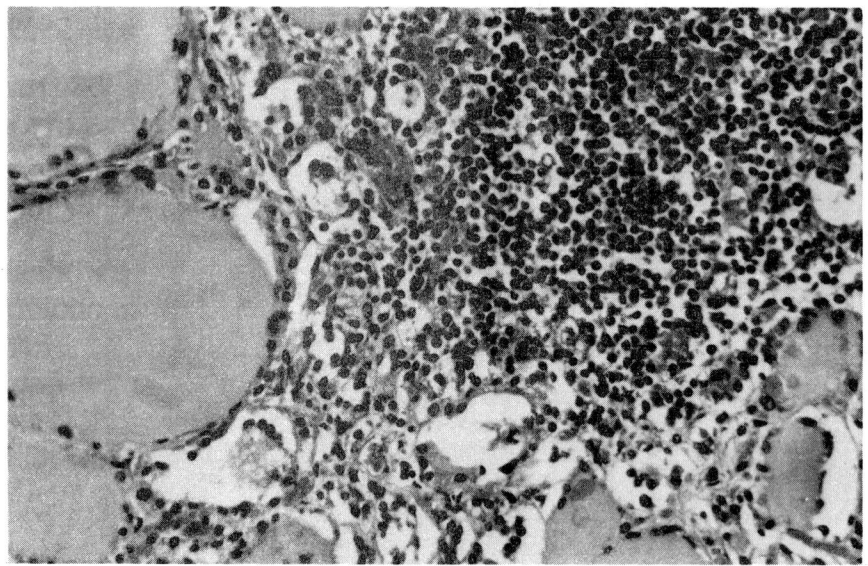

FIGURE 2. Same case as Figure 1. Infiltrate (right) is all lymphocytes. (Hematoxylin-eosin; magnification × 250.)

thyroiditis in this case. However, although temporal associations are impressive, no proof of reversion of thyroid histology is given, and there remains no method of ascertaining the pre-Dilantin® therapy status of the thyroid.

If Kuiper's patient indeed had Dilantin®-induced thyroiditis, one must include this case as an example of an idiosyncratic reaction to the drug. That Dilantin® can produce changes in the immune system has been adequately documented.[33-40] Hypersensitivity reactions and lymphoproliferative disorders described as pseudolymphoma,[33-35] immunoblastic lymphadenopathy,[36,37] and immunoblastic sarcomas of B-cells[36,37] (formerly called reticulum cell sarcomas[38-40]), and Hodgkin's disease[40] have been reported. The occurrence of these phenomena cannot be predicted. Affected individuals may possess a specific genetic composition involving their immune response to particular antigens, in this case Dilantin®.

In immunoblastic lymphadenopathy, the postulated mechanism includes a hyperimmune proliferation of B-cells with exaggeration of lymphocyte transformation to immunoblasts and plasma cells,[36,37] resulting from an impairment of T-cell (suppressor cell) regulation,[37,41] i.e., an autoimmune reaction. One may speculate that in Kuiper's patient[32] a similar sequence of events took place, i.e., the Dilantin® evoked an "autoimmune" reaction with the thyroid as the target organ. The development and persistence of thyroid cytotoxic antibody in this case supports this possibility (see also Chapter 6).

Further elucidation of Dilantin®-induced immunologic effects involving the thyroid and lymphoid systems awaits evaluation of these patients by sophisticated immunological techniques.

C. Iodine

The incidence of lymphocytic thyroiditis has been increasing since the 1930s. If one excludes Graves' disease, the likelihood of noting lymphocytes in the thyroid, removed surgically or at necropsy in patients without clinically diagnosed thyroiditis, has risen.[42-46]

Reasons for this change remain unclear, but several authors postulate that the addition of iodide to the diet (e.g., iodized salt), which occurred around 1925 to 1930 in the U.S., might somehow be related to this trend.[42-45] Volpe[43] noted that the incidence of clinically overt lymphocytic thyroiditis (Hashimoto's thyroiditis) has risen tenfold since 1935; the increase of the occult form is unknown. A recent study from Japan[47] also links iodine ingestion to the development of thyroiditis. This report, which encompasses 10,000 children (ages 6 to 18), showed an incidence of biopsy-proven lymphocytic thyroiditis of 5.3 per 1000 in a seaside area (high iodine) compared to a 1.4 per 1000 rate in an urban setting.[47]

Evans et al.[48] demonstrated that, in animals prone to develop thyroiditis, the incidence of thyroiditis increases as iodine intake is augmented. Braverman et al.[49] studied patients with Hashimoto's disease and found them more susceptible to iodine-induced hypothyroidism than controls. Volpe suggests that, in both animal and human disease, the subject with chronic lymphocytic thyroiditis may show extreme sensitivity to the effects of iodine; the latter may unmask the thyroiditis, rather than cause it.[43]

Adams et al.[50] found the addition of iodine as iodate to bread in Tasmania produced overt hyperthyroidism in individuals with a latent form of thyrotoxicosis. Evaluation of these patients demonstrated the development of thyroid autoantibodies in 80%.[49] Similarly, hyperthyroidism may ensue when iodide is added to the diet of patients with endemic or sporadic goiter.[51-52] In all of these studies, the effect of the iodine has been superimposed upon an abnormal (at least physiologically) gland,[51-53] either one that is iodine-deficient or one in which autonomous nodules are present. Mechanisms invoked for this iodine-induced hyperthyroidism include abnormal iodide-concentrating capacity[52] or increased iodine supply to unregulated thyroid tissue.[50] Hence, either subclinical Graves' disease or toxic nodular goiter was present.

Iodine inhibits thyroid hormone release and, temporarily, its synthesis in both euthyroid and hyperthyroid subjects.[54] Occasionally because of failure of intrathyroid compensatory mechanisms, goiter and hypothyroidism occur.[55,56] Patients with chronic lymphocytic thyroiditis[57] or treated Graves' disease[55,58] show exquisite sensitivity to iodine and hypothyroidism occurs readily with small doses. Circulating antithyroid antibodies can be detected in these cases;[59] similar antibodies can occur after radioiodine therapy.[60] Wolff[55] notes that subjects with minor disturbances of thyroid function tend to be more sensitive to iodine.

Iodine administered during pregnancy may cause goiterous hypothyroidism and cretinism in the child.[55] A similar effect has been noted in rats.[61] Similarly, iodide may induce hypothyroidism in children with cystic fibrosis.[62] Borel and Reddy[63] noted gross brown pigmentation of the thyroid in patients with mucoviscidosis. They attributed lipofuscin pigmentation to chronic vitamin E deficiency with autooxidation of lipids.

Glatstein et al.[64] caution that iodine sensitizes the thyroid to external radiation; even small doses associated with neck X-rays can induce hypothyroidism in patients receiving iodine.

All these reports indicate that the effect of iodine is greater if the thyroid is abnormal. Thus, by extrapolation, Volpe's[43] hypothesis of iodine (or iodide) unmasking an underlying thyroid anomaly appears valid.

The mode of action of the iodine "thyroiditis" is unknown. If excess iodine is causative, it may, by mechanisms still to be determined, function as a hapten and invoke an antigen-antibody response. This is reflected in the tissue by lymphocytic infiltration. Whether this occurs is debatable, but if it or a similar situation ensues, it appears likely that the reaction is not universal. A predisposition to this effect of iodide is probably necessary (? specific HLA type). The presence of occult thyroiditis may represent this predisposition.[43]

A note of caution should be added here. Blaming iodide for this changing incidence of lymphocytic infiltration of the thyroid may not be justified. Reflecting on the many environmental, therapeutic, socioeconomic, and nutritional alterations which have taken place in this country since 1935, iodine may be the scapegoat. Increases in background radiation, widespread use of drugs of many types (for medicinal or illegal purposes), and necessity for additives to preserve food taste and color for long distance shipping — these are but a few of the possibilities that need to be considered as related to changes in thyroid histopathology. In addition, common use of biopsy and cytology, as well as more extensive examination of surgical specimens, might influence incidence rates.

The answer to the question of whether an etiologic relationship exists between iodide and thyroiditis appears to be affirmative. However, the magnitude of this problem remains unknown. Unmasking of preexisting thyroiditis may account for a large part of this increased incidence. It is hoped that utilizing more refined and sensitive techniques to diagnose thyroiditis, especially in iodine-deficient populations, may offer answers to these question.

D. Minocycline

Minocycline, a tetracycline antibiotic, has been reported to produce a grossly coal-black thyroid in man and animals.[65] Attwood and Dennett[65] reported such a case and showed that minocycline interferes with iodide peroxidase and is degraded to a black, insoluble pigment within follicular epithelial cells. In their patient, Attwood and Dennett described nuclear pyknosis and epithelial damage although no evidence of functional derangement was documented. They refer to animal data[66] suggesting that minocycline has an antithyroid action and caution monitoring of thyroid function in patients receiving the drug.

III. SUMMARY

This chapter has reviewed thyroiditis associated with drugs and has discussed three major substances: lithium, Dilantin® and iodine. Possible mechanisms of action of these drugs and their relationship to thyroid lesions have been covered.

Other drugs have produced or enhanced the production of thyroiditis in animal models,[67] also.

REFERENCES

1. **Mehbod, H., Swartz, C. D., and Brest, A. N.** The effect of prolonged thiazide administration on thyroid function, *Arch. Int. Med.*, 119, 283, 1967.
2. **Hunton, R. B., Wills, M. V., and Skipper, E. W.**, Hypothyroidism in diabetes treated with sulphonylurea, *Lancet*, 2, 449, 1965.
3. **Burke, G., Silverstein, G. E., and Sorkin, A. I.**, Effect of long-term sulfonylurea therapy on thyroid function in man, *Metabolism*, 16, 651, 1967.
4. Specialized Diagnostic Laboratory Tests, *Bio-science Laboratories*, Van Nuys, California, 1972.
5. **Baldessarini, R. J. and Lipinski, J. F.**, Lithium salts: 1970-1975, *Ann. Intern. Med.*, 83, 527, 1975.
6. **Cade, J. F. J.**, Lithium salts in the treatment of psychotic excitement, *Med. J. Aust.*, 36, 349, 1949.
7. **Singer, I. and Rotenberg, D.**, Mechanisms of lithium action, *N. Engl. J. Med.*, 289, 254, 1973.
8. **Aronoff, M. F., Evens, R. G., and Durell, J.**, Effects of lithium salts on electrolyte metabolism, *J. Psychiatr. Res.*, 8, 139, 1971.
9. **Schou, M.**, Biology and pharmacology of the lithium ion, *Pharmacol. Rev.*, 9, 17, 1957.
10. **Tasaki, I., Lerman, L., and Watanabe, A.**, Analysis of excitation process in squid giant axons under bi-ionic conditions, *Am. J. Physiol.*, 216, 130, 1969.
11. **Baldessarini, R. J. and Yorke, C.**, Effects of lithium and of pH on synaptosomal metabolism of noradrenaline, *Nature*, 228, 1301, 1970.
12. **Rosenbaum, A. H., Maruta, T., and Richelson, J.**, Drugs that alter mood. II. Lithium, *Mayo Clin. Proc.*, 54, 401, 1979.
13. **Hansen, H. E. and Andersen, A.**, Lithium intoxication, *Q. J. Med.*, 67, 123, 1978.
14. **Schou, M.**, Lithium: Elimination rate, dosage, control, poisoning, goiter mode of action, *Acta Psychiatr. Scand.*, 207 (Suppl.), 49, 1969.
15. **Thomsen, K.**, Renal lithium elimination in man and active treatment of lithium poisoning, *Acta Psychiatr. Scand.*, 207 (Suppl.), 83, 1969.
16. **Hestbech, J., Hansen, H. E., Amdisen, A., and Olsen, S.**, Chronic renal lesions following long-term treatment with lithium, *Kidney Int.*, 12, 205, 1977.
17. **Perrild, H., Madsen, A., and Hansen, R.**, Irreversible myxedema after lithium carbonate, *Br. Med J.*, 1, 1108, 1978.
18. **Berens, S. C., Bernstein, R. S., Robbins, J., and Wolff, J.**, Antithyroid effects of lithium, *J. Clin. Invest.*, 49, 1357, 1970.
19. **Shopsin, B.**, Effects of lithium on thyroid function: A review, *Dis. Nerv. Syst.*, 31, 237, 1970.
20. **Gershon, S. and Shopsin, B., Eds.**, *Lithium: Its Role in Psychiatric Research and Treatment*, Plenum Press, New York, 1973.
21. **Lauridsen, U. B., Kirkegaard, C., and Nerup, J.**, Lithium and the pituitary-thyroid axis in normal subjects, *J. Clin. Endocrinol. Metab.*, 39, 383, 1974.
22. **Temple, R., Berman, M., Carlson, H. E., Robbins, J., and Wolff, J.**, The use of lithium in Graves' disease, *Mayo Clin. Proc.*, 47, 872, 1972.
23. **Segal, R. L., Rosenblatt, S., and Eliasoph, I.**, Endocrine exophthalmos during lithium therapy of manic depressive disease, *N. Engl. J. Med.*, 289, 136, 1973.
24. **Gharib, H. and Munoz, J. M.**, Endocrine manifestations of diphenylhydantoin therapy, *Metabolism*, 23, 515, 1974.
25. **Oppenheimer, J. H., Fisher, L. V., Nelson, K. M., and Jailer, J. W.**, Depression of the serum protein-bound iodine level by diphenylhydantoin, *J. Clin. Endocrinol. Metab.*, 21, 252, 1961.

26. Wolff, J., Standaert, M. E., and Rall, J. E., Thyroxine displacement from serum proteins and depression of serum protein-bound iodine by certain drugs, *J. Clin. Invest.*, 40, 1373, 1961.
27. Oppenheimer, J. H., Role of plasma proteins in the binding, distribution and metabolism of the thyroid hormones, *N. Engl. J. Med.*, 278, 1153, 1968.
28. Lightfoot, R. W. and Christian, C. L., Serum protein binding of thyroxine and diphenylhydantoin, *J. Clin. Endocrinol. Metab.*, 26, 305, 1966.
29. Larsen, P. R., Atkinson, A. J., Wellman, H. N., and Goldsmith, R. E., The effect of diphenylhydantoin on thyroxine metabolism in man, *J. Clin. Invest.*, 49, 1266, 1970.
30. Mendoza, D. M., Flock, E. V., Owen, C. A., and Paris, J., Effect of 5, 5'-diphenylhydantoin on the metabolism of L-thyroxine ^{131}I in the rat, *Endocrinology*, 79, 106, 1966.
31. Hansen, J. M., Skovsted, L., Lauridsen, U. B., Kirkegaard, C., and Siersbaek-Nielsen, K., The effect of diphenylhydantoin on thyroid function, *J. Clin. Endocrinol. Metab.*, 39, 785, 1974.
32. Kuiper, J. J., Lymphocytic thyroiditis possibly induced by diphenylhydantoin, *JAMA*, 210, 2370, 1969.
33. Saltzstein, S. L. and Ackerman, L. V., Lymphadenopathy induced by anticonvulsant drugs and mimicking clinically and pathologically malignant lymphomas, *Cancer*, 12, 164, 1959.
34. Dorfman, R. F. and Warnke, R., Lymphadenopathy simulating the malignant lymphomas, *Hum. Pathol.*, 5, 519, 1974.
35. Bellido, P. D., Ciria, M. D., Mujals, D. R., and Morell, A. R., Lymphadenopathies and phenytoin, *Lancet*, 1, 1372, 1977.
36. Lukes, R. J. and Tindle, B. H., Immunoblastic lymphadenopathy, *N. Engl. J. Med.*, 292, 1, 1975.
37. Frizzera, G., Moran, E. M., and Rappaport, H., Angio-immunoblastic lymphadenopathy, *Am. J. Med.*, 59, 803, 1975.
38. Gams, R. A., Neal, J. A., and Conrad, F. G., Hydantoin-induced pseudo-pseudolymphoma, *Ann. Intern. Med.*, 69, 557, 1968.
39. Anthony, J. J., Malignant lymphoma associated with hydantoin drugs, *Arch. Neurol.*, 22, 450, 1970.
40. Hyman, G. A. and Sommers, S. C., The development of Hodgkin's disease and lymphoma during anticonvulsant therapy, *Blood*, 28, 416, 1966.
41. Waldmann, T. A., Blaese, R. M., Broder, S., and Krakauer, R. S., Disorders of suppressor immunoregulatory cells in the pathogenesis of immunodeficiency and autoimmunity, *Ann. Intern. Med.*, 88, 226, 1978.
42. Beierwaltes, W. H., Iodine and lymphocytic thyroiditis, *Bull. All India Inst. Med. Sci.*, 3, 145, 1969.
43. Volpe, R., Lymphocytic thyroiditis, in *The Thyroid*, Werner, S. C., and Ingbar, S. H., Eds., Harper and Row, New York, 1978, 996.
44. Asamer, H., Riccabonna, G., and Holthaus, N., Immunohistologische Befunde bei Schilddrusenerkrankungen in einer endemische Kropfebiet, *Arch. Klin. Med.*, 215, 270, 1968.
45. Headington, J. T. and Tantajumroon, T. T., Surgical thyroid disease in Northern Thailand, *Arch. Surg.*, 95, 157, 1967.
46. Weaver, D. K., Batsakis, J. G., and Nishiyama, R. H., Relationship of iodine to "lymphocytic goiter", *Arch. Surg.*, 98, 183, 1969.
47. Inoue, M., Taketani, N., Sato, T., and Nakayima, H., High incidence of chronic lymphocytic thyroiditis in apparently healthy school children: Epidemiological and clinical study, *Endocrinol. Jpn.*, 22, 483, 1975.
48. Evans, T. C., Beierwaltes, W. H., and Nishiyama, R. H., Experimental canine Hashimoto's thyroiditis, *Endocrinology*, 84, 641, 1969.
49. Braverman, L. E., Ingbar, S. H., Vagenakis, A. G., Adams, L., and Maloof, F., Enhanced susceptibility to iodine myxedema in patients with Hashimoto's disease, *J. Clin. Endocrinol. Metab.*, 32, 515, 1971.
50. Adams, D. D.,Kennedy, T. H., Stewart, J. C., Utiger, R. D., and Vidor, G. I., Hyperthyroidism in Tasmania following iodide supplementation: Measurements of thyroid stimulating autoantibodies and thyrotropin, *J. Clin. Endocrinol. Metab.*, 41, 221, 1975.
51. Connolly, R. J., Vidor, G. I., and Stewart, J. C., Increase in thyrotoxicosis in endemic goiter area after iodation of bread, *Lancet*, 1, 500, 1970.
52. Vagenakis, A. G., Wang C., Burger, A., Maloof, F., Braverman, L. E., and Ingbar, S. H., Iodine-induced thyrotoxicosis in Boston, *N. Engl. J. Med.*, 287, 523, 1972.
53. Croxson, M. S., Gluckman, P. D., and Ibbertson H. K., The acute thyroidal response to iodized oil in severe endemic goiter, *J. Clin. Endocrinol. Metab.*, 42, 926, 1976.
54. Lamberg, B. A., Aetiology of hypothyroidism, *Clin. Endocrinol. Metab.*, 8, 3, 1979.
55. Wolff, J., Iodide goiter and the pharmacologic effects of excess iodide, *Am. J. Med.*, 47, 101, 1969.
56. Bernecker, C., Intermittent therapy with potassium iodide in chronic obstructive disease of the airways: A review of 10 years experience, *Acta Radiol.*, 56, 275, 1969.

57. **Paris, J., McConahey, W. M., Tauxe, W. N., Woolner, L. B., and Bahn, R. C.**, The effect of iodide in Hashimoto's thyroiditis, *J. Clin. Endocrinol. Metab.*, 21, 1037, 1961.
58. **Braverman, L. E., Woever, K. A., and Ingbar, S. H.**, Induction of myxedema by iodide in patients euthyroid after radioiodine or surgical treatment for diffuse toxic goiter, *N. Engl. J. Med.*, 281, 816, 1969.
59. **Hall, R., Turner-Warwick, M., and Doniach, D.**, Autoantibodies in iodide goiter and asthma, *Clin. Exp. Immunol.*, 1, 285, 1966.
60. **Einhorn, J., Fagraeus, A., and Jonsson, J.**, Thyroid antibodies in euthyroid subjects after iodine-131 therapy, *Radiat. Res.*, 28, 296, 1966.
61. **Theodoropoulos, T., Braverman, L. E., and Vagenakis, A. G.**, Iodide-induced hypothyroidism: A potential hazard during perinatal life, *Science*, 206, 502, 1979.
62. **Rosenstein, B. J., Plotnick, L. P., and Blasco, P. A.**, Iodide induced hypothyroidism without a goiter in an infant with cystic fibrosis, *J. Pediatr.*, 93, 261, 1978.
63. **Borel, O. M. and Reddy, J. K.**, Excessive lipofuscin accumulation in the thyroid gland in mucoviscidosis, *Arch. Pathol.*, 96, 269, 1973.
64. **Glatstein, E., McHardy-Young S., Brast, N., Eltringham, J. R., and Kriss, J. P.**, Alterations in serum thyrotropin (TSH) and thyroid function following radiotherapy in patients with malignant lymphoma, *J. Clin. Endocrinol. Metab.*, 32, 833, 1971.
65. **Attwood, H. D. and Dennett, X.**, A black thyroid and minocycline treatment, *Br. Med. J.*, 2, 1109, 1976.
66. **Benitz, K. F. et al.**, *Toxic Appl. Pharm.*, 11, 150, 1967, cited by Attwood and Dennett (ref. 65).
67. **Silverman, D. A. and Rose, N. R.** Neonatal thymectomy increases the incidence of spontaneous and methylcholanthrene-enhanced thyroiditis in rats, *Science*, 184, 162, 1974.

Chapter 9

RADIATION-ASSOCIATED THYROIDITIS

Virginia A. LiVolsi

TABLE OF CONTENTS

I.	Introduction	110
II.	Effects of Radiation — General Aspects	110
III.	External Radiation and the Thyroid	112
IV.	Radioiodine and the Thyroid.	112
V.	Clinical Aspects of Radiation Thyroiditis	113
VI.	Pathological Aspects of Radiation Thyroiditis.	113
VII.	Radiation in Animal Thyroids	114
VIII.	Summary	115
References		115

I. INTRODUCTION

The recently discovered association between childhood head and neck radiation and the development of thyroid cancer has elicted considerable public concern — newspaper references, television programs, etc. have been warning the public of the risks of thyroid carcinoma in radiation-exposed individuals. More recently, the possible hazards of radiation leakage from nuclear-powered, energy-generating plants has produced public furor.

The relationship between radiation and the thyroid needs to be viewed from several standpoints.

1. What is the effect of *external* ionizing radiation?
2. What changes are noted following radioiodine therapy, i.e., *internal* radiation?
3. What are the clinical and physiologic changes associated with thyroid radiation?
4. What pathologic changes are identified in the thyroid gland in radiated individuals?
5. What is the evidence for radiation-producing thyroid tumor particularly carcinoma?
6. Are any other lesions attributed to thyroid or neck radiation?
7. Do lesions similar to human disorders develop in animals exposed to radiation?

This chapter will explore these questions, summarize the available data, and attempt to illustrate and correlate the pathological and clinical evidence of radiation's effect on the thyroid gland.

II. EFFECTS OF RADIATION — GENERAL ASPECTS

It is beyond the scope of this discussion to detail the known or postulated molecular sequences involved in the biological (cellular) effects of radiation. A brief summary of the known cellular events will be given as a background to understanding the thyroid's reaction to radiation.

In considering the effects of radiation on cells, one has to remember that most research in this area has been done on in vitro tissue culture systems.[1] Such systems, almost certainly, do not reflect entirely the in vivo situation. However, information so obtained provides us with an initial understanding of the cellular events that occur.

Little[1] outlined the development of radiation injury. Either wave or particulate radiation produces ionization or excitation by ejecting fast electrons from cell atoms. These electrons interact with other atoms and molecules causing further ionization. In this process, heat is formed and most of the latter is dissipated into the surrounding medium. Whether the rise in temperature fosters some of the ensuing chemical reactions is unclear but certainly possible.

The ionization events produce *free radicals,* powerful, unstable oxidative compounds which lead to numerous chemical reactions involving biologic macromolecules (proteins, enzymes, nucleic acids).[1] Tievsky[2] points out that one sensitive chemical group in many of the biologically important molecules is the sulfhydryl group; oxidation of such groups by free radicals can so alter molecular structure or stoichiometry as to inactivate entire enzyme systems and produce cell derangement or even cell death.[1,2] Various factors influence these events:[1-4] radiation dose, method of administration (one or divided doses), length of recovery periods between doses, phase of cell cycle, and age of animal (fetus, infant or adult).

Concentrated high dose radiation is more likely to produce necrosis and cell death with collapse of cellular organelles representing the morphologic expression of enzymatic paralysis.[5] Radiation of lesser dosage such as that in the therapeutic range (500 to 5000 rads) produces less dramatic changes. When one views the long-term effects of sublethal ionizing radiation in intact animals, one sees changes reflecting vascular (endothelial cell) damage. Fajardo and Stewart[6] evaluated the process of radiation damage in rabbit hearts and described endothelial cell disruption, occlusion of capillaries, ischemia, and finally fibrosis. Attempt at repair and regeneration of endothelial and uncommitted mesenchymal cells (? myofibroblasts) are thwarted by radiation damage to these elements.[6]

The effects of irradiation on individual cells can be appreciated by reconsidering tissue culture studies. Little[1] discusses "division delay" wherein a cell radiated in the premitotic (G_2) phase of its cycle cannot undergo mitosis for a variable period of time because of chemical damage to its DNA. Experiments have shown that cells surviving radiation demonstrate delayed growth rates in succeeding generations.[7,8] Such DNA (genetic) damage may lead eventually to malignant transformation.[1]

Aggarwal[9] described various chromosomal aberrations which may occur naturally. This author stresses that exposure to radiation increases the *number* but not the *variety* of chromosomal aberrations. These abnormalities may comprise the major genetic damage caused by radiation. The incidence of chromosome damage and of tumor increases as radiation dose increases.[9]

White[10] has emphasized the degrees of radiosensitivity of various groups of cells. Stem cells and the most immature of differentiating progenitor cells appear most sensitive to radiation which produces immediate death or delayed death due to mitotic abnormalities. Radiation induces mitotic inhibition in proliferating cells and this effect is dose related. Cells which are nonproliferative, or proliferate only under stress, show little effect of biologic importance when they are radiated. However, proliferating cells (marrow, gastrointestinal, and skin cells) by nature undergo continuous attrition and must be replenished. These elements share short generative cycles and are very reactive during sensitive portions of these cycles. Most of the cell damage (related to numerous mitoses), leads to severe depletion of these cells since radiation inhibits mitoses.[10]

From the morphologic standpoint, Graham[11] indicates that nuclear size enlargement, multinucleation, and cytoplasmic vacuolization result after radiation therapy. These changes indicate interference with nucleic acid metabolism and mitoses. Changes in availability of the folic acid derivative, tetrahydrofolic acid inhibits DNA formation leading to decreased cell division, multinucleation, and cytomegaly.[11-14]

The neoplastic potential of tissues surviving radiation injury is real, but its incidence and estimation vary in different studies, depending on host, organ studied, and dose given.[15,16] As with many emotionally and politically dynamic issues, many questions remain to be answered. The Japanese Atomic Bomb Casualty Commission studies have disclosed several facts about (a) the acute effects of high-dose radiation with marrow, and gastrointestinal damage leading to death by infection and/or hemorrhage, and (b) the long term effects of shorter life span, premature aging, decreased fertility, and, most widely publicized, development of neoplasms.[17,18] Anderson[18] summarized the known data on irradiated human populations including the Japanese atomic bomb survivors, patients radiated for ankylosing spondylitis, radium dial workers, and children radiated for enlarged thymuses or tonsils.[18]

Carcinomas and sarcomas of various organs and tissues have been reported in patients receiving therapeutic external radiation[19-23] as well as inhaling radioactive dusts.[24] Fibrosing injuries affecting bowel,[25] heart,[6] and other organs have been reported as well. Having these generalized effects, the remainder of this chapter will consider the thyroid gland's reactions to radiation.

III. EXTERNAL RADIATION AND THE THYROID

The most widely publicized effect of external radiation on the thyroid is the development of carcinoma.[26-59] Incidence rates vary, and the identification and/or differentiation of clinical nodules from the cancer produces problems in interpretation.[29,31,34-36,40,45,46] An estimate of 5 to 7% is usually given,[34] i.e., 5 to 7% of exposed patients will develop thyroid cancer. Whether each palpable nodule in the glands of radiated patients represents the cancer, or whether the malignancy is found incidentally in a thyroid removed for a nodule which pathologically was benign, is not always clearly noted.[31,34,46-48] Despite these discrepancies regarding the magnitude of the risk, there remains little doubt that thyroid cancer is increased in patients whose glands were radiated. The risk appears greatest for individuals radiated in infancy and childhood[26,33-36,38-40,43,45,46] although radiated adults show higher incidences of thyroid neoplasms than nonirradiated subjects.[30,31,42]

Most tumors which arise in radiated glands are low-grade papillary neoplasms.[24-60] Those follicular cancers which have been described[28,31,34,35,37,41,45,46,48] appear to represent follicular variants of papillary cancer and not true angioinvasive follicular carcinomas.[39,41,48,49] Rare instances of anaplastic carcinoma following radiation (usually of low-grade tumors) have been reported.[50-53] These latter cases may reflect radiation-associated transformation of benign or low-grade tumors.

Benign nodules appear with increased frequency in radiated patients.[60,61] Again, the incidence of this is difficult to ascertain, since irradiated individuals are recalled, carefully examined, tested, and followed. Controls in the general population are not easily obtained.[31,34,37,39-41,45-47,61] Hempelman and Furth[62] have postulated the mechanisms involved in radiation-associated thyroid neoplasia. Sublethal radiation initiates neoplastic mutation in thyroid cells, which, by the influence of thyroid-stimulating hormone as the effector allowing thyroid follicular cells to divide, promotes the development of a neoplasm.

Another possibility should be considered. Radiation can produce a relative hypothyroidism with depression of thyroid hormone level, thus eliciting increase in thyroid-stimulating hormone. The latter by its action on thyroid epithelial proliferation may lead to the production of an autonomous tumor, either benign or malignant.[63-66] Indeed, experimentally neoplasms can be produced by excessive stimulation of the gland.[62-64]

As will be discussed below, besides an increased incidence of tumors, irradiated thyroids show fibrosis, follicular atrophy, and chronic inflammatio;[61] in some cases, overt clinical hypothyroidism is seen.

IV. RADIOIODINE AND THE THYROID

Both ^{131}I and ^{125}I have found clinical usefulness in the treatment of hyperthyroidism.[67-73] Benign and malignant nodules arising in glands so treated have been described, but the incidence appears far lower than with external radiation.[73-79] Reasons for this include (a) different types of ionized particles involved, and (b) extensive glandular destruction and fibrosis is more likely to occur with internal radiation because of concentration of the radioiodine within the gland.[29,58,61,80,81]

Indeed, the major long term effect of therapeutic radioiodine appears to be the development of hypothyroidism.[70,72,73,80-83] Various studies have indicated that ^{125}I produces less hypothyroidism than ^{131}I, but not all reports support this.[69-71] The pathologic features of radioiodine effect on the thyroid are discussed below.

V. CLINICAL ASPECT OF RADIATION THYROIDITIS

Hypothyroidism represents the major clinical consequence of radiation thyroiditis. The incidence of this serious complication varies. For external radiation, the frequency of hypothyroidism appears dose related.[15,84-86] With radioiodine exposure, the likelihood of developing hypothyroidism seems to increase with time and is less dependent on dose received.[72,73,80-83]

Hurley[87] has described the acute effects of internal radiation which resemble subacute thyroiditis clinically. Thus, with 4 days of treatment, pain radiating to the jaws or ears, tenderness, and neck swelling are noted. Mild hyperthyroidism is found with elevations of T_3, T_4, and radioiodine uptake. Edema of the neck may be mild or severe, the latter necessitating steroids or even tracheostomy.[88,89] This thyroiditis subsides within 3 to 4 weeks.[87] Several authors suggest that the thyroid's response to radioiodine depends on the functional state of the gland.[87,90,91]

The long term effect of irradiation is the development of hypothyroidism.[80-83,86] The longer the followup of treated patients, the greater the incidence of hypothyroidism.[80,86] Although this development is somewhat dose-related and dependent on thyroid functional state at time of radiation, this result has serious metabolic consequences. (Careful followup of patients treated with radioiodine is mandatory.) Slingerland et al.[92] have summarized four types of thyroid function changes (both clinical and chemical) following radioiodine therapy. Thus, of 160 treated patients, 74% were clinically euthyroid and 26% hypothyroid. These patients fell into one of the following groups:[92]

1. Euthyroid clinically and chemically with normal thyrotropin (TSH) and TSH response
2. Clinically euthyroid and chemically, but with no response to TSH and high endogenous TSH
3. Clinically euthyroid but chemically hypothyroid
4. Myxedematous clinically and by lab test

The mechanism of hypothyroidism following radioiodine has been described by Malone and Cullen[81] as twofold: early and late onset. The former is dose dependent and accounts for 5 to 40% of cases. Thyroid cell death appears responsible for this type of hypothyroidism.[93] Late hypothyroidism seems non-dose-dependent and may be related to the presence of autoimmune factors especially if present before therapy,[81] thyroid nodularity, individual sensitivity, heterogeneous distribution of isotope,[94] and initial size of gland.[95,96] Relative importance of these and other factors in the pathogenesis of the thyroid dysfunction requires further studies.

VI. PATHOLOGICAL ASPECTS OF RADIATION THYROIDITIS

Both acute and chronic histologic changes have been described. Acute changes, occurring in the first few weeks after therapy, correspond to the clinically noted symptoms. These alterations include follicular disruption, neutrophilic infiltration, cellular necrosis, and edema; subsequently, vascular damage with thrombosis, hemorrhage, and further gland destruction take place.[88,90,91,97] The changes seen are not found uniformly in the gland and are not recognized in all treated patients. Differences result from variations in dose, nodularity of gland, size of gland, and poorly understood host response factors.[98]

Changes which occur months or years after radioiodine therapy, and which are as-

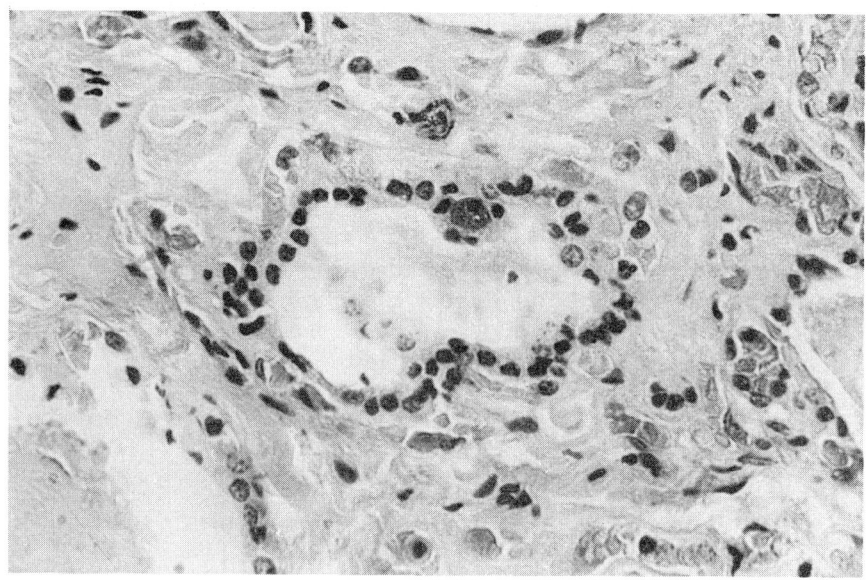

FIGURE 1. Section of residual thyroid from patient who 3 yr before had been treated with ^{131}I for Graves' disease. Note fibrosis and central follicle with bizarre nucleus (above center). (Hematoxylin-eosin; magnification × 300.)

sociated with hypothyroidism, include a grossly small, fibrotic gland.[29,48,61,90,91,97-101] Histologically, fibrosis, follicular disruption, atrophic and microfollicles, attenuated epithelium, oxyphilic change, and nuclear abnormalities are found. Associated vascular changes include arteriolar intimal thickening and hyalinization.[15,29,61,90,91,97-101] Squamous metaplasia may be seen.[102] Atypia in stromal and endothelial cells may be identified also;[11] lymphocytic infiltration may be seen also.[90,91,98] The entire picture is not unlike that of the histopathology of idiopathic myxedema (see Chapter 7).

The nuclear abnormalities[100] seen in these radioiodine treated thyroids resemble the nucleomegaly described by Graham[11] in her studies on radiated tissues. However, Kennedy and Thomson[100] point out that such abnormal nuclei are also seen in the thyroid remnant following surgery. The present author notes such nuclei sparsely distributed in glands surgically resected for Graves' disease.

Pathologic alterations described in thyroids which have received external radiation occur with remarkably high frequency — up to 76% of these glands show microscopic abnormalities.[29,41,49,61] These include:[49] focal hyperplasia (88%), thyroiditis (67%), adenomas (51%), Hurthle cell changes (42%), fibrosis (25%) and colloid nodules (51%) and finally, thyroid cancer (as described above).

VII. RADIATION IN ANIMAL THYROIDS

Experimental radiation in various animals has resulted in histopathologic alterations similar to those encountered in man.[97,98]

Bower and Clark[103] implanted radium needles in dog thyroids and after 2 weeks noted microscopically a central necrotic zone bordered by an infarcted area and then an inflammatory and hemorrhagic zone. The thyroid tissue showed swollen cuboidal cells, dark nuclei, and sparse colloid. After 3 weeks, fibrosis of the gland with decreased size was found.

Freedberg et al.[97] demonstrated that ^{131}I administration to animals showed within

12 hr, the presence of edema, congestion, and follicular cell vacuolization. This progressed to cellular and follicular degeneration, leukocytic infiltration and vascular damage with thrombosis. Within 6 to 8 weeks, fibrosis and atrophy of the gland were found. Frantz et al.[104] recognized atrophy and fibrosis in rats given ^{131}I whereas neoplasms were identified in externally radiated animals.

Doniach[105] described the effects of 1000 rads on rat thyroids which showed shrinkage of the gland, inhibition of goiter formation, and tumor induction. Lindsay[106] induced benign and malignant neoplasms in rats by administering radioiodine. These tumors were identified as low-grade papillary lesions and resembled those tumors induced by iodine deficiency or goiterogens, suggesting the intervention of thyrotropin as either a promoter or by another mechanism.[107,108]

VIII. SUMMARY

This chapter has reviewed the effects of radiation on the thyroid gland in man stressing the high incidence of pathologic abnormalities, including carcinoma, especially following external radiation. Radioiodine produces less tumor development, but presents the problem of concentrated high-dose radiation in the thyroid. Following initial, short term "subacute" thyroiditis, there eventuates permanent hypothyroidism in a large percentage of cases so treated. This is reflected pathologically by atrophy and fibrous replacement of the thyroid. Animal experiments adding some understanding to the problem are discussed briefly.

REFERENCES

1. **Little, J. B.**, Cellular effects of ionizing radiation, *N. Engl. J. Med.*, 278, 307, 369, 1968.
2. **Tievsky, G.**, *Ionizing Radiation*, Charles C Thomas, Springfield, Ill., 1962.
3. **Barone, R. M. and Das Gupta, T. K.**, Effects of irradiation on malignant cell cytoplasm, *J. Surg. Oncol.*, 3, 274, 1972.
4. **Eisenbrandt, D. L. and Phemister, R. D.**, Radiation injury in the neonatal canine kidney, *Lab. Invest.*, 37, 437, 1977.
5. **Jordan, S. W., Dean, P. N., and Ahlquist, J.**, Early ultrastructural effects of ionizing radiation, *Lab Invest.*, 27, 538, 1972.
6. **Fajardo, L. F. and Stewart, J. R.**, Pathogenesis of radiation-induced myocardial fibrosis, *Lab. Invest.*, 29, 244, 1973.
7. **Puck, T. T. and Marcus, P. I.**, Action of x-rays on mammalian cells, *J. Exp. Med.*, 103, 653, 1956.
8. **Dewey, W. C., Humphrey, R. M., and Cork, A.**, Comparison of cell-multiplication and colony-formation as criteria for radiation damage in cells grown in vitro, *Int. J. Radiat. Biol.*, 6, 463, 1963.
9. **Aggarwal, R. K.**, Automatic recognition of irradiated chromosomes, *J. Histochem. Cytochem.*, 22, 561, 1974.
10. **White, D. C.**, *An Atlas of Radiation Histopathology*, U.S. Energy Research and Development Administration, Washington, D.C., 1975.
11. **Graham, R. M.**, *The Cytologic Diagnosis of Cancer*, W. B. Saunders, Philadelphia, 1972.
12. **Whitehead, N., Reyner, F., and Lindenbaum, J.**, Megaloblastic changes in cervical epithelium, *JAMA*, 226, 1421, 1973.
13. **van Niekleik, W. A.**, Cervical cytologic abnormalities caused by folic acid deficiency, *Acta Cytol.*, 10, 67, 1966.
14. **Boschann, H. W.**, Radiation changes in benign cells, in *Compendium on Diagnostic Cytology*, Wied, G. L., Koss, L. G., and Reagan, J. W., Eds., The Tutorials of Cytology, Chicago, 1974, 226.

15. **Hempelmann, L. H., Pifer, J. W., Burker, G. J., Terry, R., and Ames, W. R.**, Neoplasms in persons treated with x-rays in infancy for thymic enlargement, *J. Nat. Cancer Inst.*, 38, 317, 1967.
16. **Pincus, R. A., Reichlin, S., and Hempelmann, L. H.**, Thyroid abnormalities after radiation exposure in infancy, *Ann. Intern. Med.*, 66, 1154, 1967.
17. **Liebow, A. A., Warren, S., and DeCoursey, E.**, Pathology of atomic bomb casualties, *Am. J. Pathol.*, 25, 853, 1949.
18. **Anderson, R. E.**, Longevity in radiated human populations with particular reference to the atomic bomb survivors, *Am. J. Med.*, 55, 643, 1973.
19. **Paik, H. H. and Wilkinson, E. J.**, Peritoneal osteosarcoma following irradiation therapy of ovarian cancer, *Obstet. Gynecol.*, 47, 488, 1976.
20. **Simon, N.**, Breast cancer induced by radiation, *JAMA*, 237, 789, 1977.
21. **Petersen, O.**, Radiation cancer. Report of twenty-one cases, *Acta Radiol.*, 42, 221, 1954.
22. **Goolden, A. W. G.**, Radiation cancer. A review with special reference to radiation tumours in the pharynx, larynx and thyroid, *Br. J. Radiol.*, 30, 626, 1957.
23. **Goolden, A. W. G. and Morgen, R. L.**, Radiation cancer of the pharynx, *Acta Radiol.*, 3, 353, 1965.
24. **Saccomanno G., Archer, V. E., Auerbach, O., Kuschner, M., Saunders, R. P., and Klein, M. G.**, Histologic types of lung cancer among uranium miners, *Cancer*, 27, 515, 1971.
25. **Newman, A., Katsaris, J., Blendis, L. M., Charlesworth, M., and Walter, L. H.**, Small-intestinal injury in women who have had pelvic radiotherapy *Lancet*, 2, 1471, 1973.
26. **Hanford, J. M., Quimby, E. H., and Frantz, V. K.**, Cancer arising many years after radiation therapy, *JAMA*, 181, 404, 1962.
27. **Tubiana, M.**, On the relationship of irradiation and thyroid cancer, *Int. Colloq., Tum. Thyr. Gland*, Marseilles, 1964, S. Karger Co., Basel, 1966, 314.
28. **Andre, P.**, Postirradiation thyroid cancers, *Int. Colloq. Tum. Thyr. Gland*, Marseilles, 1964, S. Karger Co., Basel, 1966, 299.
29. **Andre, P.**, *Pathological Effects of Thyroid Irradiation*, U.S. Federal Radiation Council, Washington, D.C., 1966.
30. **Block, M. A., Miller, M. J., and Horn, R. C.**, Carcinoma of the thyroid after external radiation to the neck in adults, *Am. J. Surg.*, 118, 764, 1969.
31. **Sampson, R. J., Key, C. R., Buncher, C. R., and Iijima, S.**, Thyroid carcinoma in Hiroshima and Nagasaki. I. Prevalence of thyroid carcinoma at autopsy, *JAMA*, 209, 65, 1969.
32. **Wilson, S. M., Platz, C., and Block, G. M.**, Thyroid carcinoma after irradiation, *Arch. Surg.*, 100, 330, 1970.
33. **Conrad, R. A., Dobyns, B. M., and Sutow, W. W.**, Thyroid neoplasia as late effect of exposure to radioactive iodine in fallout, *JAMA*, 214, 316, 1970.
34. **DeGroot, L. and Paloyan, E.**, Thyroid carcinoma and radiation. A Chicago epidemic, *JAMA*, 225, 487, 1973.
35. **Hempelmann, L. H.**, Radiation-induced thyroid neoplasms in man, in *Thyroid Neoplasia*, Young, S. and Inman, D. R., Eds., Academic Press, New York, 1968, 267.
36. **Hempelmann, L. H.**, Radiation exposure and thyroid cancer in man, in *Thyroid Cancer*, Hedinger, E., Ed., Springer-Verlag, Berlin, 1969, 103.
37. **Modan, B., Baidatz, D., Mart, H., Steinitz, R., and Levin, S. G.**, Radiation-induced head and neck tumours, *Lancet*, 1, 277, 1974.
38. **Rallison, M. L., Dobyns, B. M., Keating, F. R., Rall, J. E., and Tyler, F. H.**, Thyroid disease in children: A survey of subjects potentially exposed to fallout radiation, *Am. J. Med.*, 56, 457, 1974.
39. **Refetoff, S., Harrison, J., Karanfilski, B. T., Kaplan, E. L., DeGroot, L. H., and Bekerman, C.**, Continuing occurrence of thyroid carcinoma after irradiation to the neck in infancy and childhood, *N. Engl. J. Med.*, 292, 171, 1975.
40. **Becker, F. O., Economou, S. G., Southwick, H. W., and Eisenstein, R.**, Adult thyroid cancer after head and neck irradiation in infancy and childhood, *Ann. Intern. Med.*, 83, 347, 1975.
41. **Favus, M. J., Schneider, A. B., Stachura, M. E., Arnold, J. E., Ryo, U. Y., Pinsky, S. M., Colman, M., Arnold, M. J., and Frohman, L. A.**, Thyroid cancer occurring as a late consequence of head and neck irradiation, *N. Engl. J. Med.*, 294, 1019, 1976.
42. **Goldschmidt, H.**, Dermatologic radiotherapy and thyroid cancer, *Arch. Dermatol.*, 113, 362, 1977.
43. **Schneider, A. B., Favus, M. J., Stachura, M. E., Arnold, J. E., Ryo, U. Y., Pinsky, S., Colman, M., Arnold, M. J., and Frohman, L. A.**, Plasma thyroglobulin in detecting thyroid carcinoma after childhood head and neck irradiation, *Ann. Intern. Med.*, 86, 29, 1977.
44. **Greenspan, F. S.**, Radiation exposure and thyroid cancer, *JAMA*, 237, 2089, 1977.
45. **Southwick, H. W.**, Radiation-associated head and neck tumors, *Am. J. Surg.*, 134, 438, 1977.
46. **DeGroot, L. J.**, Ed., *Radiation-Associated Thyroid Carcinoma*, Grune and Stratton, New York, 1977.

47. **Sampson, R. J.,** Thyroid carcinoma, *N. Engl. J. Med.,* 295, 340, 1976.
48. **Sampson, R. J.,** Prevalence and significance of occult thyroid cancer, in *Radiation-Associated Thyroid Carcinoma,* DeGroot, L. J., Ed., Grune and Stratton, New York, 1977 137.
49. **Straus, F. H. and Spitalnik, P. F.,** Histologic parenchymal changes in the human thyroid after low dose childhood irradiation, in *Radiation-Associated Thyroid Carcinoma,* DeGroot L. J., Ed., Grune and Stratton, New York, 1977, 183.
50. **Baker, H. W.,** Anaplastic thyroid cancer twelve years after radiation therapy, *Cancer,* 23, 885, 1963.
51. **Levene, M. B. and Vickery A. L.,** Case records of the Massachusetts General Hospital-2-1977, *N. Engl. J. Med.,* 296, 94, 1977.
52. **Komorowski, R. A., Hanson, G. A., and Garancis, J. C.,** Anaplastic thyroid carcinoma following low-dose irradiation, *Am. J. Clin. Pathol.,* 70, 303, 1978.
53. **Getaz, E. P., Shimaoka K., and Rao, U.,** Anaplastic carcinoma of the thyroid following external irradiation, *Cancer,* 43, 2248, 1979.
54. **Duffy, B. J. and Fitzgerald, P. J.,** Thyroid cancer in childhood and adolescence: Report on 28 cases, *Cancer,* 3, 1018, 1950.
55. **Clark, D. E.,** Association of irradiation with cancer of the thyroid in children and adolescents, *JAMA,* 159, 1007, 1955.
56. **Simpson, C. L. and Hempelmann, L. H.,** The association of tumours and roentgen-ray treatment of the thorax in infancy, *Cancer,* 10, 42, 1957.
57. **Simpson, C. L., Hempelmann, L. H. and Fuller, L. M.,** Neoplasia in children treated with x-rays in infancy for thymic enlargement, *Radiology,* 64, 840, 1955.
58. **Goolden, A. W. G.,** The effect of radiation on the thyroid gland, in *Modern Trends in Endocrinology,* Vol. 4, Prunty, F. T. G. and Hardiner-Hill, H., Eds., Appleton-Century-Crofts, New York, 1972, 250.
59. **Fukunago, F. H. and Lockett, L. J.,** Thyroid carcinoma in the Japanese in Hawaii, *Arch. Pathol.,* 92, 6, 1971.
60. **Wagner, D. H., Recant, W. M., and Evans, R. H.,** A review of one hundred and fifty thyroidectomies following prior irradiation to the head, neck and upper part of the chest, *Surg. Gynecol. Obstet.,* 147, 903, 1978.
61. **Komorowski, R. A. and Hanson, G. A.,** Morphologic changes in the thyroid following low-dose childhood radiation, *Arch. Pathol.,* 101, 36, 1977.
62. **Hempelmann, L. and Furth, J.,** Etiology of thyroid cancer in *Thyroid Cancer,* Greenfield, L., Ed., CRC Press, Boca Raton, Fla., 1978, 37.
63. **Meier, D. A. and Hamburger, J. A.,** An autonomously functioning thyroid nodule, cancer and prior radiation, *Arch. Surg.,* 103, 759, 1971.
64. **Meissner, W. A. and Adler, A.,** Papillary carcinoma of the thyroid: A study of the pathology of two hundred twenty-six cases, *Arch. Pathol.,* 66, 518, 1958.
65. **Olen, E. and Klinck, G. H.,** Hyperthyroidism and thyroid cancer, *Arch. Pathol.* 81, 531, 1966.
66. **Williams, E. D., Doniach, I., Bjarnson, O., and Michie, W.,** Thyroid cancer in an iodide rich area, *Cancer,* 39, 215, 1977.
67. **Hagen, G. A., Ouellette, R. P., and Chapman, E. M.,** Comparison of high and low dosage levels of ^{131}I in the treatment of thyrotoxicosis, *N. Engl. J. Med.,* 277, 559, 1967.
68. **Goldsmith, R. E.,** Radioisotope therapy for Graves' disease, *Mayo Clin. Proc.,* 47, 953, 1972.
69. **Reynolds, L. R. and Kotchen T. A.,** Antithyroid drugs and radioactive iodine, *Arch. Intern, Med.,* 139, 651, 1979.
70. **McDougall, I. R., Greig, W. R., Gray, H. W., and Gillespie, F. C.,** Iodine-125 treatment for thyrotoxicosis, *Lancet,* 2, 840, 1970.
71. **Werner, S. C., Johnson, P. M., Goodwin, P. N., Wiener, J. D., and Lindeboom, G. A.,** Long-term results with iodine-125 treatment for toxic diffuse goitre, *Lancet,* 2, 681, 1970.
72. **Weidinger, P., Johnson, P. M., and Werner, S. C.,** Five-years' experience with iodine-125 therapy of Graves' disease, *Lancet,* 2, 74, 1974.
73. **McDougall, I. R. and Greig, W. R.,** ^{125}-I therapy in Graves' disease: Long-term results in 355 patients, *Ann. Intern. Med.,* 85, 720, 1976.
74. **Pilch, B. Z., Kahn, C. R., Ketcham, A. S. and Henson, D.,** Thyroid cancer after radioactive iodine diagnostic procedures in childhood, *Pediatrics,* 51, 898, 1973.
75. **Kreps, E. M., Kreps, S. M., and Kreps, S. I.,** Treatment of hyperthyroidism with sodium iodide I-^{131} Carcinoma of the thyroid after 20 years, *JAMA,* 226, 774, 1973.
76. **Mc Dougall, I. R.,** Thyroid cancer after I-^{131} therapy, *JAMA,* 227, 438, 1974.
77. **Burke, G., Levinson, M. J., and Zitman, I. H.,** Thyroid carcinoma ten years after sodium iodide-I^{131} treatment, *JAMA,* 199, 247, 1967.
78. **Karlan M. S., Pollock, W. F., and Snyder, W. H.,** Carcinoma of the thyroid following treatment of hyperthyroidism with radioactive iodine, *Calif. Med.,* 101, 196, 1964.

79. Sheline, G. E., Lindsay, S., McCormack, K. R., and Golante, M., Thyroid nodules occurring late after treatment of thyrotoxicosis with radioiodine *J. Clin. Endocrinol. Metab.*, 22, 8, 1962.
80. Safa, A. M., Schumacher, P., and Rodriquez-Antunez, A., Long-term follow-up result in children and adolescents treated with radioactive iodine (I^{131}) for hyperthyroidism, *N. Engl. J. Med.*, 292, 167, 1975.
81. Malone, J. F. and Cullen, M. J., Two mechanisms for hypothyroidism after ^{131}-I therapy, *Lancet*, 2, 73, 1976.
82. Burke, G. and Silverstein, G. E., Hypothyroidism after treatment with sodium iodide I-^{131}, *JAMA*, 210, 1051, 1969.
83. Glennon, J. A., Gordon, E. S., and Sawin, C. T., Hypothyroidism after low dose ^{131}-I treatment of hyperthyroidism, *Ann. Intern. Med.*, 76, 721, 1972.
84. Glatstein, E., McHardy-Young, S., Brast, N., Eltringham, J. R., and Kriss, J P., Alterations in serum thyrotropin (TSH) and thyroid function following radiotherapy in patients with malignant lymphoam, *J. Clin. Endocrinol. Metab.*, 32, 833, 1971.
85. Shafer, R. B., Nuttall, F. Q., Pollak, K., and Kuisk, H., Thyroid function after radiation and surgery for head and neck cancer, *Arch. Intern. Med.*, 135, 843, 1975.
86. Rosenthal, M. B. and Goldfine, I. D., Primary and secondary hypothyroidism in nasopharyngeal carcinoma, *JAMA*, 236, 1595, 1976.
87. Hurley, J. A., Thyroiditis, *Disease-A-Month*, Vol. 24, December 3, 1977.
88. Andrews, G. A., Kniseley, R. M., Bigelow, R. R., Root, S. W., and Brucer, M., Pathologic changes in normal human thyroid tissue following large doses of I^{131}. *Am. J. Med.*, 16, 372, 1954.
89. Becker, D. V. and Hurley, J. R., Complications of radioiodine treatment of hyperthyroidism, *Semin. Nucl. Med.*, 1, 442, 1971.
90. Dobyns, B. M., Vickery, A. L., Maloof, F., and Chapman, E. M., Functional and histologic effect of therapeutic doses of radioactive iodine on thyroid of man, *J. Clin. Endocrinol. Metab.*, 13, 548, 1953.
91. Dailey, M. E., Lindsay, S., and Miller, E. R., Histologic lesions in thyroid glands of patients receiving radioiodine for hyperthyroidism, *J. Clin. Endocrinol. Metab.*, 13, 1513, 1953.
92. Slingerland, D. W., Dell, E. S., and Burrows, B. A., The spectrum of thyroid function after radioiodine treatment, *Further Adv. Thyroid Res.*, 13, 993, 1971.
93. Smith, R. N. and Wilson, G. M., Clinical trial of different doses of ^{131}-I treatment of thyrotoxicosis, *Br. Med. J.*, 1, 129, 1967.
94. Lamberg, B. A., Aetiology of hypothyroidism, *J. Clin. Endocrinol. Metab.*, 8, 3, 1979.
95. Glanzmann, C., Kaestner F., and Horst, W. Therapie der Hyperthyreose mit Radioiosotopen des Jods, *Klin. Wochinschr.*, 53, 669, 1975.
96. Roudelbush, C. P., Hoye, K. E., and DeGroot, L. J., Compensated low-dose ^{131}-I therapy of Graves' disease, *Ann. Intern. Med.*, 87, 441, 1977.
97. Freedberg, A. S., Kurland, G. S., and Blumgart, H. L., The pathologic effects of I^{131} on the normal thyroid gland of man, *J. Clin. Endocrinol.*, 12, 1315, 1952.
98. Hazard, J. B., Thyroiditis: A review, *Am. J. Clin. Pathol.*, 25, 289, 399, 1955.
99. Lindsay, S., Dailey, M. E., and Jones, M. E., Histologic effects of various types of ionizing radiation on normal and hyperplastic human thyroid glands, *J. Clin. Endocrinol. Metab.*, 14, 1179, 1954.
100. Kennedy, J. S. and Thomson, J. A., The changes in the thyroid gland after irradiation with ^{131}I or partial thyroidectomy for thyrotoxicosis, *J. Pathol.*, 112, 65, 1974.
101. Curran, R. C., Eckert, H., and Wilson, G. M., The thyroid gland after treatment of hyperthyroidism by partial thyroidectomy or iodine-^{131}, *J. Pathol. Bacteriol.*, 76, 541, 1958.
102. LiVolsi, V. A. and Merino, M. J., Squamous cells in the human thyroid gland, *Am. J. Surg. Pathol.*, 2, 139, 1978.
103. Bower, J. O. and Clark, J. H., The resistance of the thyroid gland to the action of radium rays, *Am. J. Roentgenol.*, 10, 632, 1923.
104. Frantz, V. K., Kligerman, M. M., Harland, W. A., Phillips, M. E., and Quimby, E. H., A comparison of the carcinogenic effects of internal and external irradiation on the thyroid gland of the male Long-Evans rats, *Endocrinology*, 61, 574, 1957.
105. Doniach, I., Damaging effect of x-irradiation of less than 1000 rads on goitrogenic capacity of rat thyroid gland, in *Thyroid Neoplasia,* Young, S. and Inman, D. R., Eds., Academic Press, New York, 1968, 259.
106. Lindsay, S., Experimental production of thyroid neoplasms in the rat by irradiation, in *Thyroid Neoplasia,* Young, S. and Inman, D. R., Eds., Academic Press, New York, 1968, 279.
107. Lindsay, S., Ionizing radiation and experimental thyroid neoplasms: A review, in *Thyroid Cancer,* Hedinger, E., Ed., Springer-Verlag, New York, 1969, 161.
108. Schaller, R. T. and Stevenson, J. K., Development of carcinoma of the thyroid in iodine deficient mice, *Cancer,* 19, 1063, 1966.

Chapter 10

THYROIDITIS ASSOCIATED WITH THYROID TUMORS

Virginia A. LiVolsi

TABLE OF CONTENTS

I.	Introduction	120
II.	Pathologic Characteristics of Tumor-Thyroiditis	120
	A. Lymphocytic Infiltrates Only	120
	B. Extensive Involvement with Germinal Center Formation	120
III.	Types of Tumors Involved	120
	A. Papillary (Mixed Papillary-Follicular) Carcinoma	120
	B. Medullary Carcinoma	123
	C. Other Epithelial Tumors	123
	D. Lymphoma	124
IV.	Pathophysiology: Immunologic Facets	125
V.	Clinical Correlations	127
VI.	Summary	128
References		128

I. INTRODUCTION

The histologic finding of chronic thyroiditis in patients with thyroid carcinoma, chiefly papillary or mixed papillary-follicular type, has produced confusion regarding both the significance of this thyroiditis and the potential of chronic thyroiditis in general as a premalignant lesion. This chapter will (a) review the pathology of lymphocytic thyroiditis found in association with thyroid tumors, (b) relate it to specific tumor subtypes, (c) discuss immunologic facets of this lesion, and (d) summarize clinical correlations.

II. PATHOLOGIC CHARACTERISTICS OF TUMOR-THYROIDITIS

A. Lymphocytic Infiltrates Only

The histopathologist encounters scattered lymphocytic and even mixed lymphocytic-plasmacytic infiltrates at the periphery of a thyroid neoplasm frequently. Especially in the vicinity of the infiltrative edges of the most common thyroid carcinoma, papillary cancer, this lymphoid infiltrate is found in the majority of cases.[1-9]

It remains debatable whether this mild degree of thyroiditis reflects nonspecific changes commonly seen in adult thyroids, or whether it is specifically tumor related. As has been discussed in Chapters 7 and 8, chronic nonspecific thyroiditis may reflect a reaction to iodide-sufficient diets and may be noted commonly in thyroids surgically removed for nonthyroid disease (e.g., laryngeal cancer) or at autopsy in patients dying of nonendocrine disorders.[10-13] It appears that this lesion is identified more commonly with increasing age. Thus it is possible that the finding of a mild lymphocytic infiltration in a thyroid harboring a tumor is merely coincidental.

However, when one recognizes the thyroiditic changes solely in the vicinity of the tumor with sparing of the noninvolved gland, speculation arises regarding an interrelationship (see below). Indeed, if one can extrapolate from carcinomas in other organs (e.g., colon, breast, lung) the finding of scattered lymphocytes at the invasive edge of such tumors is not uncommon.[14-17] The presence of large infiltrates around some neoplasms has been correlated with a favorable prognosis.[15,16]

B. Extensive Involvement with Germinal Center Formation

Less often, a thyroid cancer may be associated with an extensive thyroiditis. Thus, the histopathology of fullblown, classical Hashimoto's disease with lymphoplasmacytic infiltrates, the formation of germinal centers, and follicular atrophy with Hurthle cell metaplasia may be found in a gland also containing a neoplasm. Indeed, the lymphoid infiltrate may become intimately admixed with the tumor, so that it involves even the fibrovascular cores of tumor papillae (Figures 1 to 3), as well as the peripheral edge of the tumor and even the entire gland.

It is florid cases of tumor-associated thyroiditis that have produced controversy regarding the premalignant potential of Hashimoto's disease. As will be discussed below, adequate serologic and clinical documentation of Hashimoto's thyroiditis in patients with thyroid carcinoma is sorely lacking.

III. TYPES OF TUMOR INVOLVED

A. Papillary (Mixed Papillary-Follicular) Carcinoma

By far the most common neoplasm of, or in, the thyroid to show this paratumor thyroiditis is the papillary carcinoma. The incidence of coexistent tumor thyroiditis and papillary cancer is unknown, since often only those cases with extensive thyroiditic

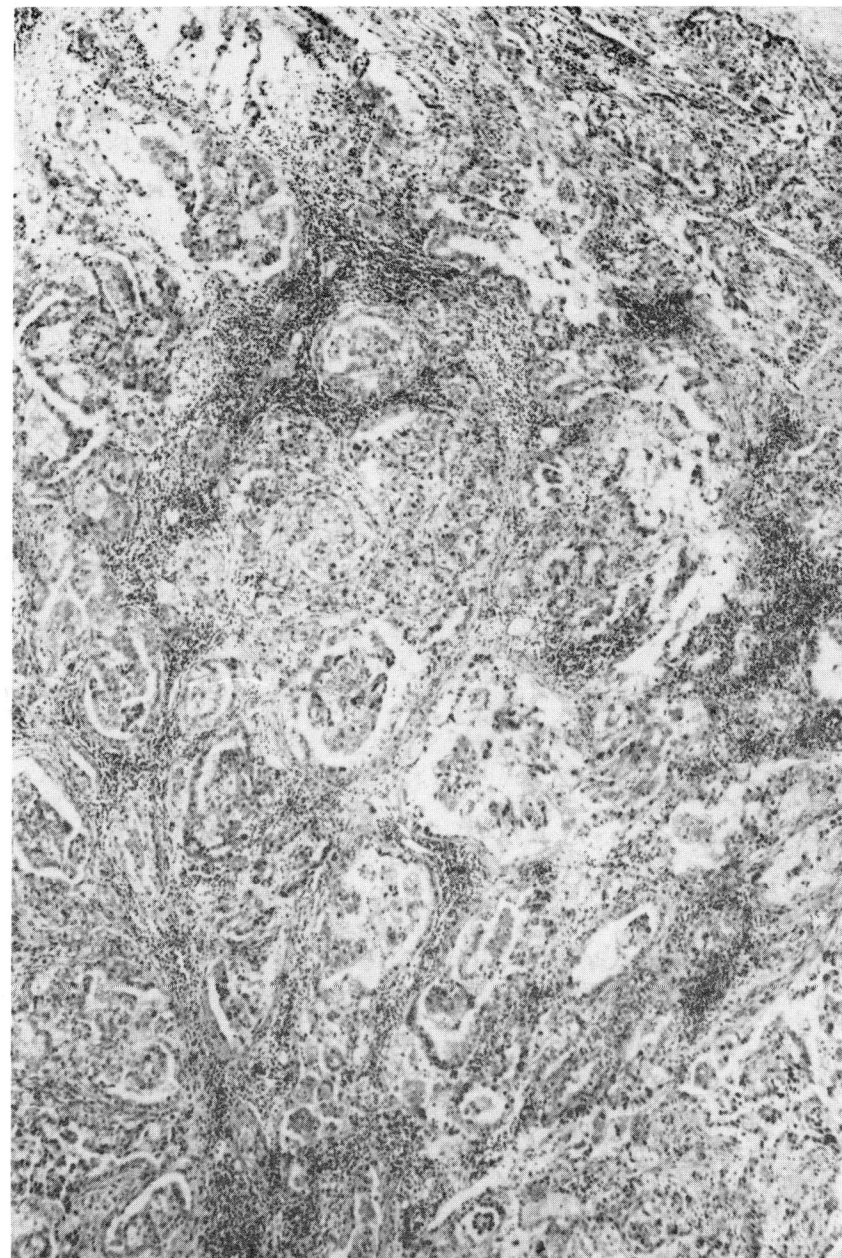

FIGURE 1. Low power view of mixed papillary-follicular carcinoma shows diffuse infiltrative nature of the lesion with associated intratumor lymphocytic infiltrate. (Hematoxylin-eosin; magnification × 100.)

changes are recorded; minor lymphocytic infiltrates may not be considered important.

Bastenie et al.[7] claim that lymphocytic infiltration is mild in most cases; it is marked in 10% and approaches that seen in Hashimoto's disease only in rare instances. Hirabayashi and Lindsay[4] identified some degree of thyroiditis in 65% of the 329 papillary cancers in their material. This type of tumor accounted for 92% of cases in which a

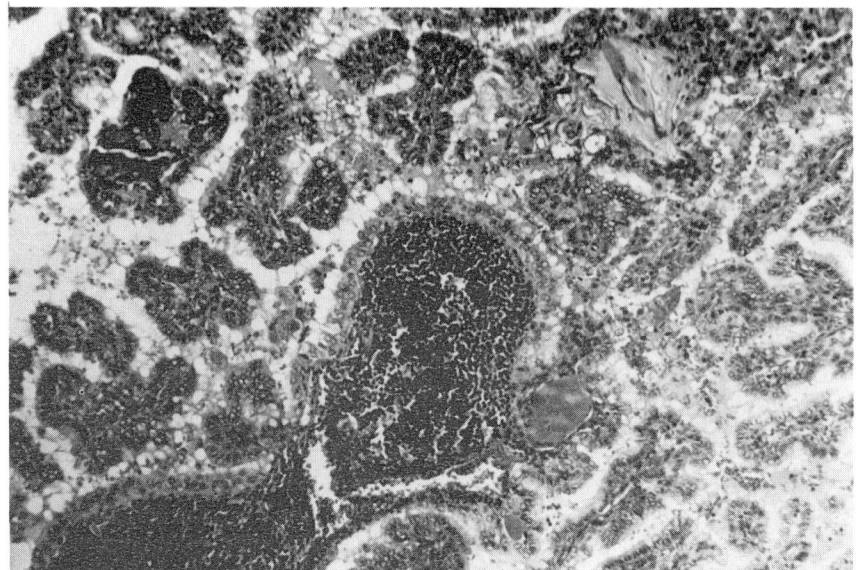

FIGURE 2. Another papillary carcinoma demonstrates lymphocytes within fibrovascular cores of papillae. (Hematoxylin-eosin; magnification × 150.)

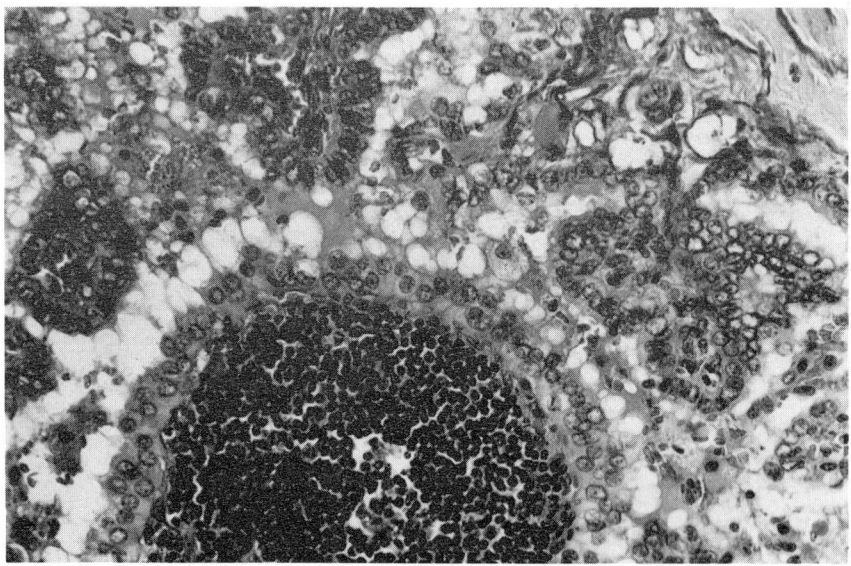

FIGURE 3.. Same case as Figure 2. Note ground-glass papillary cancer nuclei in epithelial cells, (Hematoxylin-eosin; magnification × 300.)

neoplasm was associated with thyroiditis. Meier et al.[5] evaluated 256 cases of thyroid cancer and found focal thyroiditis in 35%, with marked reactions in 10% of their cases. Dailey et al.[1] examined the question of tumor thyroiditis and found 35 examples of carcinoma associated with thyroiditis compared to 85 carcinomas without thyroiditis and 110 cases of Hashimoto's disease without neoplasm. Unfortunately, in these

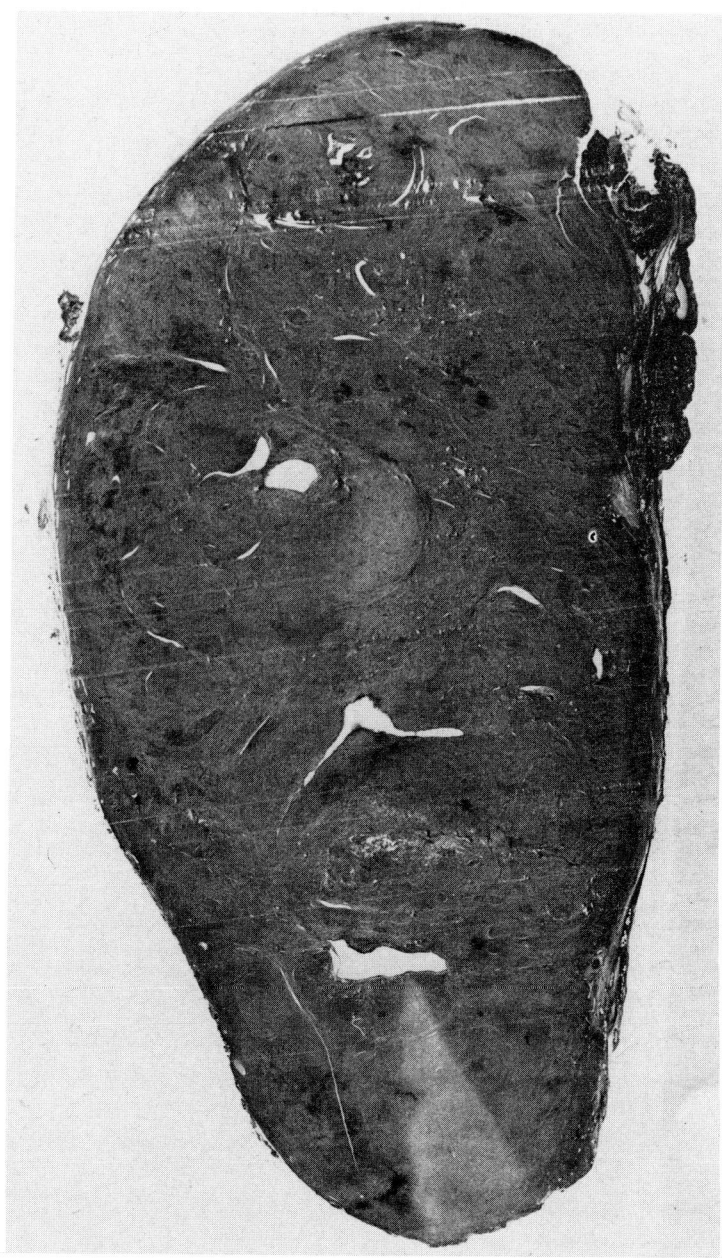

FIGURE 4. Cross section of thyroid lobe in patient with history of Hashimoto's thyroiditis and recent rapid growth. Note replacement of lobe by diffusely infiltrating tumor. (Hematoxylin-eosin; magnification × 4.)

arising in Hashimoto's disease, but rather an inflammatory reaction reflecting a secondary host response to the carcinoma.[8,35]

IV. PATHOPHYSIOLOGY: IMMUNOLOGIC FACETS

The presence of circulating antithyroid antibodies has been observed in from 2 to 45% of patients with thyroid cancer.[3,41,42] In addition, occasionally long acting thyroid

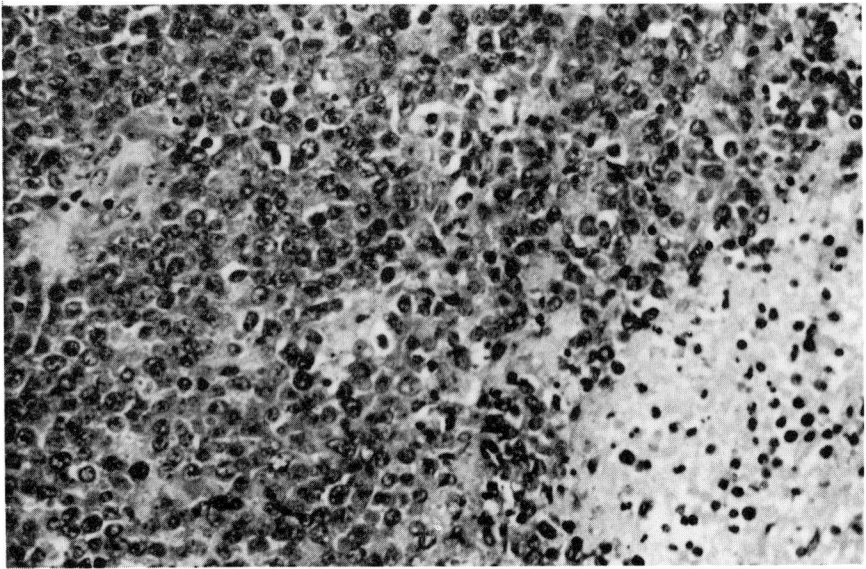

FIGURE 5. Malignant lymphoma with area of tumor necrosis (lower right). (Hematoxylin-eosin; magnification × 200.)

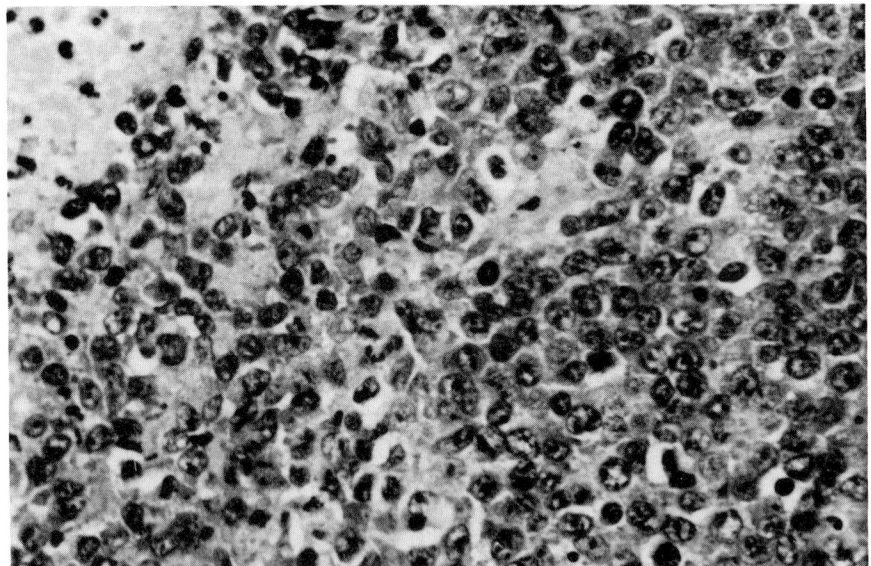

FIGURE 6. Higher power view of lymphoma shows malignant character of cells. (Hematoxylin-eosin; magnification × 300.)

stimulator (LATS)[43] and thyroid-stimulating immunoglobulin have been reported.[44] Goudie noted that human thyroid cancers in vitro showed depletion of microsomal autoantigen which he postulated might be involved in immunologic reactions associated with thyroid tumors.[45] Following extirpation of the tumor, the antibodies disappear.[46]

Recent studies have disclosed the presence of circulating thyroglobulin in athyroid patients with recurrent thyroid cancer.[47-49] Thyroglobulin has been identified immunohistochemically in follicular-cell derived (papillary, follicular) thyroid cancer.[50-51] Apparently, this protein can be secreted into the circulation by the tumors which produce it; normally, thyroglobulin is circulated in very small amounts.[47-53] Perhaps the tumor thyroglobulin may be abnormal, but it retains an intact, immunologically reactive site common to the normal human protein.[48,49] In animal thyroid cancer also, abnormal thyroglobulin is found suggesting a similar condition in human thyroid neoplasms.[54]

Hence, the peritumor thyroiditis can be explained by two possible mechanisms: (a) denaturation or alteration of the neoplastic thyroid tissue may allow access to the circulation of thyroid antigens not normally found in serum[7] and (b) similarly, elaboration of tumor thyroglobulin may elicit an immune response, including antibody formation.[7] This situation strongly resembles many of the animal models of induced autoimmune thyroiditis in that the thyroiditic lesion is produced by immunization with thyroid extract or chemically altered thyroglobulin[55-58] (see Chapter 15).

Savel[59] has shown that human tumor extracts can indeed stimulate lymphocytes in vitro; this author suggested that the greater the stimulation, te better the prognosis. Major efforts at defining the mechanisms of this reaction occupy many immunologists,[60,61] and new data and interpretations are reported almost daily. For the present discussion, it suffices that thyroid cancers, predominantly papillary ones, elicit an immune response to some thyroid antigen(s) and this is manifested histologically as thyroiditis.

V. CLINICAL CORRELATIONS

The diagnosis of peritumor thyroiditis is most frequently made only after examination of the tissue. Preoperative predictions of the presence and extent of the thyroiditis are difficult, if not impossible, since antithyroid antibodies are generally low and are measurable in about 20 to 40% of cases.[3,41,62-64] These are of low titer and can be found in such diverse other conditions as subacute thyroiditis, true Hashimoto's, and Graves' disease.[62-64] In addition, the clinical situation usually dictates attention to the thyroid nodule and the peritumor inflammation is considered of minor import.

Meier et al.[5] noted that for papillary carcinoma, the greater the lymphoid infiltration in and around the tumor, the lower the incidence of regional node metastases. Franssila[26] however did not find that lymphoid reaction was prognostically significant. Nevertheless, it is noteworthy that papillary thyroid cancer tends to behave in an indolent manner.

The controversy which has arisen over the premalignant potential of Hashimoto's thyroiditis has led to the advocation of total thyroidectomy as treatment for this condition.[4,20,65,66] Incidences of carcinoma associated with thyroiditis in surgical series[20,65-70] have ranged from 8.3 to 24% (Table 1). Hence, the recommendation for total thyroid extirpation is understood.[20] However, serologic, indeed, even preoperative evidence for autoimmune thyroiditis is lacking in these reports; most of the operations were performed for nodules.

It is the present author's belief that total thyroidectomy is unjustified in Hashimoto's thyroiditis since most modern evidence indicates that cancer-associated thyroiditis represents a secondary host-immune reaction to tumor, and not a neoplastic transformation of epithelium in Hashimoto's disease.[7] Goudie[71] suggests that some thyroid cancers are slightly autoantigenic (for unknown reasons), and that they evoke an autoimmune response which attacks predominantly, but not exclusively, the thyroid surrounding the carcinoma.

Table 1
HASHIMOTO'S THYROIDITIS AND THYROID CARCINOMA[a]

% Coincidence of both disorders	Ref.
0.5	66
3	25
7	68
8.3	70
8.7	67
11	65
11.1	19
17.7	1
22.5	4
23.7	69
24	20
10-35 (depending on severity of infiltration by lymphocytes)	5

[a] Excludes lymphoma.

VI. SUMMARY

Lymphocytic thyroiditis of varying degrees of severity occurs in many cases of thyroid cancer either within, or surrounding, the tumor or both. Papillary tumors are involved most often. This type of thyroiditis is believed to represent an autoimmune reaction to the tumor and, in this fashion, it resembles animal models of thyroiditis.

Controversy over the thyroiditis representing a preexisting lesion upon which carcinoma is superimposed remains, but most modern studies do not support a premalignant significance for autoimmune thyroiditis. Indeed, serologic documentation of Hashimoto's disease is rarely found in cases of peritumor thyroiditis. In addition, long-term followup studies of individuals with clinically and serologically proven Hashimoto's lesions fail to disclose an increased frequency of epithelial tumor development.

Some studies have disclosed that malignant lymphoma may supervene upon a Hashimoto's lesion, although this too is unusual. However, the converse does appear valid, i.e., when malignant lymphoma does arise in the thyroid, it occurs only in the setting of Hashimoto's thyroiditis.

REFERENCES

1. **Dailey, M. E., Lindsay, S., and Skahen, R.,** Relation of thyroid neoplasms to Hashimoto's disease of the thyroid gland, *Arch. Surg.,* 70, 291, 1955.
2. **Hazard, J. B.,** Neoplasia, in *The Thyroid,* Hazard, J. B., and Smith, D. E., Eds., Williams and Wilkins, Baltimore, 1964, 243.
3. **Doniach, D. and Roitt, I. M.,** Autoimmune thyroid disease, in *Textbook of Immunopathology,* Miescher, P. A., and Müller-Eberhard, H. J., Eds., Grune & Stratton, New York, 1969, 516.
4. **Hirabayashi, R. N. and Lindsay, S.,** Thyroid carcinoma and chronic thyroiditis of the Hashimoto type: A statistical study of their relationship, *Int. Coll. Tum. Thyroid Gland,* Marseille, 1964, S. Karger, Basel, 1966, 272.

5. Meier, D. W., Woolner, L. B., Beahrs, O. H., and McConahey, W. M., Parenchymal findings in thyroidal carcinoma; pathologic study of 256 cases, *J. Clin. Endocrinol. Metab.*, 19, 162, 1959.
6. Prior, J. T. and Fairchild, R. D., Thyroid neoplasms and coexistent thyroiditis: Observations in 15 cases, *Am. J. Surg.*, 106, 57, 1963.
7. Bastenie, P. A., Ermans, A. M., and Delespesse, G., Chronic lymphocytic thyroiditis and cancer of the thyroid, in *Thyroiditis and Thyroid Function: Clinical, Morphological and Physiopathologic Studies*, Bastenie, A. and Ermans, A. M., Eds., Pergamon Press, Oxford, 1972, 159.
8. Hawk, W. A. and Hazard, J. B., The many appearances of papillary carcinoma of the thyroid, *Cleveland Clin. Q.*, 43, 207 1976.
9. Franssilla, K., Value of histologic classification of thyroid cancer, *Acta Pathol. Microbiol. Scand. Suppl.*, 225, 5, 1971.
10. Beierwaltes, W. H., Iodine and lymphocytic thyroiditis, *Bull. All India Inst. Med. Sci.*, 3, 145, 1969.
11. Volpe, R., Lymphocytic thyroiditis, in *The Thyroid*, Werner, S. C. and Ingbar, S. H., Eds., Harper and Row, New York, 1978, 996.
12. Asamer, H., Riccabonna, G., and Holthaus, N., Immunohistologische Befunde bei Schilddrusenerkrankungen in einer endemische Kropfebiet, *Arch. Klin. Med.*, 215, 270, 1968.
13. Headington, J. T. and Tantajumroon, T. T., Surgical thyroid disease in Northern Thailand, *Arch. Surg.*, 95, 157, 1967.
14. Morson, B. C. and Dawson, I. M. P., *Gastrointestinal Pathology*, Blackwell Scientific, Oxford, 1972.
15. Haagensen, C. D., *Diseases of the Breast*, W. B. Saunders, Philadelphia, 1971.
16. Fisher, E. R., Gregorio, R. M., and Fisher, B., The pathology of invasive breast cancer, *Cancer*, 36, 1, 1975.
17. Black, M. M., Cellular and biologic manifestations of immunogenicity in precancerous mastopathy, *Nat. Cancer Inst. Monogr.*, 35, 73, 1972.
18. Ayala, A., Sloane, J., and Wolma, F. J., Coexistent lymphoma, adenocarcinoma and struma lymphomatosa, *JAMA*, 204, 829, 1968.
19. Chesky, V. E., Hellwig, C. A., and Welsh, J. W., Cancer of the thyroid associated with Hashimoto's disease: An analysis of 48 cases, *Am. Surg.*, 28, 678, 1962.
20. Perzik, S. L., *Surgery in Thyroid Disease*, Stratton Medical Book, New York, 1976.
21. Pencea, V., Dobrescu, G., Gneazdovischi, V., Rusu, M., and Cernea, M., Association of autonomous thyroid adenoma with chronic thyroiditis, *Endocrinologie*, 15, 271, 1977.
22. Wegelin, C., Die Entzundungen der Schilddruse, *Arztl. Mh. Fortbild.*, 5, 3, 1949.
23. Senhauser, D. A., Immune pathologic correlations in thyroid diseases, in *The Thyroid*, Hazard, J. B. and Smith, D. E., Eds., William & Wilkins Co., Baltimore, 1964, 167.
24. Buchanan, W. W., Harden, R. M., and Clark, D. H., Hashimoto's thyroiditis: A differentiation from simple goiter, thyroid neoplasm, drug-induced goiter and dyshormonogenesis, *Br. J. Surg.*, 52, 430, 1965.
25. Woolner, L. B., McConahey, W. M., and Beahrs, O. H., Struma lymphomatosa (Hashimoto's thyroiditis and related thyroidal disorders), *J. Clin. Endocrinol.*, 19, 53, 1959.
26. Franssila, K. O., Is the differentiation between papillary and follicular thyroid carcinoma valid? *Cancer*, 32, 853, 1973.
27. Woolner, L. B., Thyroid carcinoma: Pathologic classification with data on prognosis, *Semin. Nucl. Med.*, 1, 481, 1971.
28. Woolner, L. B., Beahrs, O. H., Black, B. M., McConahey, W. M., and Keating, F. R., Classification and prognosis of thyroid carcinoma, *Am. J. Surg.*, 102, 354, 1961.
29. Russell, W. O., Ibanez, M. L., Clark, R. L., and White E. C., Thyroid carcinoma: Classification, intraglandular dissemination and clinicopathological study based upon whole organ sections of 80 glands, *Cancer*, 16, 1425, 1963.
30. Lindsay, S., Papillary thyroid carcinoma revisited, in *Thyroid Cancer*, C. E., Hedinger, Ed., Springer-Verlag, Heidelberg, 1969, 29.
31. Noguchi, S., Noguchi, A., and Murakami, N., Papillary carcinoma of the thyroid. I. Developing patterns of metastasis, *Cancer*, 26, 1053, 1970.
32. Russell, W. O., Ibanez, M. L., Clark R. L., Hill, G. S., and White, E. C., Follicular (organoid) carcinoma of the thyroid gland. Report of 84 cases, in *Thyroid Cancer*, Hedinger, C. E., Ed., Springer-Verlag, Heidelberg, 1969, 14.
33. Chen, K.T.K. and Rosai, J., Follicular variant of papillary thyroid carcinoma: A clinicopathologic study of 6 cases, *Am. J. Surg. Pathol.*, 1, 123, 1977.
34. LiVolsi, V. A., Pathology of thyroid cancer, in *Thyroid Cancer*, Greenfield, L., Ed., CRC Press, Boca Raton, Fla., 1978, 85.
35. Woolner, L. B., McConahey, W. M., Beahrs, O. H., and Black, B. M., Primary malignant lymphoma of the thyroid, *Am. J. Surg.*, 111, 502, 1966.

36. Kenyon, R. and Ackerman, L. V., Malignant lymphoma of the thyroid gland apparently arising in struma lymphomatosa, *Cancer*, 8, 964, 1955.
37. Lindsay, S. and Dailey, M. E., Malignant lymphoma of the thyroid gland and its relation to Hashimoto's disease: A clinical and pathological study of 8 patients, *J. Clin. Endocrinol.*, 15, 1332, 1955.
38. Meissner, W. A. and Warren, S., *Tumors of the Thyroid Gland,* Fascicle No. 4, 2nd Series, Armed Forces Institute of Pathology, Washington, D.C., 1969.
39. Saltenstein, S. L., Extranodal malignant lymphoma and pseudolymphomas, *Pathol. Annu.*, 4, 159, 1969.
40. Fu, Y. S. and Perzin, K. H., Lymphosarcoma of the small intestine: A clinicopathologic study, *Cancer*, 29, 645, 1972.
41. Anderson, J. R., Buchanan, W. W., and Goudie, R. B., *Autoimmunity: Clinical and Experimental,* Charles C Thomas, Springfield, Ill., 1967.
42. Whaley, K. and Buchanan, W. W., Aspects cliniques de l'auto-immunite, *Triangle,* 9, 61, 1969.
43. Valena, L. LeMarchand-Beraud, T., and Vannotti, A., Plasma TSH and LATS in patients treated for thyroid carcinoma, *Eur. J. Cancer,* 6, 139, 1970.
44. Snow, M. H., Davies, T., Smith, B. R., Ross, W. M., Evans, R. G. B., Teng, C. S., and Hall, G., Thyroid stimulating antibodies and metastatic thyroid carcinoma, *Clin. Endocrinol.*, 10, 413, 1979.
45. Goudie, R. B., Autoantigen loss in human thyroid carcinoma, in *Thyroid Neoplasia,* Young S. and Inman, R., Eds., Academic Press, New York, 1968, 363.
46. Fujimoto, Y., Suzuki, H., Abe, K., and Brooks, J. R., Autoantibodies in malignant lymphoma of the thyroid gland, *N. Engl J. Med.,* 276, 380, 1967.
47. VanHerle, A. J. and Uller, R. P., Elevated serum thyroglobulin: A marker of metastases in differentiated thyroid carcinomas, *J. Clin. Invest.*, 56, 272, 1975.
48. Owen, C. A., McConahey, W. M., Childs, D. S., and McKenzie, B. F., Serum thyroglobulin in thyroid carcinoma, *J. Clin Endocrinol.*, 20, 187, 1960.
49. LoGerfo, P., Stillman, T., Colacchio, D., and Feind, C., Serum thyroglobulin and recurrent thyroid cancer, *Lancet*, 1, 881, 1977.
50. LoGerfo, P., LiVolsi, V., Colacchio, D., and Feind, C., Thyroglobulin production by thyroid cancers, *J. Surg. Res.,* 24, 1, 1978.
51. LoGerfo, P., Colacchio, T., Colacchio, D., and Feind, C., Thyroglobulin in benign and malignant disease, *JAMA,* 241, 923, 1979.
52. Nakamura, R. M., *Mechanisms of Autoimmune Disease,* American Society of Clinical Pathologists, Chicago, 1979.
53. DeGroot, L. J., Hove, K., Refetoff, S., VanHerle, A. J., Asteris, G. T., and Rochman, H., Serum antigens and antibodies in the diagnosis of thyroid cancer, *J. Clin. Endocrinol. Metab.*, 45, 1220, 1977.
54. Robbins, J., Abnormal thyroglobulin in experimental thyroid tumors, in *Thyroid Neoplasia,* Young, S. and Inman, R., Eds., Academic Press, New York 1968, 405.
55. Witebsky, E., Experimental thyroiditis, in *The Thyroid,* Hazard, J. B. and Smith, D. E., Eds., Williams & Wilkins, Baltimore, 1964, 143.
56. Weigle, W. O., Experimental autoimmune thyroiditis, *Pathol. Annu.*, 8, 329, 1973.
57. Bocker, W. and Lietz, H., Suppression of experimental allergic thyroiditis in guinea pigs by homologous and heterologous thyroglobulin, *Virchows Arch. A.,* 361, 307, 1973.
58. Mangkornkanok, M., Markowtiz, A. S., and Battifora, H. A., Chronic thyroiditis in the rabbit induced with homologous thyroid microsomes, *Science,* 178, 316, 1972.
59. Savel, H., Effect of autologous tumor extracts on cultured human peripheral blood lymphocytes, *Cancer,* 24, 56, 1969.
60. Twomey, J. J. and Good, R. A., Eds., *The Immunopathology of Lymphoreticular Neoplasms,* Plenum Press, New York, 1978.
61. Good, R. A., Cancer and Immunity: The progress, the disappointments, the lesions of both. I. Antigenicity, *Hosp. Practice,* 14, 11, 1979.
62. Hurley, J. R., Thyroiditis, *Disease-A-Month,* Vol. 24, December 1977.
63. Doniach, D., Bottazzo, G. F., and Russell, R. C. G., Goitrous autoimmune thyroiditis (Hashimoto's disease), *J. Clin. Endocrinol. Metab.*, 8, 63, 1979.
64. Doniach, D. and Roitt, I. M., Thyroid autoallergic disease, in *Clinical Aspects of Immunology,* Gell, P. G. H., Coombs, R. R. A., and Lachman, P. J., Eds., Blackwell Scientific, Oxford, 1975, 1355.
65. Pollock, W. F. and Sprong, D. H., The rationale of thyroidectomy for Hashimoto's thyroiditis, *West J. Surg. Obstet. Gynecol.*, 66, 17, 1958.
66. Crile, G. and Hazard, J. B., Incidence of cancer in struma lymphomatosa, *Surg. Gynecol. Obstet.,* 115, 101, 1962.
67. Schlicke, C. P., Hill, J. E., and Schultz, G. F., Carcinoma in chronic thyroiditis, *Surg. Gynecol. Obstet.,* 111, 552, 1960.

68. **Shands, W. C.**, Carcinoma of the thyroid in association with struma lymphomatosa (Hashimoto's disease), *Ann. Surg.,* 151, 675, 1960.
69. **Catz, B., Perzik, S. L., Friedman, N. B., and Sacks, H.**, Association of lymphocytic thyroiditis with other lesions of the thyroid, *Surg. Gynecol. Obstet.,* 136, 47, 1973.
70. **Holmes, H. B., Kreutner, A., and O'Brien, P. H.**, Hashimoto's thyroiditis and its relationship to other thyroid diseases, *Surg. Gynecol. Obstet.,* 144, 887, 1977.
71. **Goudie, R. B.**, Thyroiditis and thyroid carcinoma, *Int. Coll. Tum. Thyr. Gland,* Marseilles, 1964, S. Karger, Basel, 1966, 292.

Chapter 11

RIEDEL'S STRUMA

Virginia A. LiVolsi

TABLE OF CONTENTS

I.	Introduction; History	134
II.	Case Report	134
III.	Incidence	137
IV.	Clinical Features	137
V.	Laboratory Data	138
VI.	Pathology	138
VII.	Diagnosis	139
VIII.	Differential Diagnosis	139
	A. Clinical	139
	B. Pathologic	139
IX.	Etiology and Pathogenesis	141
X.	Association of Riedel's Disease with Other Conditions	142
	A. Thyroid	142
	B. Nonthyroid	143
XI.	Therapy	143
XII.	Course and Prognosis	143
XIII.	Summary	143
References		144

I. INTRODUCTION; HISTORY

Although a similar disorder had been described by Bowlby in 1885,[1] the thyroid lesion which bears his name was detailed by Riedel in 1896[2] and 1897,[3] and reviewed by him in 1910.[4]

Riedel[2,4] summarized the clinical features of three patients: two men (one 42, another 29 yr old) and a 23-yr old woman. Each presented with goiter of recent, rapid onset associated with dyspnea seemingly excessive for the degree of thyroidomegaly. At surgery, the author noted dense iron-hard tumor[2] tissue infiltrating thyroid, cervical soft tissues, trachea, vessels, and nerves. Although no evidence of infection was identified, dense scar and chronic inflammation characterized the lesion microscopically. Of interest, was Professor Riedel's description of an associated endarteritis which he attributed to the inflammation.[4]

Riedel admonished clinicians not to misdiagnose this lesion as a neoplasm because of its rapid growth, extreme hardness, and infiltrative nature.[4] The patient described initially was reevaluated by the author 15 yr later. After merely small-wedge resection of the thyroid mass to relieve obstruction, this patient's lesion regressed, recurred several years later, and then regressed again. A true neoplasm would not behave in this manner.[4]

Following this classic description, and until the entity of Hashimoto's thyroiditis was recognized in 1912,[5] numerous cases of chronic thyroiditis were diagnosed as Riedel's disease.[6] Subsequently, pathologists including James Ewing,[7] suggested that Hashimoto's thyroiditis represented an early form of Riedel's struma. Graham and McCullagh[8] separated the two disorders and recognized that they were distinct. Despite this latter work, however, the confusion continued with Hashimoto's and Riedel's lesions classified as a spectrum of chronic thyroiditis. In fact, the fibrosing variant of Hashimoto's disease has been misdiagnosed as Riedel's struma.[6,9]

An additional source of confusion has occurred since some workers have classified Riedel's struma as the endstage of those instances of subacute granulomatous (de Quervain's) thyroiditis that do not completely resolve.[6]

In this chapter, I will attempt to describe the Riedel's lesion and separate it from the more usual forms of thyroiditis. Following a representative case report, arguments will be summarized for Riedel's struma representing a lesion involving the thyroid and not *of* the thyroid.

II. CASE REPORT

This 49 yr old black female was admitted to Yale-New Haven Hospital after successful cardiopulmonary resuscitation in the Emergency Room. The patient, who had suffered a left-sided cerebrovascular accident 6 yr ago and a myocardial infarct 1 yr ago, had a history of hypertension treated with thiazides and alphamethyldopa. Five years before, splenectomy had been performed for idiopathic thrombocytopenic purpura. However, she had done well following this. A goiter noted 10 months prior to admission was treated by thyroid replacement. Ultrasound of the neck demonstrated a cystic mass which was cold on radioiodine scan. Thyroid function tests showed the patient was euthyroid. No thyroid antibodies were detected.

One month before admission, the patient noted malaise and became easily fatigued. The goiter had enlarged and became tender in the 4 days prior to hospitalization. On the day of admission, the patient suddenly clutched her neck and complained of shortness of breath. She began wheezing and collapsed. For 3 to 5 min, the patient was apneic. On arrival at the hospital, she was pulseless; electrocardiogram was flat. She was successfully resuscitated.

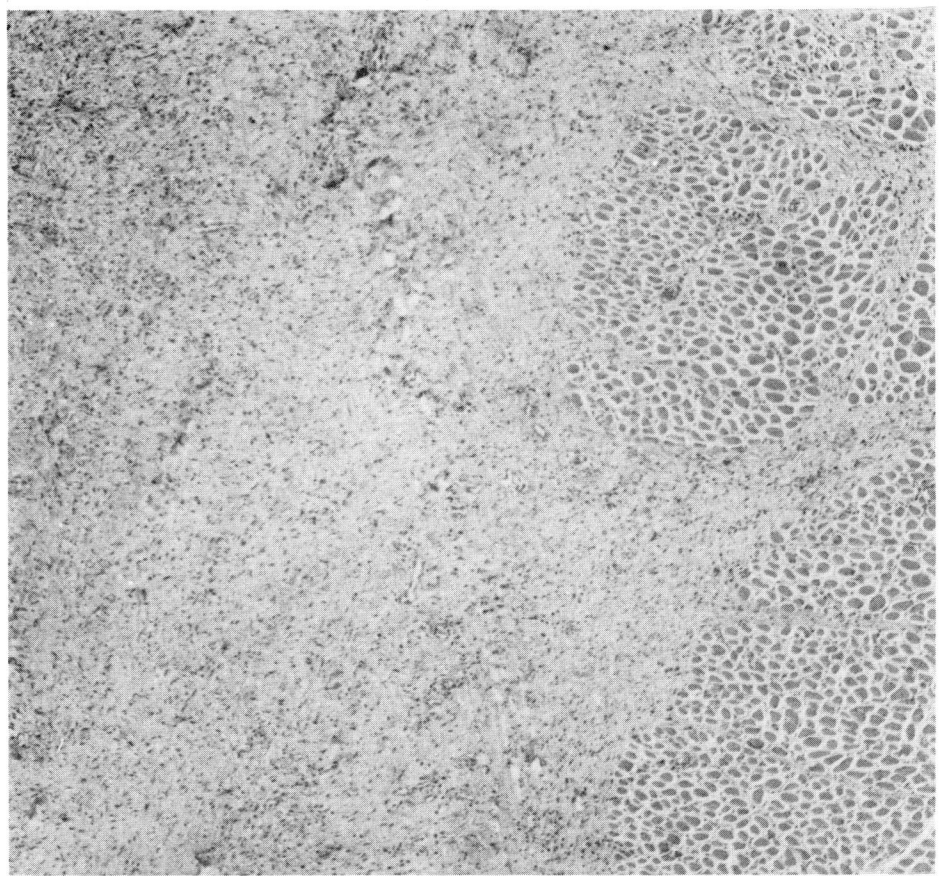

FIGURE 1. Low power view of Riedel's struma shows fibrous tissue and associated chronic inflammatory cell infiltrate invading neck muscles (right). (Hematoxylin-eosin; magnification × 100.)

Physical examination on admission to the Intensive Care Unit disclosed a comatose black female on a respirator with a blood pressure of 190/80, pulse of 80, temperature 100.9°F. The neck was supple and the thyroid was grossly enlarged. The chest was clear. Neurological examination revealed pupils unreactive to light, positive corneal and gag reflexes, no facial asymmetry, and a dysconjugate gaze with a positive doll's eyes sign. There was flaccid quadriplegia without response to deep pain. Seizure activity in the form of right focal myoclonic movements was noted.

The impression on admission was that the patient had experienced acute upper airway obstruction, secondary to acute thyroiditis with rapidly enlarging goiter, and that the resultant hypoxemia had resulted in cardiopulmonary arrest and anoxic encephalopathy, which produced the neurological signs and seizures. Supportive therapy was given and on the third hospital day, the patient died.

At autopsy, the upper poles of the thyroid emerged from a ball-shaped symmetric mass, which replaced the lower halves of the gland and infiltrated the anterior strap muscles. Compression on the trachea with notching was noted. Cross section showed a central cystic lesion containing 100 cc of serosanguinous fluid. Fresh hemorrhage was also seen.

Microscopically, a proliferation of fibrous tissue was noted infiltrating skeletal muscle and thyroid gland, which appeared otherwise normal (Figures 1 and 2). Patchy collections of lymphocytes were noted in the fibrous mass. Associated arterial and

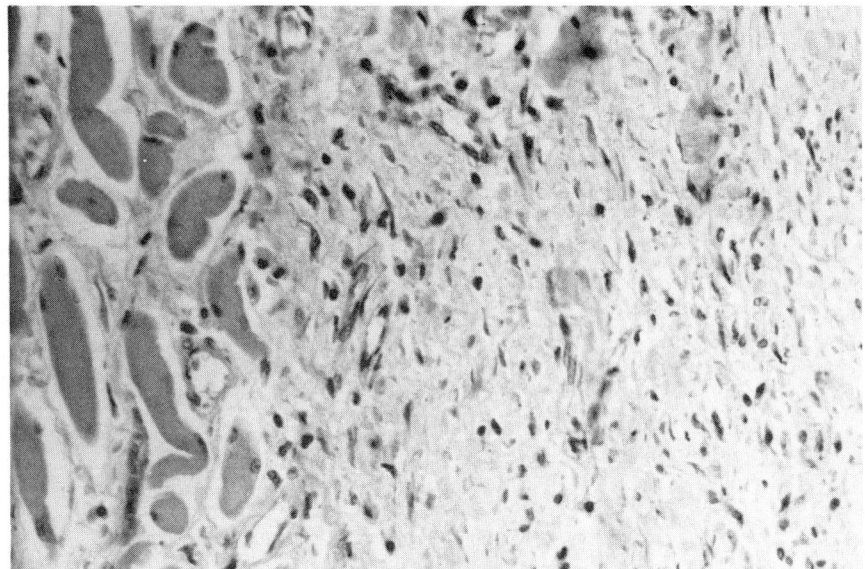

FIGURE 2. Higher power of Figure 1 shows muscle fibers (left) being "choked" by fibrous tissue proliferation (Hematoxylin-eosin; magnification × 250.)

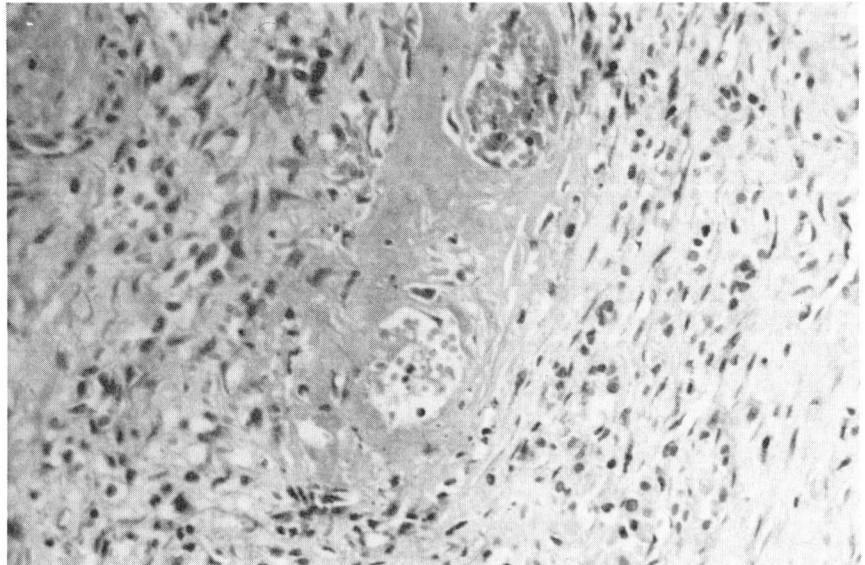

FIGURE 3. Perithyroidal vessel shows fibrinoid degeneration of its wall. (Hematoxylin-eosin; magnification × 150.)

venous thrombosis and focal fibrinoid necrosis of vessel walls was seen in the vicinity of the mass (Figures 3 and 4).

Additional findings included healed infarcts of cerebrum and heart, anoxic encephalopathy, and several acute microinfarcts of the myocardium. Vasculitis with thrombosis of both arteries and veins (small to medium caliber) was identified in the duodenal wall, adrenals, and one ovary, as well as in the neck region.

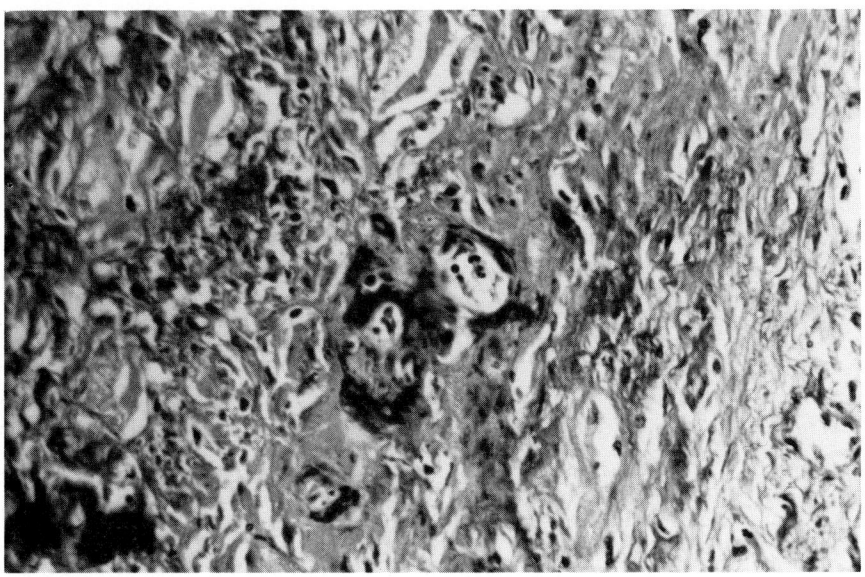

FIGURE 4. Stain for fibrin demonstrates this substance as dark staining material in vessel wall. (Hematoxylin-eosin; magnificaton × 150.)

III. INCIDENCE

Riedel's disease (Riedel's struma, invasive fibrous thyroiditis, invasive fibrosclerosis) is an extremely rare entity. Following Riedel's review in 1910,[4] Graham[10] accepted only 41 authentic cases in the literature up to 1929. Schilling[11] found two cases among 3750 patients with thyroid disease and Lindsay et al.[12] recognized only two instances of Riedel's struma in 6571 thyroidectomies over a 30 yr period. The experience of others supports this frequency.[13-15]

The classic review by Woolner et al.[16] of the Mayo Clinic experience described 20 cases of Riedel's disease in 42,000 thyroidectomies, an incidence of 0.05%. Levitt[17] and Joll[18] calculated an operative incidence of 0.03 to 0.14%.

Comparison to other thyroiditis by Lindsay et al.[12] indicated that one case of Riedel struma is found for each 100 patients with Hashimoto's. Oberdisse[19] suggests that the incidence of Riedel's disease is lower in a general population than is reflected from surgical data, since symptoms of Riedel's struma frequently lead to operative intervention.

IV. CLINICAL FEATURES

Age — The reported age incidences vary from 23 to 78 yr,[20-24] but most cases are diagnosed in the fourth to sixth decades with an average age of 50.[23,24] Some of the cases in younger patients may reflect diagnostic confusion with Hashimoto's thyroiditis.[6]

Sex — Although men and women can be affected, a female predominance is noted with ratios of 2:1 to 4:1.[6,16,20-24] Woolner et al.[16] found 16 of their 20 patients with Riedel's struma were women.

Symptoms — Characteristically, the patient presents with a goiter of months to years duration with slow, or sometimes rapid, recent enlargement.[12,16-18,22-24] The mass produces pressure symptoms and rarely is painful or tender. Dyspnea which may progress to stridor is often out of proportion to the size of the goiter.[24] Rare instances of unilateral vocal cord paralysis with hoarseness have been described.[18,21] Few if any systemic complaints are reported; fever is absent.[22]

Physical Findings — Classically, the thyroid-associated mass is described as stony-hard or woody in consistency[2-4,12,15,16,18,23,24] and fixed to surrounding structures. The goiter may not be very large and a clue to the diagnosis noted by Volpe[24] is the disproportionate severity of symptoms related to size of the mass. In one-third of cases, the involvement is totally or predominantly unilateral.[20,21,23,24] Local lymphadenopathy may be seen,[20,21] and this finding associated with the extremely hard consistency and infiltrative growth pattern has led to diagnoses of carcinoma.[6,16,22-24] If the lesion is confined to the neck, no systemic abnormalities are seen; however, in those cases in which the thyroid mass represents part of a systemic fibrosing process, signs and symptoms referrable to other areas may be identified (mediastinum, orbit, retroperitoneum)[24] (see below).

V. LABORATORY DATA

The white blood cell count may be elevated as can the sedimentation rate, but the latter is not increased to the degree seen in subacute thyroiditis.[23,24] Usually, thyroid function tests give normal results and the patient is clinically euthyroid.[6,24] Occasionally, massive replacement of the gland by fibrous tissue may produce hypothyroidism.[16,18] Indeed, 5 of Woolner's 20 cases (25%) were described as myxedematous.[16] Thyroid antibodies are not identified[23,24] or are present in low titer.[15,24] Scans may demonstrate decreased uptake in affected areas of the gland[15] or a "cold" nodule[15,24] lending credence to a malignant diagnosis. This finding is recognized most often in those cases associated with an adenoma of the thyroid.[6,16] Hypoparathyroidism has been reported rarely, presumably caused by replacement of parathyroid tissue.[22]

VI. PATHOLOGY

Gross — Woolner et al.[16] have listed the two major gross findings in Riedel's disease. Characteristically, a fibrosing process involves part or all of the thyroid lobe, may be uni- or bilateral, and is described as woody, and very hard. Most importantly, extension of the fibrous lesion beyond the capsule of the thyroid into surrounding structures of the neck is found. Indeed, the surgeon finds it impossible to define the thyroid capsule from the extrathyroidal lesion, i.e., there is no tissue plane.[6] Although rarely recognized by the operating surgeon, an adenoma may be found at the center of the fibrous mass.[16,23]

Histopathology — (Figures 1 to 4) Woolner et al.[16] enumerated the microscopic criteria for the diagnosis of Riedel's struma: complete destruction of involved thyroid tissue with absence of normal lobulation, lack of granulomatous reaction, and extension of fibrosis beyond the thyroid into adjacent tissues, surrounding nerves, blood vessels, fat, and skeletal muscle. Bastenie[23] added several other features for distinguishing the Riedel's lesion from other thyroiditides. Hence, lymhocytes are sparse as are Hurthle cells. In addition, a number of acceptable cases of Riedel's struma are associated with a central adenoma. Most important is the recognition of an associated arteritis and phlebitis[11,23,25] with intimal proliferation, medial destruction, adventitial inflammation, and frequent thrombosis.

Table 1
CLINICAL FEATURES[a]

	Riedel's disease	Subacute thyroiditis	Hashimoto's thyroiditis
Age incidence	30-70 yr (most 50 yr or over)	Any age (most 30-50 yr)	Any age (most 20-50 yr)
Sex incidence (F/M)	2-4/1	~4/1	4-10/1
Symptoms	Pressure, goiter	Pain, tenderness, goiter	± goiter, may be hyper-, eu-, or hypothyroid
Thyroid involvement	Unilateral 30%	Bilateral (one side may be more affected)	Focal or diffuse
Thyroid antibodies	None or very low	±	+
Followup	Hypothyroidism rare. May recur following treatment, stabilize or regress	Thyroid function reverts to normal in almost all cases	Usually progresses to hypothyroidism

[a] Adapted from References 6, 15, 16, 23, and 24.

VII. DIAGNOSIS

Although the presence of Riedel's disease may be suspected clinically, its rarity and imitation by carcinoma make histologic proof of disease essential.[6,23,24] Clinically, Riedel's struma may be considered in a middle-aged to elderly patient with an indolent goiter of very hard consistency, adhesions to cervical tissues, and symptoms of tracheal compression. However, all these criteria mimic carcinoma which is far more common.[23,24]

Laboratory tests and scans are not helpful in diagnosis. Needle biopsy may show only fibrous tissue which is nonspecific[15] although some authors have been successful with this technique and with cytology.[15,26] Wedge resection or lobectomy is needed for histologic diagnosis and such surgery may represent a therapeutic, as well as a diagnostic, modality.

VIII. DIFFERENTIAL DIAGNOSIS

A. Clinical

The major entities which must be distinguished from Riedel's disease include the fibrosing variant of Hashimoto's thyroiditis,[9,16] subacute thyroiditis,[6,16,23] and carcinoma. (Table 1.)

Hashimoto's thyroiditis is clinically different because in this disorder, antithyroid antibodies are elevated, and in the fibrosing variant are markedly so.[9,23] In addition, infiltration of surrounding tissue is not found and usually large goiters are encountered, especially in the fibrous type.[9]

Subacute (granulomatous) thyroiditis is distinguished from Riedel's by containment within the gland, symptoms of pain, tenderness, often fever, and more rapidly evolving course.[6,16,23,24] Elevation of sedimentation rate and leukocytosis are common in subacute thyroiditis[6,16,23,24]

Carcinoma — distinction of thyroid carcinoma from Riedel's disease is usually not possible solely on clinical criteria or even surgical evaluation.

B. Pathologic

Diagnostic confusion arises histologically between Riedel's disease and fibrosing Hashimoto's thyroiditis, anaplastic thyroid carcinoma and fibrosarcoma of the neck. (Table 2.)

Table 2
PATHOLOGIC FEATURES[a]

	Riedel's disease	Fibrosing Hashimoto's thyroiditis	Subacute thyroiditis	Anaplastic carcinoma	Fibrosarcoma
Gross					
Color	White	White-tan	Grey-white	White-tan	Tan
Consistency	Very hard, woody	Firm	Smooth	Fleshy, hard	Fleshy, firm
Lobulated	No	Yes	Yes	No	No
Extrathyroid	Yes	No	No	Yes	Yes
Extent necrosis	±	No	No	Common	Yes
Microscopic					
Adenoma	Yes (25-50%)	No	No	Yes (or low-grade carcinoma) common	N/A[b]
Colloid	Normal in uninvolved areas	Depleted	Usually decreased	N/A	N/A
Oxyphils	No	Yes	±	N/A	N/A
Lymphocytes	Sparse	Marked	Yes	N/A	N/A
Squamous metaplasia	No	Yes	Rare	N/A	N/A
Stroma	Fibrosis	Fibrosis	Fibrosis	N/A	±
Giant cells	No	No	Yes	Yes	± to marked
Pleomorphism of cells	No	No	No	Marked	± to Yes (depending on degree of differentiation)
Mitoses	No	No	No	Yes	N/A
Blood vessels	Vasculitis	Adventitial fibrosis may be seen	Adventitial fibrosis may be seen	N/A	N/A

[a] Adapted from References 6, 16, 23, 24, 28, 30, 31, 39, and 43-47.
[b] N/A = Not applicable.

Fibrosing Hashimoto's thyroiditis — as described in Chapter 7, this is distinguished by absence of extracapsular spread, uniform thyroid involvement, accentuation of lobular architecture, prominent lymphoid aggregates with germinal centers, and oncocytic (Hurthle cell) and squamous metaplasia associated with follicular atrophy.[9] Riedel's struma shows, in uninvolved areas, preservation of normal thyroid. Characteristically, violation of the thyroid capsule by the fibrous process is seen.[6,9,16,23]

Anaplastic carcinoma — anaplastic thyroid carcinoma of the spindle cell type comprises about 10% of all thyroid malignancies,[27-34] occurs in elderly individuals more commonly in women,[27-34] and represents one of the most rapidly fatal of all cancers. A history of goiter is common[27-34] and may represent, histologically, an adenoma or low-grade papillary or follicular carcinoma in proximity to which a highly malignant lesion has arisen.[27,30,34,35] Grossly, these tumors are large masses and they share with Riedel's struma the capacity to infiltrate extra-thyroidal tissues, such as trachea or lymph nodes.[27-34] These lesions appear white to tan and demonstrate necrosis. An encapsulated nodule, representing a preexisting low-grade lesion may be noted[28,30,33] and represents another similarity to the gross appearance of Riedel's thyroiditis. At the microscopic level, the distinction becomes clear. The anaplastic carcinoma shows dense cellularity with foci of necrosis; the tumor is composed of obviously malignant spindle cells, often admixed with pleomorphic giant cells.[28,30-33] Numerous and often abnormal mitoses are easily identified.[28,33] In addition, the epithelial nature of this lesion can be inferred by the presence of epithelial nests[28] or by ultrastructural studies.[36-38] In contrast, Riedel's struma shows relatively uniform cellularity with normal appearing fibroblasts and dense intercellular collagen deposition.[6,16,23] Mitoses are sparse and never abnormal. Electron microscopy demonstrates fibroblasts and collagen fibers without epithelial features.[39]

Fibrosarcoma — (fibromatosis, extraabdominal desmoid tumor) may occur in the neck.[40-48] Grossly, this lesion may be distinguished from Riedel's disease or anaplastic carcinoma by its location — usually in the lateral neck removed from the thyroid.[45] Histologically, poorly differentiated fibrosarcomas resemble anaplastic carcinoma showing obviously malignant features of hypercellularity, pleomorphism, or mitoses.[41,48] It is the well-differentiated desmoid-like fibrosarcoma which produces diagnostic problems with the Riedel's lesion. The two resemble each other in their cellularity, bland cellular detail, and focal keloid-like collagen bands.[40,43-48] However, fibromatoses lack the focal lymphocytic infiltration and the vasculitic changes of Riedel's struma.

IX. ETIOLOGY AND PATHOGENESIS

The etiology of Riedel's struma remains unknown.[6,16,23,24] Initially considered infectious,[2-4] this condition is no longer believed to be etiologically related to a specific microorganism. Bacteriologic studies have given negative results.[6,16,23,24] In isolated thyroid involvement, no drug has been consistently implicated as have ergot alkaloids in retroperitoneal fibrosis.[49-52]

The possibility of an autoimmune reaction also has been raised, but remains speculative.[24] In view of the absent or low antithyroid antibodies in these patients, humoral immune factors appear uninvolved.[24] Whether cellular immunity participates in the development of Riedel's struma is unknown;[23,24,53-55] occasional patients have a polyclonal gammopathy but this most likely represents a nonspecific reaction to illness and is not etiologic.[55] Some authors suggest it represents a collagen disease[54-56] but Kay[57] admonishes against linking a group of conditions of obscure etiology together.

It is presently recognized that Riedel's struma does not represent an endstage of

Hashimoto's or subacute thyroiditis.[6,7,9,10,15,16,20,21,23,24] Indeed, one should view this disorder not as a lesion *of* the thyroid but one *involving* the thyroid. Comings et al.[55] have stated that the fibrosing process involves the soft tissues of the neck and since the thyroid is the largest structure in the area, it has elicited the most attention. Certainly, this view is justified since in no other thyroid disease except Riedel's struma can one find a similar concomitant process occurring in other body areas — as in the mediastinum or retroperitoneum.[23,24,55]

The stimulus to fibrosis is not known, but rare instances of familial occurrence have led a few authors to propose a genetic basis[24,54] in some cases. When mediastinal fibrosis occurs also, the possibility of fungal infection (*Aspergillus* or Histoplasmosis) must be considered*.[58-61] The role of ergot-like drugs must be raised in those patients with retroperitoneal and thyroid fibrosis; however, no clear cut evidence has been presented to support this.[49-51,70-72]

The significance of the vasculitis is not known;[2-4,16] whether this represents a causative factor or is the result of a fibrous lesion impinging upon vessels remains an area for future study.[23,25,73-75] Mitchinsen[73] studied the pathologic features of 40 patients with retroperitoneal fibrosis and found aortic inflammation as well as vasculitis of small arteries and veins in about 25% of cases. This author suggested the possibility of vascular damage releasing an antigen through the vessel wall and evoking an immune response with resulting fibrosis. He postulates that this leakage phenomenon may represent the common pathway whereby fibrosis occurs in drug-induced damage, or collagen disease.[73] Meyer and Hausman[74,75] considered the common finding of occlusive phlebitis in Riedel's disease and retroperitoneal fibrosis, and speculated on the possibility of this producing the fibrous lesion. However, although an attractive suggestion, i.e., that a form of immunologically mediated vasculitis is causative in Riedel's disease, it seems as likely that these vascular changes are the result and not the cause of the disorder. Recent studies in our laboratory attempting to localize immunoglobulins in vascular walls in a Riedel's lesion merely reflected serum concentrations.[39] Zabetakis et al.[76] reported a patient with retroperitoneal fibrosis and associated immune complex glomerulonephritis.

X. ASSOCIATION OF RIEDEL'S DISEASE WITH OTHER CONDITIONS

A. Thyroid

As has been noted in several studies, benign follicular adenomas of the thyroid may be found at the center of the Riedel's lesion.[6,16,22-24] In the Mayo Clinic series, Woolner et al.[16] recognized such an adenoma in 5 of 20 cases (25%). Crile[78] noted such a lesion in 7 of his 11 patients. The relationship of the adenoma to the Riedel's struma is unclear. In the case described at the beginning of this chapter, an adenoma with old and recent hemorrhage was identified. The possibility exists that in our case and perhaps in others,[6,16,23,24] acute hemorrhage into an adenoma led to sudden enlargement of the mass compressing the trachea, decreased functional breathing capacity, and produced death by asphyxiation. Another mechanism for respiratory arrest in such patients has been offered by Downing and Lee.[79] These authors suggest that compression of laryngeal nerve fibers could produce reflex laryngospasm via a central nervous system mechanism.[79] Further studies are needed to answer this question.

---

* Retroperitoneal fibrosis may be mimicked by the desmoplastic reaction accompanying carcinomas (especially breast, stomach, kidney, pancreatic cancer) and malignant lymphoma involving the retroperitoneum.[62-69] Obviously, diagnostic tissue must be obtained; the prognosis in cases of fibrosis-associated malignancies is markedly different from that of idiopathic fibrosis.

One patient with Riedel's lesion and isolated thyroid amyloidosis has been reported.[80] Chopra et al.[81] recorded a patient with clinical subacute thyroiditis and histological Riedel's disease. The concurrence of these two disorders in an isolated case should not be considered evidence for a causal relationship between these diseases.

B. Nonthyroid

As has been alluded to above, Riedel's disease affecting the thyroid may occur as an isolated lesion or may reflect one manifestation of a systemic multifocal fibrosing process.[15,23,24,54,55,70,74-76,82-89] Thus, patients with Riedel's struma may also have, alone or in combination, fibrosing lesions of any of the following: orbit,[55,71,84-86,88] bile ducts,[55] retroperitoneum,[15,55,72,73,75,82,83,89] mediastinum,[78] salivary glands,[70] and subcutaneous tissue.[82]

These cases strongly suggest that Riedel's thyroiditis represents one end of the spectrum of a multisystem fibrosing disorder.[72,73,76]

XI. THERAPY

Surgery remains the mainstay of diagnosis and therapy.[16,24] Volpe[24] states that there are two reasons for operative intervention in Riedel's disease: to allow obtaining of tissue for diagnosis and to relieve tracheal compression.

No nonsurgical therapy has resulted in success, universally. However, several authors have reported relief of symptoms and decrease in goiter size by steroid treatment.[15,70,71] Indeed, in some instances, withdrawal of steroids has resulted in recurrences.[15,70,71] These successes have been anecdotal and Volpe[24] cautions against extrapolation to all cases.

XII. COURSE AND PROGNOSIS

Most authors[6,16,22-24,90,91] including Riedel[2-4] believe that the course of this lesion is slowly progressive, but it may stabilize or spontaneously remit.[4,22,23] Recurrences have been reported;[4,22,23] Eisen[20] recorded a 16% recurrence rate. Mortality ranges from 6 to 10%.[10,20] Death results from asphyxia due to tracheal compression,[6,16,23,24] or laryngospasm.[79]

Complications if the disorder is limited to the neck include hypothyroidism and hypoparathyroidism,[6,23,81] but these are rare.

In those cases of fibrosing thyroiditis associated with mediastinal fibrosis,[55] sclerosing cholangitis,[55,84,87] or retroperitoneal fibrosis,[15,55,73,75,82] the prognosis is dependent upon the latter conditions and usually not on the neck mass.

XIII. SUMMARY

This chapter has reviewed that rare form of "thyroiditis" called Riedel's struma, its clinical and pathologic features, its association with other conditions, and theories of pathogenesis. Evidence for including this lesion as a manifestatin of systemic fibrosclerosis is presented and the viewpoint of considering Riedel's disease as a disorder *involving* the thyroid but not *of* the thyroid is espoused.

REFERENCES

1. **Bowlby, A. A.,** Diseases of the ductless glands. I. Infiltrating fibroma (? sarcoma) of the thyroid gland, *Trans. Pathol. Soc. London,* 36, 420, 1885.
2. **Riedel, B. M. C. L.,** Die chronische, zur Bildung eisenharter Tumoren fuhrende Entzundung der Schilddruse, *Verh. Dtsch. Ges. Chir.,* 25, 101-105 1896.
3. **Riedel, B. M. C. L.,** Vorstellugn eines Kranken mit chronischer Strumitis, *Vehr Dtsch. Ges. Chir.,* 26, 127-129, 18 97.
4. **Riedel, B. M. C. L.,** Ueber Verlauf und Ausgang der Strumitis chronica, *Muench. Med. Wochenschr.,* 57, 1946-1947, 1910.
5. **Hashimoto, H.,** Zur Kenntniss der lymphomatosen Veranderung der Schilddruse (Struma lymphomatosa), *Arch. Klin. Chir.,* 97, 219, 1912.
6. **Hazard, J. B.,** Thyroiditis: A review, Part II, *Am. J. Clin. Pathol.,* 25, 399, 1955.
7. **Ewing, J.** *Neoplastic Diseases,* W. B. Saunders, Philadelphia, 1922, 908.
8. **Graham, A. and McCullagh, E. P.,** Atrophy and fibrosis associated with lymphoid tissue in the thyroid, *Arch. Surg.,* 22 548-567, 1931.
9. **Katz, S. M. and Vickery, A. L.,** The fibrosing variant of Hashimoto's thyroiditis, *Hum. Pathol.,* 5, 161, 1974.
10. **Graham, A.,** Riedel's struma in contrast to struma lymphomatosa (Hashimoto), *West J. Surg.,* 39, 681-689, 1931.
11. **Schilling, J. A.,** Struma lymphomatosa, struma fibrosa and thyroiditis, *Surg. Gynecol. Obstet.,* 81, 533-550, 1945.
12. **Lindsay, S., Dailey, M. E., Friedlander, J., Yee, G., and Soley, M. H.,** Chronic thyroiditis: A clinical and pathologic study of 354 patients, *J. Clin. Endocrinol.,* 12, 1578, 1952.
13. **Cooke, R. W.,** Riedel's thyroiditis, in *Current Topics in Thyroid Research,* Cassano, C. and Andreoli, M., Eds., Academic Press, London, 1965, 944.
14. **Greene, R.,** Riedel's disease, *Br. J. Clin. Pract.,* 23, 261, 1969.
15. **Katsikas, D., Shorthouse, A. J., and Taylor, S.,** Riedel's thyroiditis, *Br. J. Surg.,* 63, 929, 1976.
16. **Woolner, L. B., McConahey, W. M., and Beahrs, O. H.,** Invasive fibrous thyroiditis (Riedel's struma), *J. Clin. Endocrinol.,* 17, 201, 1957.
17. **Levitt, T.,** *The Thyroid,* E & S Livingstone, London, 1954.
18. **Joll, C. A.,** The pathology, diagnosis and treatment of Hashimoto's disease (struma lymphomatosa), *Br. J. Surg.,* 27, 351, 1939.
19. **Oberdisse, K.,** Thyroiditis, in *Die Krankheiten der Schilddruse,* Oberdisse, K. and Klein E., Eds., Thieme Verlag, Stuttgart, 1967.
20. **Eisen, D.,** Riedel's struma, *Am. J. Med. Sci.,* 192, 673, 1936.
21. **Gilchrist, R. K.,** Chronic thyroiditis, *Arch. Surg.,* 31, 429, 1935.
22. **Crile, G.,** Thyroiditis, *Ann. Surg.,* 127, 640, 1948.
23. **Bastenie, P. A.,** Invasive fibrous thyroiditis (Riedel), in *Thyroiditis and Thyroid Function. Clinical, Morphological and Physiopathological Studies,* Pergamon Press, Oxford, 1972, 99.
24. **Volpe, R.,** Riedel's struma (struma fibrosa), in *The Thyroid,* Werner, S. C. and Ingbar, S. H., Eds., Harper and Row, New York, 1978, 1009.
25. **Hardmeier, T. and Hedinger, C.,** Die eisenharte Struma Riedel, un primarl Gefarzerkrankung, *Virchows Arch.,* 337, 547, 1964.
26. **Persson, P. S.,** Cytodiagnosis of thyroiditis, *Acta Med. Scand. Suppl.,* 143, 7, 1967.
27. **Woolner, L. B.,** Thyroid carcinoma: Pathologic classification with data on prognosis, *Sem. Nucl. Med.,* 1, 481, 1971.
28. **Meissner, W. and Warren, S.,** *Tumors of the Thyroid Gland,* AFIP Fascicle No. 4, 2nd Series, Washington, D.C., 1969.
29. **Frantz, V. K. and Yannopoulos, K.,** Carcinoma of the thyroid: A clinicopathologic study of 216 cases with a ten-year followup, *Advan. Thyroid Res.,* 9, 337, 1961.
30. **Hutter, R. V. P., Tollefsen, H. R., DeCosse, J. J., Foote, F. W., and Frazell, E. L.,** Spindle and giant cell metaplasia in papillary carcinomata of the thyroid, *Am. J. Surg.* 110, 660, 1965.
31. **Nishiyama, R. H., Dunn, E. L., and Thompson, N. W.,** Anaplastic spindle cell and giant cell tumors of the thyroid gland, *Cancer,* 30, 113, 1972.
32. **Kyriakides G. and Sosin, H.,** Anaplastic carcinoma of the thyroid, *Ann. Surg.,* 179, 295, 1974.
33. **Franssila, K.,** Value of histologic classification of thyroid cancer, *Acta Pathol. Microbiol. Scand. Suppl.,* 225, 5, 1971.
34. **Thomas, C. G. and Buckwalter, J. A.,** Poorly differentiated neoplasms of the thyroid gland, *Ann. Surg.,* 177, 632, 1973.

35. **Maloof, F. and Vickery, A. L.**, Case records of the Massachusetts General Hospital Case 37-1979, *N. Engl. J. Med.*, 301, 600, 1979.
36. **Graham, H. and Daniel, C.**, Ultrastructure of an anaplastic carcinoma of the thyroid, *Am. J. Clin. Pathol.*, 61, 690, 1974.
37. **Fisher, E. R., Gregorio, R., Shoemaker, R., Horvat, B., and Hubay, C.**, The derivation of so-called "giant cell" and "spindle cell" undifferentiated thyroid neoplasms, *Am. J. Clin. Pathol.*, 61, 680, 1974.
38. **Jao, W. and Gould, V. E.**, Ultrastructure of anaplastic (spindle and giant cell) carcinoma of the thyroid gland, *Cancer*, 35, 1280, 1975.
39. **Dise, C. A. and LiVolsi, V. A.**, Unpublished observations.
40. **Stout, A. P.**, Fibrous tumors of the soft tissues, *Minn. Med.*, 43, 455, 1969.
41. **Chung, E. B. and Enzinger, F. M.**, Infantile fibrosarcoma, *Cancer*, 38, 729, 1976.
42. **Dehner, L. P. and Askin, F. B.**, Tumors of fibrous tissue origin in childhood, *Cancer*, 38, 888, 1976.
43. **Fleischmajer, R., Nedwick, A., and Reeves, J. R. T.**, Juvenile fibromatoses, *Arch. Dermatol.*, 107, 574, 1973.
44. **Stout, A. P.**, Juvenile fibromatoses, *Cancer*, 7, 953, 1954.
45. **Conley, J., Healey, W. V., and Stout, A. P.**, Fibromatosis of the head and neck, *Am. J. Surg.*, 112, 609, 1966.
46. **DasGupta, T., Brasfield, R. D., and O'Hara, J.**, Extra-abdominal desmoids, *Ann. Surg.*, 170, 109, 1969.
47. **Stout, A. P.**, The fibromatoses, *Clin. Orthoped.*, 19, 11, 1961.
48. **Stout, A. P. and Lattes, R.**, *Tumors of the Soft Tissues*, AFIP Fascicle 1, 2nd Series, Washington, D.C., 1966.
49. **Ormond, J. K.**, Idiopathic retroperitoneal fibrosis: Ormond's syndrome, *Henry Ford Hosp. Med. Bull.*, 10, 13, 1962.
50. **Utz, D. C., Rooke, E. D., Spittell, J. A., and Bartholemew, L. G.**, Retroperitoneal fibrosis in patients taking methysergide, *JAMA*, 191, 983, 1965.
51. **Conley, J. E., Boulanger, W. J., and Mendeloff, G. L.**, Aortic obstruction associated with methysergide maleate therapy for headaches, *JAMA*, 198, 808, 1966.
52. **Graham, J. R.**, Methysergide for prevention of headache; Experience in 500 patients over three years, *N. Engl. J. Med.*, 270, 67, 1964.
53. **Que, G. S. and Mandema, E.**, A case of idiopathic retroperitoneal fibrosis presenting as a systemic collagen disease, *Am. J. Med.*, 36, 320, 1964.
54. **Turner-Warwick, R., Nabarro, J. D. N., and Doniach, D.**, Riedel's thyroiditis and retroperitoneal fibrosis, *Proc. R. Soc. Med.*, 59, 596, 1966.
55. **Comings, D. E., Skubi, K. B., VanEyes, J., and Motulsky, A. G.**, Familial multifocal fibrosclerosis, *Ann. Intern. Med.*, 66, 884, 1967.
56. **Pugh, R. C. B.**, Pathology of fibrotic lesions, *Proc. R. Soc. Med.*, 53, 685, 1960.
57. **Kay, R. G.**, Retroperitoneal vasculitis with perivascular fibrosis, *Br. J. Urol.*, 35, 284, 1963.
58. **Salyer, J. M., Harrison, H. N., Winn, D. F., and Taylor, R. R.**, Chronic fibrous mediastinitis and superior vena caval obstruction due to histoplasmosis, *Dis. Chest*, 35, 364, 1959.
59. **Goodwin, R. A., Nickell, J. A., and DesPrez, R. M.**, Mediastinal fibrosis complicating healed pulmonary histoplasmosis and tuberculosis, *Medicine*, 51, 227, 1972.
60. **Cohen, D. M. and Goggan E. A.**, Sclerosing mediastinitis and terminal valvular endocarditis caused by fungus suggestive of Aspergillus species, *Am. J. Clin. Pathol.*, 56, 91, 1971.
61. **Puri, S., Factor, S. M. and Farmer, P.**, Sclerosing mediastinitis presumed to be due to primary Aspergillosis, *N. Y. S. J. Med.*, 77, 1774, 1977.
62. **Scully, R. E., Goldabini, J. J., and McNeely, B. U.**, Case records of the Massachusetts General Hospital, *N. Engl. J. Med.*, 293, 1034, 1975.
63. **Grabstald, H. and Kaufman, R.**, Hydronephrosis secondary to ureteral obstruction by metastatic breast cancer, *J. Urol.*, 102, 569, 1969.
64. **Usher, S. M., Brendler, H., and Ciavarra, V. A.**, Retroperitoneal fibrosis secondary to metastatic neoplasm, *Urology*, 9, 191, 1977.
65. **Kendall, A. R. and Lakey, W. H.**, Sclerosing Hodgkin's diseases versus idiopathic retroperitoneal fibrosis, *J. Urol.*, 86, 217, 1961.
66. **Nitz, G. L., Hewitt, C. B., Straffon, R. A., Kiser W. S., and Stewart, B. H.**, Retroperitoneal malignancy masquerading as benign retroperitoneal fibrosis, *J. Urol.*, 103, 46, 1970.
67. **Rosas-Uribe, A. and Rappaport, H.**, Malignant lymphoma, histiocytic type with sclerosis (sclerosing reticulum cell sarcoma), *Cancer*, 29, 946, 1972.
68. **Webb, A. J. and Dawson-Edwards, P.**, Malignant retroperitoneal fibrosis, *Br. J. Surg.*, 54, 505, 1967.

69. **Morin, L. J. and Zuerner, R. T.**, Retroperitoneal fibrosis and carcinoid tumor, *JAMA*, 216, 1647, 1971.
70. **Hines, R. C., Scheuermann, H. A., Royster, H. P., and Rose, E.**, Invasive fibrous (Riedel's) thyroiditis with bilateral fibrous parotitis, *JAMA*, 213, 869, 1970.
71. **Amorosa, L. F., Shear, M. K., and Spiera, H.**, Multifocal fibrosis involving the thyroid, face and orbits, *Arch. Intern. Med.*, 136, 221, 1976.
72. **Lepor, H. and Walsh, P. C.**, Idiopathic retroperitoneal fibrosis, *J. Urol.*, 122, 1, 1979.
73. **Mitchinson, M. J.**, The pathology of idiopathic retroperitoneal fibrosis, *J. Clin. Pathol.*, 23, 681, 1970.
74. **Meyer, S. and Hausman, R.**, Occlusive phlebitis in multifocal fibrosclerosis, *Am. J. Clin. Pathol.*, 65, 274, 1976.
75. **Meijer, S. and Hausman, R.**, Occlusive phlebitis, a diagnostic feature in Riedel's thyroiditis, *Virchows Arch.*, 377, 339, 1978.
76. **Zabetakis, P. M., Novich, P. K., Matarese, R. A., and Michelis, M. F.**, Idiopathic retroperitoneal fibrosis: A systemic connective tissue disease? *J. Urol.*, 122, 100, 1979.
77. **Christian, C. L. and Sergent, J. S.**, Vasculitis syndromes: Clinical and experimental models, *Am. J. Med.*, 61, 385, 1976.
78. **Crile, G.**, *Practical Aspects of Thyroid Disease*, W. B. Saunders, Philadelphia, 1949.
79. **Downing, S. E. and Lee, J. C.**, Laryngeal chemosensitivity: A possible mechanism for sudden infant death, *Pediatrics*, 55, 640, 1975.
80. **Melato, M. and Mlac, M.**, Riedel's thyroiditis and isolated thyroid amyloidosis, *Pathologica*, 70, 33, 1978.
81. **Chopra, D., Wool, M. S., Crosson, A., and Sawin, C. T.**, Riedel's struma associated with subacute thyroiditis, hypothyroidism and hypoparathyroidism, *J. Clin. Endocrinol. Metab.*, 46, 869, 1978.
82. **Coopersmith, N. H. and Appelman, H. D.**, Multifocal fibrosclerosis with subcutaneous involvement, *Am. J. Clin. Pathol.*, 55, 369, 1971.
83. **Hellstrom, H. R. and Perez-Stable, E. C.**, Retroperitoneal fibrosis with disseminated vasculitis and intrahepatic sclerosing cholangitis, *Am. J. Med.*, 40, 184, 1966.
84. **Schneider, R. J.**, Orbital involvement in Riedel's struma, *Can. J. Ophthalmol.*, 11, 87, 1976.
85. **Andersen, S. R., Seedorff, H., and Halberg, P.**, Thyroiditis with myxoedema and orbital pseudotumor, *Acta Ophthalmol.*, 41, 120, 1963.
86. **Arnott, E. J. and Greaves, O. P.**, Orbital involvement in Riedel's thyroiditis, *Br. J. Ophalmol.*, 49, 1, 1965.
87. **Bartholomew, L. G., Cain, J. C., Woolner, L. B., Utz, D. C., and Ferris, D. O.**, Sclerosing cholangitis: Its possible association with Riedel's struma and fibrous retroperitonitis: Report of two cases, *N. Engl. J. Med.*, 269, 8, 1963.
88. **Sclare, G. and Luxton, W.**, Fibrosis of the thyroid and lacrimal glands, *Br. J. Ophthalmol.*, 51, 173, 1967.
89. **Woolner, L. B.**, Thyroiditis: Classification and clinicopathologic correlation, in *The Thyroid*, Hazard, J. B. and Smith, D. E., Eds., Williams and Wilkins, Baltimore, 1964.
90. **Eisen, D.**, Riedel's struma with report of 7 cases, *Can. Med. Assoc. J.*, 31, 144, 1934.
91. **Goodman, H. I.**, Riedel's thyroiditis: Review and report of 2 cases, *Am. J. Surg.*, 54, 472, 1941.

Chapter 12

LABORATORY DIAGNOSTIC METHODS IN THYROIDITIS

Hannibal Edwards

TABLE OF CONTENTS

I.	Introduction		148
II.	Tests of Thyroid Function		148
	A.	Protein Bound Iodine (PBI)	148
	B.	Butanol-Extractable Iodine (BEI)	149
	C.	Thyroid Hormone Measurements	149
		1. Thyroxine (T_4)	149
		2. Triiodothyronine (T_3)	149
	D.	Thyroid Function Tests in Thyroiditis	150
	E.	Thyroid-Stimulating Hormones	150
	F.	Thyroid-Stimulating Hormones in Thyroiditis	150
		1. Acute Thyroiditis	150
		2. Subacute Thyroiditis	150
		3. Hashimoto's Thyroiditis	151
		4. Riedel's Struma	151
	G.	Thyroid Antibodies	151
	H.	Thyroid Antibodies in Thyroiditis	152
		1. Acute Thyroiditis	152
		2. Subacute Thyroiditis	152
		3. Hashimoto's Thyroiditis	152
		4. Riedel's Struma	153
III.	The Role of Nuclear Medicine		153
	A.	Radionuclide Scanning	153
	B.	Fluorescent Scanning	153
	C.	Perchlorate Discharge Test	153
	D.	Scanning in Thyroiditis	154
		1. Acute Thyroiditis	154
		2. Subacute Thyroiditis	154
		3. Hashimoto's Thyroiditis	154
		4. Riedel's Struma	154
IV.	The Role of Ultrasound		154
V.	Other Techniques		156
References			156

I. INTRODUCTION

This chapter will review the major diagnostic laboratory tests utilized in the diagnosis of thyroiditis. A brief summary of the indiviual tests and the principles involved in each will be given. Then the results and uses of these tests in the diagnosis of the major forms of thyroiditis will be presented. (Since the individual chapters on the thyroiditides covered these laboratory test values in detail, this chapter will attempt only to summarize and compare test results for each form of the disorder.)

It is not my intention to exhaustively review specific methodologies involved in thyroid function evaluation; the reader is referred to specific texts and reviews of these topics.[1-7] Rather, this chapter will discuss measurements of thyroid hormones, thyroid stimulating hormones, and thyroid antibodies as well as nuclear medicine techniques and ultrasonography as these relate to the diagnosis and differentiation of thyroiditis. (Needle biopsy and cytology in the evaluation of the patient with thyroiditis will be presented in Chapter13.)

The number and variety of thyroid function tests available indicates that each has limitation; indeed, in most cases, several different examinations are performed as a backdrop against which, by comparison of test results, a diagnosis can be established.

II. TESTS OF THYROID FUNCTION

Iodine is used normally in the synthesis of thyroid hormone. Four steps are involved and may be divided into: (a) thyroid stimulating hormone (TSH) stimulates the follicular epithelium to actively concentrate iodine, (b) via a peroxidase dependent reaction, inorganic iodide is oxidized to an organic form, (c) this iodide is incorporated into tyrosine, producing mono- and di-iodotyrosines, and (d) these substances are coupled to form the major thyroid hormones: triiodotyrosine (T_3) and thyroxine (T_4).[2] The hormone is stored in colloid bound to the glycoprotein, thyroglobulin. Release of thyroid hormone involves the entry of thyroglobulin into follicular cells, hydrolysis, and release of T_3 and T_4. This step also produces di- and mono-iodotyrosines from which iodide is released within the gland and reused normally.

In the circulation, T_4 and T_3 are found. Most of the hormone T_4 circulates bound to specific proteins. T_3, believed by most to be the more active hormone, is produced by coupling in the gland and by deiodination of T_4 in the periphery. The latter method accounts for most of the T_3 present; in disease, the thyroid's fraction of T_3 increases.[2,8-10] With this background, we can review the most commonly used thyroid function tests.

A. Protein-Bound Iodine (PBI)

Normally, iodine in serum reflects that present in thyroid hormones. Thus measuring iodine measures thyroid hormone.[1-7,11] Normally thyroid hormones T_4 and T_3, after release into the circulation, are bound to specific proteins: thyroxin-binding globulin (TBG), albumin, and prealbumin (TBPA).[12,13]

In the PBI test, the serum proteins are precipitated and the iodine content of the precipitate is measured, usually by colorimetric methods.[1,3] Since in normal man, almost all circulating organic iodine (99.5%) occurs in T_4,[1,2,5-7,14-16] the PBI reflects the concentration of T_4. PBI is decreased in hypothyroidism and increased in hyperthyroidism reflecting depressed or elevated hormone levels respectively.[1-7,14,15]

Little non-hormonal iodine is found in the serum normally, although in some thyroid diseases, iodoproteins may be released.[4,14,16] As noted above, most of the hormonal iodine is protein-bound (mostly to TBG); the thyroid status of the patient is related to free (unbound) hormone. Hence, it can be easily recognized (and clinical experience supports this) that many things can produce falsely high or low PBI:[4,15,16]

1. The serum TBG may be abnormal.
   (a) Increased: pregnancy, oral contraceptives, estrogen therapy, and congenital abnormality.
   (b) Decreased: kidney disease, liver disease, androgen therapy, congenital abnormality, and drugs that compete for binding sites, e.g., aspirin.
2. Iodinated compounds or drugs; especially certain radiologic dyes.
3. Elevated levels of iodoproteins or iodotyrosines as result of thyroid disease.

B. Butanol-Extractable Iodine (BEI) [1,2,7,17,18]

Similar in principle to PBI, but more specific especially in patients who have taken inorganic iodine, this test uses acid-butanol extraction to isolate all serum iodine, then via alkaline treatment, removes nonthyroxine iodine. The residue in the butanol is thyroxine-bound iodine. The latter is measured.

C. Thyroid Hormone Measurement

1. Thyroxine (T_4)

Both PBI and BEI measure thyroid hormone indirectly; both are influenced by organic iodides and serum protein alterations.[15-18] Since these measure iodine and not the hormone directly, they are being replaced by methods to evaluate T_4 in serum. Thus, by competitive protein binding or radioimmunoassay, total T_4 can be measured. Total T_4 is elevated in 90% of hyperthyroid and decreased in 85% of hypothyroid patients.[19-25]

However, since this test still measures all T_4, including the major fraction which is protein bound, alterations in TBG will influence the result. As noted above TBG is increased in pregnancy and estrogen therapy and depressed in liver and kidney disorders.[1,4,7,14]

Attempts at assaying free T_4 were unsuccessful until very recently. Thus, other tests were developed.[25,26] The resin triiodothyronine uptake (RTU) depends on the binding of labeled T_3 to TBG and to an artificial resin. The extent of the T_3-binding is inversely related to the number of unoccupied TBG sites. To obtain the free T_4, a mathematical trick involving multiplying the RTU by the total T_4 yields the free thyroxine value.[1,7,14,25-28] Recently, development of direct free T_4 measurement assays have begun to replace other tests. Commercially, available kits will eventually make indirect tests obsolete.[25]

2. Triiodothyronine (T_3)

Direct measurement of T_3 is available.[7,20,21,23] Initially used to distinguish those patients with hyperthyroidism and normal T_4 (i.e., T_3-toxicosis,[7,29-32]) this test has found use in the evaluation of many thyroid disorders.

T_3 measurement may give spurious values (a) in euthyroid patients with liver disease or malnutrition since conversion of T_4 and T_3 is decreased*,[33-40] and (b) in 50% of hypothyroid patients, T_3 may be normal since the thyroid attempts to compensate by producing more T_3 (the more potent hormone) than T_4.[5,7,14,25]

---

* In these circumstances, it is believed that T_4 is preferentially converted to reverse T_3 (a molecular isomer of normal T_3) but inactive.[38-40]

D. Thyroid Function Tests in Thyroiditis

Acute thyroiditis—tests of thyroid function tend to remain normal and the patient is clinically euthyroid unless the gland is totally involved.[41-44] Mild increases in PBI, T_4, and T_3 may be noted as a result of release of stored hormone.[41,45-47] The PBI is invariably elevated to a greater degree than T_4 and T_3, probably as a result of iodotyrosines and iodoproteins expelled from the damaged gland.[41-44,46] These changes are of short duration and may be missed by random serum samples.

Subacute thyroiditis—thyroid function test results are altered as the phase of the disease changes. In the initial or thyrotoxic phase, PBI is increased markedly as are the BEI, T_3, and T_4;[48,50] these changes reflect damage to the thyroid gland with release of stored hormone and iodoproteins. The euthyroid phase is accompanied by a return of these circulating hormone levels to normal as stored hormone is being used up. As though to overshoot the mark, however, PBI, T_3, and T_4 fall to hypothyroid levels in phase three. These alterations are produced by glandular destruction and absence of hormone synthesis. With regeneration of follicular epithelium and recovery of function (phase four) comes restoration of thyroid hormone synthesis; PBI, T_3, and T_4 return to normal.[51-66]

Hashimoto's thyroiditis—in this disease, in which thyroid function ranges from hyper- to hypothyroidism, PBI, T_3 and T_4 generally reflect the clinical course. Thus in Hashitoxicosis, hyperthyroid (elevated) indices are found (less than 10% of Hashimoto's patients fall into this group).[4,58,67-74] Initially, about 50% of patients with this disease are euthyroid. Hypothyroidism, often not the presenting symptom complex, develops later in many individuals with classic and fibrosing Hashimoto's disease;[67,68] at this stage, low PBI, T_3, and T_4 values are found.[67-74] PBI (but rarely BEI) may be misleadingly high, especially in early phases of the disorder as a result of iodinated organic compounds released as the gland is destroyed.[70,71]

Riedel's struma—in this condition, the overwhelming majority (75%) of patients are euthyroid.[45,75-77] When the majority of the gland is replaced, hypothyroidism will occur and thyroid function tests will reflect this.[45,75-77]

E. Thyroid-Stimulating Hormones

Thyroid-stimulating hormone (TSH)—this pituitary hormone which is a sensitive assay to evaluate the pituitary-thyroid axis, can be measured by radioimmunoassay.[2,78-82] Hypothyroid patients in whom the disease process is of thyroid origin, will invariably show elevated TSH levels. Obviously pituitary or hypothalamic lesions producing hypothyroidism will demonstrate low TSH.[2]

Thyrotropin-releasing hormone (TRH)—since the availability of TRH, it has become possible to distinguish hypothalmic from pituitary hypothyroidism and each from a primary thyroid lesion.[25,83-85] Following an intravenous, intramuscular or oral bolus of TRH, serum TSH levels are monitored over time (about 3 hours). In normal individuals, a brisk rise in TSH is seen, which is followed by an increase in thyroid hormones.[86-89] Patients with hypothyroidism display an exaggerated response to TRH administration.[90-92]

F. Thyroid-Stimulating Substances in Thyroiditis

1. Acute Thyroiditis

This disease is so rare that large series of patients evaluated by modern techniques are not available.

2. Subacute Thyroiditis

Typically, TSH is low in the early phase of subacute thyroiditis and the response to

TRH is depressed.[59,61,63,93-100] It has been suggested that high levels of circulating thyroid hormone and iodoproteins released from the damaged thyroid are responsible.[59] Alternatively, the partly destroyed gland may be incapable of response to TSH; this latter must be at least partially correct since exogenous TSH fails to elicit an increase in thyroid hormone output.[48,49] During the hypothyroid phase, TSH levels are elevated and return to normal on recovery.[61,97,101]

3. Hashimoto's Thyroiditis

In this group of disorders, thyroid function may be normal, hyper- or hypothyroid. In many cases, even though chemically and clinically euthyroid, TSH is elevated and/or hyperresponds to exogenous TRH.[2,4,102] These findings indicate subclinical hypothyroidism. Evered et al.[102] caution that the abnormal TSH level or response may be the only clue to disturbed thyroid function; circulating antibodies are commonly identified in these individuals, indicating that they have autoimmune thyroiditis.[102]

Hurley[46] has divided patients with Hashimoto's thyroiditis into four groups according to thyroid function:

1. Normal thyroid function with normal function tests including TSH- and TRH-stimulation test.
2. Low thyroid reserve. These subjects show normal to low normal thyroid hormone levels, with slightly elevated TSH and an exaggerated response to TRH.
3. Mildly hypothyroid patients demonstrate low levels of serum T_3 and T_4 with high TSH and an overactive response to TRH.
4. Severely hypothyroid individuals have low thyroid hormones, markedly elevated TSH and hyperresponsiveness to TRH.

In all these patients, antithyroid antibodies are detectable (see below) confirming the diagnosis of autoimmune thyroiditis.[46]

4. Riedel's Struma

Except in those cases in which large areas of the thyroid are replaced by the fibrous tissue proliferation producing hypothyroidism, thyroid function tests give normal results.[46,75,76]

The above discussion has not included a review of LATS (long-acting thyroid stimulator) or thyroid stimulating immunoglobulin (TSI_g). The role of these substances is small, if not nonexistent, in distinguishing thyroiditis from other thyroid lesions or the thyroiditides from each other.

G. Thyroid Antibodies

Ingbar and Woeber[2] and Hall[103] summarize four types of circulating antibodies which occur in thyroid disease: antithyroglobulin antibodies,[2,25,43,46,58,103,104] antimicrosomal antibodies[2,25,58,103,104] (an antibody directed against a nonthyroglobulin colloid antigen), so-called second colloid antigen,[2,25,103] and antinuclear antibodies.[2,58,103] These substances belong to the gammaglobulin class of antibody (usually IgG) and are organ-specific (except for antinuclear antibody).[2]

Various techniques can demonstrate these antibodies: Ouchteriony diffusion techniques, competitive binding radioimmunoassay,[105] complement fixation,[25,104] tanned red-cell agglutination,[25,46,105-108] and immunofluorescence.[46,109,110] The most commonly measured of these antibodies in patients with thyroiditis include antithyroglobulin and antimicrosomal antibodies.

In the tanned red cell agglutination test, sheep or turkey red cells are coated with either human thyroglobulin (TG) or solubilized thyroid cytoplasmic (MC) proteins; serial dilutions of test serum are added. Agglutination of red cells occurs if antibodies, specific to either TG or MC respectively, are present in the serum.[2,25,43,46,58,103-110]

In some cases of autoimmune thyroiditis, anti-TG antibodies are not found. However, circulating antibodies to other thyroid components can be identified. Thus, antibodies to colloid antigen may be detected in some cases by immunofluorescence.[2,111]

At the research or specialized laboratory level, circulating antibodies to T_4 and T_3 may be present.[112] Thyroid-stimulating globulins (such as long-acting thyroid stimulator (LATS) or thyroid-stimulating immunoglobulin (TSI_g)) may be identified in a few patients with thyroiditis, although they are primarily associated with Graves' disease.[2,5,7,25,113]

H. Thyroid Antibodies in Thyroiditides

1. Acute Thyroiditis

Thyroid autoantibodies usually do not appear during the course of acute thyroiditis.[41,46]

2. Subacute Thyroiditis

Antithyroid antibodies of various types may occur during the course of subacute thyroiditis (in about 50% of cases), although the titers of these substances are, in general, low.[46,56-60] Disappearance of antibodies is the rule in this disorder. The antithyroid antibody findings suggest strongly that a short-term immunologic reaction occurs when various thyroid cellular, colloid, and thyroglobulin antigens are released as glandular destruction takes place during subacute thyroiditis.[46,56-60]

The studies of Volpe[58,59] and others[56,57,114] have disclosed a variety of antiviral antibodies during subacute thyroiditis, occurring in 50 to 70% of affected individuals. Although this may reflect an etiologic relationship in some cases, the variety of such antibodies has led several authors[58,59,115,116] to postulate that this reaction represents a generalized, nonspecific anamnestic response to inflammation of the thyroid (see also Chapter 4).

3. Hashimoto's Thyroiditis

The various forms of this disorder, also known as autoimmune thyroiditis, share as their common diagnostic and purported etiologically related manifestation, the presence in serum of affected patients of a variety of antibodies to thyroid antigens.[46,58,67,68,117,119] Hurley[46] contends that, since antithyroglobulin or antimicrosomal antibodies are detectable at some point in the course of all patients with Hashimoto's disease, "persistently negative results effectively rule out the disease".

Antibody titers may remain low in about 15% of cases and confusion with other lesions associated with low antibody titers may occur: subacute thyroiditis, Graves' disease, and thyroid carcinoma.[46,68,110] Antithyroglobulin titers of 1:32 or greater, or antimicrosomal antibodies of 1:1600 obtained by the tanned red cell hemagglutination technique, are considered diagnostic of Hashimoto's disease.[46,68,120]

Doniach et al.[68] have defined the ranges of antibody titers (considering only the two commonly measured ones) as they are found in the three major forms of autoimmune thyroiditis:

Antibody	Juvenile form	Usual or oxyphil form	Fibrous variant
Antimicrosomal	Low to moderate	Moderate to high	High
Antithyroglobulin	Trace to absent	Positive in 70% of cases	High

Antibodies to colloid antigen or nuclear antigen frequently are found, but are used less often because of difficulty in test performance and degree of specificity. Also, since the diagnostic accuracy of antimicrosomal and antithyroglobulin antibody tests is good and technically more feasible, these have become the standard commonly employed laboratory tests for autoimmune thyroiditis.[68,108]

4. Riedel's Struma

Antithyroid antibodies are rarely, if ever, detectable in this disorder.[46,75,76]

III. THE ROLE OF NUCLEAR MEDICINE

Radioimmunoassays are used in the measurement of thyroid hormones and have been discussed above. This section will review the use of radionuclide scans in thyroiditis.

A. Radionuclide Scanning

Radionuclides normally concentrated by thyroid tissue include iodide isotopes (^{131}I, ^{125}I, ^{123}I) and ^{99}technetium. However, iodide partakes normally in thyroid physiology, is taken up by the gland and incorporated. Indeed, measurement of radioiodide uptake over time indicates capacity of the gland: low uptake is seen in hypothyroidism and an increased percentage of the administered radioisotope is taken up by the hyperfunctioning gland.[2,25,121-125] ^{131}I with a longer half-life subjects the patient to greater radiation exposure than the other radioiodides. It is believed more useful in the evaluation of nodules. Thus hypofunctioning nodules, such as cancers or cysts, will not take up the radioiodide.[2,14,25,121-125] ^{99}Technetium offers advantages over iodine-131 because of shorter half-life and lower radiation dose; it can be given in patients who have taken iodides. However, ^{99}technetium may be concentrated by some carcinomas and is less useful than the iodide scan.[14,25]

Various instruments for imaging are available;[14,25,121-125] newer ones are developed annually to improve imaging, analysis, or recording. Other isotopes have been tried in efforts to distinguish benign from malignant diseases of the thyroid. Their number bespeaks the less than adequate results with any one of them: ^{75}Selenomethionine,[122,126] ^{131}Cesium,[127] and ^{67}Gallium.[128]

B. Fluorescent Scanning

Fluorescent scanning[14,129,130] is a new technique in which radioisotopes are not administered. It involves focal irradiation of the thyroid with gamma rays from an ^{241}Americum source. It interacts with intraglandular stable iodine, producing a characteristic fluorescent X-ray. The result is an estimate of the amount and distribution of iodine in the gland. Since this test does not require concentration of iodine in the gland, patients with excess iodide ingestion can be tested accurately.[14,129,130] Safety is another feature since isotopes are not administered.

C. Perchlorate Discharge Test

This test detects defects in organification of iodide, since normally, iodide is trapped by the gland, organified, and bound to proteins, especially thyroglobulin. The perchlorate ion inhibits this trapping step (other substances act similarly to perchlorate, e.g., thiocyanite, thiouracil, but practically, perchlorate is used in this test),[25] and thus nonbound intrathyroidal iodide is released into the circulation.

Practically, radioiodide is administered and accumulates in the gland; after 2 hr, perchlorate ion is given and counts are taken over the thyroid gland at 15 min intervals for 2 hr. Normally, since the radioiodide is trapped into colloid, little is unbound to be available for release following perchlorate administration. If greater than 5% of the radionuclide dose is extruded within the test period, a defect in organification is present.[25,131,132]

D. Scanning in Thyroiditis
1. Acute Thyroiditis

Depending upon the focal or diffuse nature of thyroid involvement, radioiodide uptake will be normal or decreased. Scans may indicate a patchy uptake if diffuse inflammation is present, or a "cold" area if the infection is localized or an abscess develops.[41]

2. Subacute Thyroiditis

As has been discussed in Chapter 4, the radioiodide uptake in subacute thyroiditis is depressed characteristically, especially in the hypothyroid phase of the disease.[44,55-60,93,133,134] This result indicates damage and destruction to the follicular epithelium so that its function is interfered with.[55-60]

Scans of the thyroid in subacute disease often demonstrate patchy uptake of the isotope since gland involvement is frequently irregular. Areas of minimally affected or normal thyroid will take up the radionuclide more avidly than the affected zones.[44,93,133,134] Fluorescent scanning shows depletion of intrathyroidal iodine stores as the gland is destroyed by inflammation.[44,129,130]

3. Hashimoto's Thyroiditis

Radioiodine uptake may be increased, decreased, or normal depending upon the functional state of the gland.[14] As the disease progresses toward hypothyroidism, uptake of iodine is decreased.[14,25,46]

Scans usually show a symmetrically enlarged gland with a patchy uptake again indicating irregular involvement of the gland, at least, in early stages.[14,25,46] Hypofunctioning nodules may be revealed in about 20% of patients with this disorder;[46,135] rarely "hot" nodules will be noted.[135,136] Thomas et al.[122] reported that in chronic thyroiditis, the radioiodide uptake may be homogeneous or heterogeneous, but the uptake of ^{75}Seleno-methionine is uniform. These authors indicated that this pattern was characteristic for this disorder. Not all authors agree, however.[14,25]

Fluorescent scanning has been useful in Hashimoto's disease,[129,130,137,138] since the technique allows one to follow the iodine content of the gland and thus the progression of the disease. Thus, this method, which is safe and not influenced by therapy or excess iodine ingestion, can be utilized as a prognostic indicator in chronic thyroiditis.[130]

The perchlorate discharge test gives abnormal results in most patients with Hashimoto's disease[25,139] since damage to follicular epithelium interferes with organification. This test is not, however, diagnostic, since similar results are obtained in Graves' disease.[139,140]

4. Riedel's Struma

Only in that minority of cases in which hypothyroidism is present will radioiodine uptake be depressed.[46,76,141] Scans will demonstrate cold areas where thyroid replacement by the fibrosing process has occurred.[44,75,76,110]

IV. THE ROLE OF ULTRASOUND

Ultrasonography or echography utilizes sound frequencies to distinguish lesions,

Table 1
THYROIDITIS: LABORATORY EVALUATION[a]

	Serum PBI	Serum T$_4$	Serum T$_3$	T$_3$ Resin uptake	Serum TSH	I-^{131}Scan
Acute thyroiditis	N[b] or slight I[c]	N or slight I	N or slight I	N	N	Patchy or cold nodule
Subacute thyroiditis						
Hyperthyroid phase	I	I	I	I	D[d]	Patchy uptake, low RaI uptake
Hypothyroid phase	D	D	D	D	I	Patchy uptake
Hashimoto's thyroiditis	I, D, or N	I, D, or N	I, D, or N	I, D, or N	N or I	Patchy uptake, RaI[e] N, I or D
Fibrous variant	D	D	D	D	I	RaI D, Patchy scan
Riedel's struma	N or D	N or D	N or D	N or D	N or I	Normal with cold areas

[a] Adapted from References 1-8, 14, and 16.
[b] N = normal.
[c] I = increased.
[d] D = decreased.
[e] RaI = radioiodine.

since interfaces between tissues of different densities transmit different sounds or echos.[142-146] This procedure is safe since no radioactive substances are given; it is simple and painless.[25,142-146]

Ultrasound techniques can be used to outline the thyroid and its lesions, especially differentiating between solid and cystic lesions.[142-146] This method has been utilized as an adjunct procedure and guide to needle biopsy.[25,147-149]

The value of this technique in the various forms of thyroiditis remains minimal; its major use is found in distinguishing cystic from solid nodules, and indicating the possibility of malignancy.[148-150]

V. OTHER TECHNIQUES

Complex radiologic techniques including angiography,[151] lymphography,[152-154] and thermography[155-157] are used chiefly in distinguishing neoplasms and cannot differentiate the various forms of thyroiditis.

REFERENCES

1. **Sunderman, F. W. and Sunderman, F. W., Jr., Eds.,** *Evaluation of Thyroid and Parathyroid Function,* J. B. Lippincott, Philadelphia, 1963.
2. **Ingbar, S. H. and Woeber, K. A.,** The thyroid gland, in *Textbook of Endocrinology,* W. B. Saunders Co., Philadelphia, 1968, 105.
3. **Hamolsky, M. W.,** *Thyroid Testing,* Lea and Febiger, Philadelphia, 1971.
4. **Evered, D.,** Diseases of the thyroid gland, *Clin. Endocrinol. Metab.,* 3, 425, 1974.
5. **Sterling, K.,** Thyroid function tests, *Adv. Intern. Med.,* 18, 345, 1972.
6. **Bartuska, D. G. and Dratman, M. B.,** Evolving concepts of thyroid function, *Med. Clin. North Am.,* 57, 1117, 1973.
7. **Sterling, K.,** *Diagnosis and Treatment of Thyroid Diseases,* CRC Press, Boca Raton, Fla., 1975.
8. **Copiferri, R. and Evered, D.,** Investigation and treatment of hypothyroidism, *Clin. Endocrinol. Metab.,* 8, 39, 1979.
9. **Lieblich, J. and Utiger, R. D.,** Triiodothyronine radioimmunoassay, *J. Clin. Invest.,* 51, 157, 1971.
10. **Wahner, H. W. and Gorman, C. A.,** Interpretation of serum triiodothyronine levels measured by the Sterling technique, *N. Engl. J. Med.,* 284, 225, 1971.
11. **Barker, S. B., Humphrey, M. J., and Soley, M. H.,** Clinical determination of protein-bound iodine, *J. Clin. Invest.,* 30, 55, 1951.
12. **Sterling, K.,** Thyroxine in blood, *Mayo Clin. Proc.,* 39, 586, 1964.
13. **Oppenheimer, J. H.,** Role of plasma proteins in the binding, distribution and metabolism of the thyroid hormones, *N. Engl. J. Med.,* 278, 1153, 1968.
14. **Braverman, L. E. and Vagenakis, A. G.,** The thyroid, in *Nuclear Medicine,* Wagner, H. N., Ed., HP Publishing Co., New York, 1975, 127.
15. **Davis, R. J.,** Factors affecting the determination of serum protein bound iodine, *Am. J. Med.,* 40, 918, 1966.
16. **Acland, J. D.,** The interpretation of protein bound iodine: A review, *J. Clin. Pathol.,* 24, 187, 1971.
17. **Benotti, J. and Pinto, S.,** A simplified method for butanol-extractable iodine and butanol insoluble iodine, *Clin. Chem.,* 12, 491, 1966.
18. **Pileggi, V. J., Lee, N. D., Golub, O. J., and Henry, R. J.,** Determination of iodine compounds in serum. I. Serum thyroxine in the presence of some iodine contaminants., *J. Clin. Endocrinol. Metab.,* 21, 1272, 1961.
19. **Abuid, J. and Larsen, P. R.,** Triiodothyronine and thyroxine in hyperthyroidism: Comparison of the acute changes during therapy with antithyroid agents, *J. Clin. Invest.,* 54, 201, 1974.

20. **Goldie, D. J., Jennings, R. D., and McGowan, G. K.,** The estimation of serum thyroxine by competitive binding analysis: A modified method, *J. Clin. Pathol.,* 27, 74, 1974.
21. **Murphy, B. E. P. and Pattee, C. J.,** Determination of thyroxine utilizing the property of protein-binding, *J. Clin. Endocrinol.,* 24, 187, 1974.
22. **Hollander, C. S.,** On the nature of the circulating thyroid hormone: Clinical studies of triiodothyronine and thyroxine in serum using gas chromatographic methods, *Trans. Assoc. Am. Physicians,* 81, 76, 1968.
23. **Chopra, I. J.,** A radioimmunoassay for measurement of thyroxines in unextracted serum, *J. Clin. Endocrinol. Metab.,* 34, 938, 1972.
24. **Odell, W. D., Wilber, J. F., and Utiger, R. D.,** Studies of thyrotropin physiology by means of radioimmunoassay, *Rec. Prog. Horm. Res.,* 23, 47, 1967.
25. **Refetoff, S.,** Thyroid function tests, in *Endocrinology,* Vol. 1. DeGroot, L. J., Cahill, G. F., Martini, L., Nelson, D. H., Odell, W. D., Potts, J. T., Steinberger, E., and Winegrad, A. I., Eds., Grune & Stratton, New York, 1979, 387.
26. **Hamolsky, M. W., Stein, M. and Freedberg, A. S.,** The thyroid hormone-plasma protein complex in man. II. A new in vitro method for study of "uptake" of labeled hormonal components by human erythrocytes, *J. Clin. Endocrinol.,* 17, 33, 1957.
27. **Gorman, C. A.,** Some problems in thyroid diagnosis, *Med. Clin. North Am.,* 56, 841, 1972.
28. **Mitchell, M. H., Harden, A. B., and O'Rourke, M. E.,** The in vitro resin sponge uptake of triiodothyronine- 131 I from serum in thyroid disease and in pregnancy, *J. Clin. Endocrinol. Metab.,* 20, 1474, 1960.
29. **Sterling, K., Bellabarba, D., Newman, E. S., and Brenner, M. A.,** Determination of triiodothyronine concentration in human serum, *J. Clin. Invest.,* 48, 1150, 1969.
30. **Sterling, K., Refetoff, S., and Selenkow, H. A.,** T_3 thyrotoxicosis: Thyrotoxicosis due to elevated serum triiodothyronine, *JAMA,* 213, 571, 1970.
31. **Nauman, J. A., Nauman, A., and Werner, S. C.,** Total and free triiodothyronine in human serum, *J. Clin. Invest.,* 46, 1346, 1967.
32. **Gharib, H. and Wahner, H. W.,** Clinical experience with assays for triiodothyronine, *Med. Clin. North Am.,* 56, 861, 1972.
33. **Carter, J. N., Eastman, C. J., Corcoran, J. M., and Lazarus, L.,** Effect of severe chronic illness on thyroid function, *Lancet,* 2, 971, 1974.
34. **Burger, A., Nicod, P., Suter, P., Vallotton, M. B., Vagenakis, A., and Braverman, L.,** Reduced active thyroid hormone levels in acute illness, *Lancet,* 1, 653, 1976.
35. **Chopra, I. J. and Smith, S. R.,** Circulating thyroid hormones and thyrotropin in adult patients with protein malnutrition, *J. Clin. Endocrinol. Metab.,* 40, 221, 1975.
36. **Wartofsky, L., Burman, K. D., Dimond, R. C., Noel, G. L., Frantz, A. G., and Earll, J. M.,** Studies on the nature of thyroidal suppression during acute falciparium malaria: integrity of pituitary response to TRH and alterations in serum T_3 and reverse T_3, *J. Clin. Endocrinol. Metab.,* 44, 85, 1977.
37. **Larsen, P. R.,** Triiodothyronine: Review of recent studies of its physiology and pathophysiology in man, *Metabolism,* 21, 1073, 1972.
38. **Chopra, I. J., Chopra, U., Smith, S. R., Reza, M., and Solomon, D. H.,** Reciprocal changes in serum concentration of 3,3',5'-triiodothyronine (reverse T_3) and 3,3',5-triiodothyronine (T_3) in systemic illness, *J. Clin. Endocrinol. Metab.,* 41, 1043, 1975.
39. **Lim, V. S., Fang, V. S., Katz, A. I., and Refetoff, B.,** Thyroid dysfunction in chronic renal failure: A study of the pituitary-thyroid axis and peripheral turnover kinetics of thyroxine and triiodothyronine, *J. Clin. Invest.,* 60, 522, 1977.
40. **Refetoff, S., DeLange, F., Berquist, H., Fang, V. S., VanHumskerke, V., Seo, H., and Ermans, A. M.,** Importance of the intracellularly formed triiodothyronine (T_3) in the regulation of cell metabolism, *Clin. Res.,* 24, 276, 1976.
41. **Volpe, R.,** Acute suppurative thyroiditis, in *The Thyroid,* Werner, S. C. and Ingbar, S. H., Eds., Harper and Row New York, 1971, 849.
42. **Volpe, R.,** The pathology of thyroiditis, *Hum. Pathol.,* 9, 429, 1978.
43. **Volpe, R.,** Etiology, pathogenesis and clinical aspects of thyroiditis, Part 2, *Pathol. Annu.,* 13, 399, 1978.
44. **DeGroot, L. J. and Stanbury, J. B.,** *The Thyroid and Its Diseases,* John Wiley and Sons, New York, 1975, 572.
45. **Hazard, J. B.,** Thyroiditis: A review, *Am. J. Clin. Pathol.,* 25, 289, 1955.
46. **Hurley, J. R.,** Thyroiditis, *Disease-A-Month,* December 1977.
47. **Himsworth, R. L. and Kark, A. E.,** Studies on a case of suppurative thyroiditis, *Acta Endocrinol.,* 85, 55, 1977.
48. **Dorta, T. and Berand, T.,** New studies on the subject of subacute thyroiditis, *Helv. Med. Acta,* 28, 19, 1961.

49. **Crile, G. and Rumsey, E. W.**, Subacute thyroiditis, *JAMA*, 142, 458, 1950.
50. **Lindsay, S. and Dailey, M. E.**, Granulomatous or giant cell thyroiditis: Clinical and pathologic study of 37 patients, *Surg. Gynecol. Obstet.*, 98, 197, 1954.
51. **Fraser, R. and Harrison, R. J.**, Subacute thyroiditis, *Lancet*, 1, 382, 1952.
52. **Volpe, R. and Johnson, M. W.**, Subacute thyroiditis: A disease commonly mistaken for pharyngitis, *Can. Med. Assoc. J.*, 77, 297, 1957.
53. **Woolner, L. B., McConahey, W. M., and Beahrs, O. W.**, Granulomatous thyroiditis (deQuervain's thyroiditis), *J. Clin. Endocrinol.*, 17, 1202, 1957.
54. **Steinberg, F. U.**, Subacute granulomatous thyroiditis: A review, *Ann. Intern. Med.*, 52, 1014, 1960.
55. **Furszyfer, J., McConahey, W. M., Wahner, H. W., and Kurland, L. T.**, Subacute (granulomatous) thyroiditis in Olmsted County, *Mayo Clin. Proc.*, 45, 396, 1970.
56. **Greene, J. N.**, Subacute thyroiditis, *Am. J. Med.*, 51, 97, 1971.
57. **Bastenie, P. A., Bonnyns, M., and Neve, P.**, Subacute and chronic granulomatous thyroiditis, in *Thyroiditis and Thyroid Function: Clinical, Morphological and Physiopathological Studies*, Bastenie, P. A., and Ermans, A.M., Eds., Pergamon Press, Oxford, 1972, 69.
58. **Volpe, R.**, Thyroiditis: Current views of pathogenesis, *Med. Clin. North Am.*, 59, 1163, 1975.
59. **Volpe, R.**, Subacute (de Quervain's) thyroiditis, *Clin. Endocrinol. Metab.*, 8, 81, 1979.
60. **DePauw, B. E. and DeRooy, H. A. M.**, De Quervain's subacute thyroiditis, *Neth. J. Med.*, 18, 70, 1975.
61. **Larson, P. R.**, Serum triiodothyronine, thyroxine, and thyrotropin during hyperthyroid, hypothyroid and recovery phases of subacute, non-suppurative thyroiditis, *Metabolism*, 23, 467, 1974.
62. **Ingbar, S. H. and Freinkel, N.**, Thyroid function and the metabolism of iodine in patients with subacute thyroiditis, *Arch. Intern. Med.*, 101, 339, 1958.
63. **Weihl, A. C., Daniels, G. H., Ridgway, E. C., and Maloof, F.**, Thyroid function tests during the early phase of subacute thyroiditis, *J. Clin. Endocrinol. Metab.*, 44, 1107, 1977.
64. **Izumi, M. and Larsen, P. R.**, Correlation of sequential changes in serum thyroglobulin, triiodothyronine and thyroxine in patients with Graves' disease and subacute thyroiditis, *Metabolism*, 27, 449, 1978.
65. **Volpe, R., Johnston, M. W., and Huber, N.**, Thyroid function in subacute thyroiditis, *J. Clin. Endocrinol.*, 18, 65, 1958.
66. **Schultz, A. L.**, Subacute diffuse thyroiditis. Clinical and laboratory findings in 24 patients and the effect of treatment with adrenal corticoids, *Postgrad. Med.*, 29, 76, 1961.
67. **Neve, P., Ermans, A. M., and Bastenie, P. A.**, Struma lymphomastosa (Hashimoto), in *Thyroiditis and Thyroid Function: Clinical, Morphological and Physiopathological Studies*, Bastenie, P. A. and Ermans, A. M., Eds., Pergamon Press, Oxford, 1972, 109.
68. **Doniach, D., Bottazzo, G. F. and Russell, R. C. G.**, Goitrous autoimmune thyroiditis (Hashimoto's) disease, *Clin. Endocrinol. Metab.*, 8, 63, 1979.
69. **Hall, R. and Evered, D. C.**, Autoimmune thyroid disease: Thyroiditis, in *Endocrinology*, Vol. 1, DeGroot, L. J., Cahill, G. F., Martini, L., Nelson, D. H., Odell, W. D., Potts, J. T., Steinberger, E., and Winegrad, A. I., Eds., Grune & Stratton, New York, 1979, 461.
70. **McConahey, W. M., Keating, F. R., Butt, H. R., and Owen, C. A.**, Comparison of certain laboratory tests in the diagnosis of Hashimoto's thyroiditis, *J. Clin. Endocrinol. Metab.*, 21, 879, 1961.
71. **Camus, M., Ermans, A. M., and Bastenie, P. A.**, Alterations of iodine metabolism in asymptomatic thyroiditis, *Metabolism*, 17, 1064, 1968.
72. **Volpe, R., Row, V. V., Webster, B. R., McAllister, W. J., Johnston, W., and Ezrin, C.**, Studies of iodine metabolism in Hashimoto's thyroiditis, *J. Clin. Endocrinol. Metab.*, 25, 593, 1965.
73. **Doniach, D. and Hudson, R. V.**, Lymphadenoid goitre: Diagnostic and biochemical aspects, *Br. Med. J.*, 1, 672, 1957.
74. **Morgans, M. E. and Trotter, W. R.**, Defective organic binding of iodine by the thyroid in Hashimoto's thyroiditis, *Lancet*, 1, 553, 1957.
75. **Bastenie, P. A.**, Invasive fibrous thyroiditis (Riedel), in *Thyroiditis and Thyroid Function: Clinical, Morphological and Physiopathological Studies*, Bastenie, P. A. and Ermans, A. M., Eds., Pergamon Press, Oxford, 1972, 99.
76. **Volpe, R.** Riedel's struma (struma fibrosa), in *The Thyroid*, Werner, S. C. and Ingbar, S. H., Eds., Harper & Row, New York, 1978, 1009.
77. **Woolner, L. B., McConahey, W. M., and Beahrs, O. H.**, Invasive fibrous thyroiditis (Riedel's struma), *J. Clin. Endocrinol.*, 17, 201, 1957.
78. **Rosenberg, I. N. and Bastomsky, C. H.**, Thyroid, *Ann. Rev. Physiol.*, 27, 71, 1965.
79. **Brown, J. R.**, The measurement of thyroid stimulating hormone (TSH) in body fluid: A critical review, *Acta Endocrinol.*, 32, 289, 1959.
80. **Wilbert, J. F.**, Thyrotropin releasing hormone: Secretion and actions, *Annu. Rev. Med.*, 24, 353, 1973.

81. Hershman, J. M. and Pittman, J. A., Utility of the radioimmunoassay of serum thyrotropin in man, *Ann. Intern. Med.*, 74, 481, 1971.
82. Mayberry, W. E., Gharib, H., Bilstad, J. M., and Sizemore, G. W., Radioimmunoassay for human thyrotropin: Clinical value in patients with normal and abnormal thyroid function, *Ann. Intern. Med.*, 74, 471, 1971.
83. Uller, R. P., VanHerle, A. J., and Chopra, I. J., Comparison of alterations in circulating thyroglobulin, triiodothyronine and thyroxine in response to exogenous (bovine) and endogenous (human) thyrotropin, *J. Clin. Endocrinol. Metab.*, 37, 741, 1973.
84. Shenkman, L., Mitsuma, T., Suphavai, A., and Hollander, C. S., Triiodothyronine and thyroid-stimulating hormone response to thyrotropin-releasing hormone, *Lancet*, 1, 111, 1972.
85. Azizi, F., Vagenakis, A. G., Portnay, G. I., Rapoport, B., Ingbar, S. H., and Braverman, L. E., Pituitary-thyroid responsiveness to intramuscular thyrotropin-releasing hormone based on analyses of serum tyrosine, triiodothyronine and thyrotropin concentration, *N. Engl. J. Med.*, 292, 273, 1975.
86. Snyder, P. J. and Utiger, R. D., Response to thyrotropin releasing hormone (TRH) in normal man, *J. Clin. Endocrinol. Metab.*, 34, 380, 1972.
87. Haigler, E. D., Pittman, J. A., Hershman, J. M., and Baugh, C. M., Direct evaluation of pituitary thyrotropin reserve utilizing synthetic thyrotropin releasing hormone, *J. Clin. Endocrinol. Metab.*, 33, 573, 1971.
88. Haigler, E. D., Hershman, J. M., and Pittman, J. A., Response to orally administered synthetic thyrotropin-releasing hormone in man, *J. Clin. Endocrinol. Metab.*, 35, 631, 1972.
89. Beckers, C., Maskens, A., and Cornette, C., Thyrotropin response to synthetic thyrotropin-releasing hormone in normal subjects and in patients with nontoxic goiter, *Eur. J. Clin. Invest.*, 2, 220, 1972.
90. Bowers, C. Y., Friesin, H. G., Hwang, P., Guyda, H. J., and Folkers, K., Prolactin and thyrotropin release in man by synthetic pyroglutamyl-histidyl-prolinamide, *Biochem. Biophys. Res. Commun.*, 45, 1033, 1971.
91. Jensen, S. E., A new way of measuring thyrotropin (TSH) reserve, *J. Clin. Endocrinol. Metab.*, 29, 409, 1969.
92. Fleischer, N., Lorente, M., Kirkland, J., Kirkland, R., Clayton, G., and Calderon, M., Synthetic thyrotropin releasing factor as a test of pituitary thyrotropin reserve, *J. Clin. Endocrinol. Metab.*, 34, 617, 1972.
93. Lewitus, W., Rechnic, J., and Lubin, E., Sequential scanning of the thyroid as an aid in the diagnosis of subacute thyroiditis, *Isr. J. Med. Sci.*, 3, 847, 1967.
94. Glinoer, D., Puttemans, N., Van Herle, A. J., Camus, M., and Ermans, A. M., Sequential study of the impairment of thyroid function in the early stage of subacute thyroiditis, *Acta Endocrinol.*, 77, 26, 1974.
95. Kamio, N., Kobayashi, I., Mori, N., Uehara, T., Fukuda, H., Tsuyusaki, K., Nakamura, Y., and Kobayashi, S., Permissive role of thyrotropin on thyroid radioiodine uptake during the recovery phase of subacute thyroiditis, *Metabolism*, 26, 295, 1977.
96. Gordin, A. and Lamberg, B. A., Serum thyrotropin response to thyrotropin releasing hormone and the concentration of free tyrosine in subacute thyroiditis, *Acta Endocrinol.*, 74, 111, 1973.
97. Ogihara, T., Yamamoto, T. Azukizawa, M., Miyai, K. and Kumahara, Y. Serum thyrotropin and thyroid hormones in the course of subacute thyroiditis, *J. Clin. Endocrinol. Metab.*, 37, 602, 1973.
98. Staub, J. J., TRH test in subacute thyroiditis, *Lancet*, 1, 868, 1975.
99. Demeester-Mirkine, N., Brauman, H., and Corvilain, J., Delayed adjustment of the pituitary response in circulating thyroid hormones in a case of subacute thyroiditis, *Clin. Endocrinol.*, 5, 9, 1976.
100. Lebacq, E. G., Therasse, G., Schmitz, A., Delannoy, A., and Destailleurs, C., Subacute thyroiditis, *Acta Endocrinol.*, 81, 707, 1976.
101. Volpe, R., Acute and subacute thyroiditis, *Pharm. Ther. C.*, 1, 171, 1976.
102. Evered, D. C., Ormston, B. J., Smith, P. A., Hall, R., and Bird, T., Grades of hypothyroidism, *Br. Med. J.*, 1, 657, 1973.
103. Hall, R., Immunologic aspects of thyroid function, *N. Engl. J. Med.*, 266, 1204, 1962.
104. Trotter, W. R., Belyavin, G., and Waddams, A., Precipitating and complement fixing antibodies in Hashimoto's disease, *Proc. R. Soc. Med.*, 50, 961, 1957.
105. Mori, T. and Kriss, J. P., Measurements by competitive binding radioassay of serum antimicrosomal and antithyroglobulin antibodies in Graves' disease and other thyroid disorders, *J. Clin. Endocrinol. Metab.*, 33, 688, 1971.
106. Fulthorpe, A. J., Roitt, I. M., Doniach, D., and Couchman, K. G., A stable sheep cell preparation for detecting thyroglobulin autoantibodies and its clinical applications, *J. Clin. Pathol.*, 14, 654, 1961.
107. Bird, R. and Stephenson, J., Evaluation of a tanned red cell technique for thyroid microsomal antibodies, *J. Clin. Pathol.*, 26, 623, 1973.

108. **Bigos, S. T., Hindson, D., and McCallum, J.**, Serum thyroid-stimulating hormone and antimicrosomal antibodies as a screen for autoimmune thyroid disease, *J. Lab. Clin. Med.*, 93, 1035, 1979.
109. **Holborow, E. J., Brown, P. C., Roitt, I. M., and Doniach, D.**, Cytoplasmic localization of complement-fixing autoantigen in human thyroid epithelium, *Br. J. Exp. Pathol.*, 40, 583, 1959.
110. **Doniach, D. and Roitt, I. M.**, Thyroid autoallergic disease, in *Clinical Aspects of Immunology*, Gell, P. G. H., Coombs, R. R. A., and Lachman, P. J., Eds., Blackwell Scientific, Oxford, 1975, 1355.
111. **Balfour, B. M., Doniach, D., Roitt, I. M., and Couchman, K. G.**, Fluorescent antibody studies in human thyroiditis: Autoantibodies to an antigen of the thyroid distinct from thyroglobulin, *Br. J. Exp. Pathol.*, 42, 307, 1961.
112. **Staeheli, V., Vallotton, M. B., and Burger, A.**, Detection of human antithyroxine and anti-triiodotyronine antibodies in different thyroid conditions, *J. Clin. Endocrinol. Metab.*, 41, 669, 1975.
113. **McKenzie, J. M., Zakarija, M., and Sato, A.**, Humoral immunity of Graves' disease, *Clin. Endocrinol. Metab.*, 7, 31, 1978.
114. **Eylan, E., Zmucky, R., and Sheba, C.**, Mumps virus and subacute thyroiditis—Evidence of a causal association, *Lancet*, 1, 1062, 1957.
115. **Strakosch, C. R., Joyner, D., and Wall, J. R.**, Thyroid stimulating antibodies in patients with subacute thyroiditis, *J. Clin. Endocrinol. Metab.*, 46, 345, 1978.
116. **Sugenoya, A., Kidd, A., Silverberg, J., Row, V. V., and Volpe, R.**, A comparison of the radioligand technique and the cellular stimulation technique for the demonstration of thyroid stimulating immunoglobulins, Abstract presented at Proc. Endocrinol. Soc., Miami, Fla., June, 1978.
117. **Volpe, R.**, Lymphocytic (Hashimoto's) thyroiditis, in *The Thyroid*, Werner, S. C., and Ingbar, S. H., Eds., Harper and Row, New York, 1978, 996.
118. **Brown, J., Solomon, D. H., Beall, G. N., Terasaki, P. I., Chopra, I. J., VanHerle, A. J., and Wu, S.-Y.**, Autoimmune thyroid disease — Graves' and Hashimoto, *Ann Intern. Med.*, 88, 379, 1978.
119. **Volpe, R.**, The role of autoimmunity in hypoendocrine and hyperendocrine function, *Ann. Intern. Med.*, 87, 86, 1977.
120. **Doniach, D.**, Humoral and genetic aspects of thyroid autoimmunity, *Clin. Endocrinol. Metab.*, 4, 267, 1975.
121. **Maisey, M. N., Moses, D. C., Hurley, P. J., and Wagner, H. N.**, Improved methods of thyroid scanning, *JAMA*, 223, 761, 1973.
122. **Thomas, C. G., Pepper, F. D., and Owen, J.**, Differentiation of malignant from benign lesions of the thyroid gland using complementary scanning with 75-selenomethionine and radioiodide, *Ann. Surg.*, 170, 396, 1969.
123. **Pittman, J. A., Dailey, G. E., and Beschi, R. J.**, Changing normal values for thyroidal radioiodine uptake, *N. Engl. J. Med.*, 280, 1431, 1969.
124. **Wong, E. T. and Schultz, A. L.**, Changing values for the normal thyroid radioactive iodine uptake test, *JAMA*, 238, 1741, 1977.
125. **Quinn, J. L. and Behinfar, M.**, Radioisotope scanning of the thyroid, *JAMA*, 199, 170, 1967.
126. **Weinstein, M. B., Ashkar, F. S., and Caron, C. D.**, 75-Se selenomethionine as a scanning agent for the differential diagnosis of the cold thyroid nodule, *Sem. Nucl. Med.*, 1, 390, 1971.
127. **Murray, I. P. C., Stewart, R. D. H., and Indyk, J. S.**, Thyroid scanning with 131-cesium, *Br. Med. J.*, 4, 653, 1970.
128. **Kaplan, W. D., Holman, B. L., Selenkow, H. A., Davis, M. A., Holmes, R. A., Isitman, A. T., and Chandler, H. L.**, 67-gallium-citrate and the nonfunctioning thyroid nodules, *J. Nucl. Med.*, 15, 424, 1974.
129. **Hoffer, H. P.**, Fluorescent thyroid scanning, *Am. J. Roentgenol.*, 105, 721, 1969.
130. **Wahner, H. W., Sweet, R. A., McConahey, W. M., and Duick, D. S.**, Fluorescent thyroid scanning, *Mayo Clin. Proc.*, 53, 151, 1978.
131. **Baschieri, L., Benedetti, G., deLuca, F., and Negri, M.**, Evaluation and limitations of the perchlorate test in the study of thyroid function, *J. Clin. Endocrinol. Metab.*, 23, 786, 1963.
132. **Stewart, R. D. H. and Murray, I. P. C.**, An evaluation of the perchlorate discharge test, *J. Clin. Endocrinol. Metab.*, 26, 1050, 1966.
133. **Marchetta, F. C. and Bender, M. A.**, Radioactive iodine uptake and localization studies with a scintiscanner in subacute thyroiditis, *N.Y. State J. Med.*, 56, 1951, 1956.
134. **Hamburger, H. I., Kadian, G., and Rossin, H. W.**, Subacute thyroiditis — Evolution depicted by serial 131-I scintigrams, *J. Nucl. Med.*, 6, 560, 1965.
135. **Fisher, D. A., Oddie, T. H., Johnson, D. E., and Nelson, J. C.**, The diagnosis of Hashimoto's thyroiditis, *J. Clin. Endocrinol. Metab.*, 40, 795, 1975.
136. **Bialas, P., Marks, S., Dekker, A., and Field, J. B.**, Hashimoto's thyroiditis presenting as a solitary functioning thyroid nodule, *J. Clin. Endocrinol. Metab.*, 43, 1365, 1976.
137. **Hoffer, P. B., Gottschalk, A., and Refetoff, S.**, Thyroid scanning techniques: The new and the old, *Curr. Probl. Radiol.*, 2, 1, 1972.

138. **Rapoport, B., Block, M. B., Hoffer, P. B., and DeGroot, L. J.**, Depletion of thyroid iodine during subacute thyroiditis, *J. Clin. Endocrinol. Metab.*, 36, 610, 1973.
139. **Takeuchi, K., Suzuki, H., Horuichi, Y., and Mashimo, K.**, Significance of iodideperchlorate discharge test for detection of iodine organification defect of the thyroid, *J. Clin. Endocrinol. Metab.*, 31, 144, 1970.
140. **Suzuki, H. and Mashimo, K.**, Significance of the iodide-perchlorate discharge test in patients with 131 I-treated and untreated hyperthyroidism, *J. Clin. Endocrinol. Metab.*, 34, 332, 1972.
141. **Katsikas, D., Shorthouse, A. J., and Taylor, S.**, Riedel's thyroiditis, *Br. J. Surg.*, 63, 929, 1976.
142. **Blum, M., Goldman, A. B., Herskovic, A., and Hermberg, J.**, Clinical application of thyroid echography, *N. Engl. J. Med.*, 287, 1164, 1972.
143. **Thijs, L. G.**, Diagnostic ultrasound in clinical thyroid investigation, *J. Clin. Endocrinol. Metab.*, 32, 709, 1971.
144. **Thijs, L. G. and Wiener, J. D.**, Ultrasonic examination of the thyroid gland, *Am. J. Med.*, 60, 96, 1976.
145. **Miskin, M., Rosen, I. B., and Walfish, P. G.**, B-mode ultrasonography in assessment of thyroid gland lesions, *Ann. Intern. Med.*, 79, 505, 1973.
146. **Blum, M.**, Enhanced clinical diagnosis of thyroid disease using echography, *Am. J. Med.*, 59, 301, 1975.
147. **Jensen, F. and Rasmussen, S. N.**, The treatment of thyroid cysts by ultrasonically guided fine needle aspiration, *Acta Chir. Scand.*, 142, 209, 1976.
148. **Walfish, P. G., Hazani, E., Strawbridge, H. T. G., Miskin, M., and Rosen, I. B.**, Combined ultrasound and needle aspiration cytology in the assessment and management of hypofunctioning thyroid nodule, *Ann. Intern. Med.*, 87, 270, 1977.
149. **Rosen, I. B., Walfish, P. G., and Miskin, M.**, The ultrasound of thyroid masses, *Surg. Clin. North Am.*, 59, 19, 1979.
150. **Himsworth, R. L. and Kark, A. E.**, Studies on a case of suppurative thyroiditis, *Acta Endocrinol.*, 85, 55, 1977.
151. **Damascelli, B., Cascinelli, N., Terno, G., Dragoni, G., and Saccozzi, R.**, Second thoughts on the value of selective thyroid angiography, *Am. J. Roentgenol. Radium Ther. Nucl. Med.*, 114, 822, 1972.
152. **Matoba, N. and Kikuchi, T.**, Thyroidolymphography, *Radiology*, 92, 339, 1969.
153. **Sachdeva, H. S., Chowdhary, G. C., Bose, S. M., Gupta, B. B., and Wig, J. D.**, Thyroid lymphography, *Arch. Surg.*, 109, 385, 1974.
154. **Ram, M. D., Archer, B. T., and Brown, H. W.**, Thyroidography and thyrolymphography, *Surg. Gynecol. Obstet.*, 138, 417, 1974.
155. **Samuels, B. I.**, Thermography: A valuable tool in the detection of thyroid disease, *Radiology*, 102, 59, 1972.
156. **Galli, G., Salvo, D., Troncone, L., and DeRossi, G.**, Combined thermography and isotope scanning in thyroid pathology, *Acta Radiol.*, 15, 656, 1974.
157. **Clark, O. H., Greenspan, F. S., Coggs, G. C., and Goldman, L.**, Evaluation of solitary cold thyroid nodules by echography and thermography, *Am. J. Surg.*, 130, 2065, 1975.

Chapter 13

NEEDLE BIOPSY AND CYTOLOGY IN THE DIAGNOSIS OF THYROIDITIS

Virginia A. LiVolsi and Paul LoGerfo

TABLE OF CONTENTS

I. Introduction 164

II. Needle Biopsy in Thyroiditis 164
    A. Techniques 164
    B. Results 165

III. Aspiration Cytology in Thyroiditis 165
    A. Techniques 166
    B. Results 168

IV. Summary 168

References 169

I. INTRODUCTION

Frable[1] claims that in the evaluation of a thyroid lump, it seems ironic to spend large sums on biochemical, angiographic, ultrasonic, and radionuclide tests to determine its nature, when a specimen obtained directly from the lesion will provide a rapid, relatively cheap, and much more cost-effective diagnosis.

Indeed, the ultimate diagnostic tests in evaluating thyroid pathology is the examination under the microscope of a specimen from the gland. This specimen may be provided by biopsy (open [surgical] or closed) for histologic interpretation or by aspiration for cytologic examination.

Evered[2] has decried the use of closed (needle) biopsy or aspiration cytology in thyroid diagnosis, citing the possibility of tumor dissemination and the inaccuracy of these diagnostic procedures as the two major contraindications. That author's experience seems overshadowed by that of others who strongly endorse both needle biopsy and aspiration cytology for diagnosis.[3-40]

This monograph has discussed the evaluation of thyroiditis and has not been concerned chiefly with thyroid masses. However, both needle biopsy and cytology can offer diagnostic information as well. This chapter will review these techniques and the results obtained by their use in the evaluation of patients with thyroiditis.

II. NEEDLE BIOPSY IN THYROIDITIS

Open (surgical) biopsy under local or general anesthesia is not performed routinely for diagnosis in thyroiditis since improvement in biopsy techniques has replaced the need for formal surgical biopsy.[18] Indeed, the place of surgery in thyroiditis has been relegated to the realm of therapy and not diagnosis (see Chapter 14).

A. Techniques

Closed (needle) biopsy is performed usually as an office procedure on outpatients. Needle biopsy entails obtaining a core of tissue from the thyroid, fixation in formalin or a similar fixative, and processing the specimen for histologic examination.[6-17]

The procedure is performed in individuals with a dominant mass, or in patients suspected of having thyroiditis, to confirm a clinical diagnosis; it is described below:[10,12,15,18]

1. The patient lies supine with the neck overextended by placing a small pillow under the shoulders.[7-9,11,12,16,17]
2. Alcohol wash of the throat is followed by the placing of sterile surgical drapes over the area.
3. Aseptic technique is observed throughout the procedure.[7,10,12,15,18]
4. Following skin infiltration with an anesthetic, a small skin incision is made.
5. The trocar and sheath are introduced through the incision tangential to the trachea toward the thyroid.
6. The trocar is removed and the needle within the sheath is inserted into the gland.
7. While the needle is held, the sheath is rotated until it completely encloses the needle, cutting the tissue.
8. Both sheath and needle are rotated together, completing the detachment of the tissue core from its surroundings. Several samples (up to three) from different areas of the gland may be obtained and are especially useful in evaluating thyroiditis.
9. The sheath and needle are withdrawn together.

10. Firm pressure is applied to the neck for 5 to 10 min to prevent the development of a hematoma.
11. The tissue core is expelled from the needle and quickly fixed.
12. If desired, the needle may be washed in saline and any material so obtained may be examined cytologically (this procedure is useful only in suspected tumors); however, if ultrasonic guidance is utilized to direct the biopsy needle into the suspected lesion, this last step is not required.

B. Results

Adequate tissue is obtained in 74% to 95% of cases; the improvement in obtaining adequate samples reflects experience with the technique.[6-17] The accuracy of diagnosis in thyroiditis may be as high as 90%.[6-17] Indeed, Maloof et al.[10] claim that the diffuse nature of the thyroiditic process and the firmness of the gland so involved ensures adequate sampling. However, the patchy nature of some forms of thyroiditis may produce difficulty in interpretation. Thus Volpe[19] suggests that certain patients with "painless" thyroiditis, who have been considered as examples of Hashimoto's disease on the basis of lymphocytic infiltration of the gland noted on needle biopsies,[19,20] may represent subacute thyroiditis in which the granulomatous areas are not sampled.

Complications of the needle biopsy procedures are rare and, if they occur, are usually minor.[6-17] Thus, bleeding with the development of hematoma, tracheal puncture, or temporary laryngeal nerve injury have been described.[6-18] In the large series from the Massachusetts General Hospital which included over 1000 biopsies, only three hematomas were encountered (a complication rate of 0.3%). No fatalities occurred.[10] In tumors, cancer cell dissemination has been reported rarely.[6,21-23]

Acute thyroiditis—needle biopsy is used in this rare condition only in order to obtain material for smears and cultures to identify the offending organism.[24-26]

Subacute thyroiditis—the finding of characteristic granulomatous inflammation should enable a correct diagnosis in these cases. However, if the sample shows fibrosis and nonspecific inflammation, a misdiagnosis of autoimmune thyroiditis may be rendered.[6,10,12,19]

Hashimoto's thyroiditis—(Figures 1 and 2.) The finding of a lymphoplasmacytic infiltrate and Hurthle cell change should be diagnostic.[6,10,12,15] However, as Boehme et al.[13] have stressed, the pathologist should not examine the specimens or render an opinion without sufficient clinical information available. The possibilities for error if a histologic picture suggests Hashimoto's disease include peritumor (papillary carcinoma) thyroiditis, and malignant lymphoma.[13,14] In fact, Wang et al.[8] underdiagnosed malignant lymphoma in five patients with concomitant Hashimoto's thyroiditis.

Riedel's struma—Biopsy of such a lesion would disclose fibrous tissue. Misinterpretation of such a biopsy as fibrosing Hashimoto's diseases[27] or underdiagnosis of anaplastic carcinoma might occur. Again, the value of specific clinical signs and symptoms in such a case cannot be overestimated.

III. ASPIRATION CYTOLOGY IN THYROIDITIS

Aspiration cytology refers to a procedure in which a small-gauge needle is inserted into a lesion; cells are obtained, which are then spread on a slide, stained, and examined as a cytologic specimen.[22,28] Aspiration cytology differs from exfoliative cytology in that the former is not used as a screening procedure but as a diagnostic tool.[22]

Although widely used in Europe, aspiration cytology has begun to increase in popularity only recently in this country. Reasons for this include (a) the reliance on histologic diagnosis by pathologists in America, (b) relative lack of training in cytopathol-

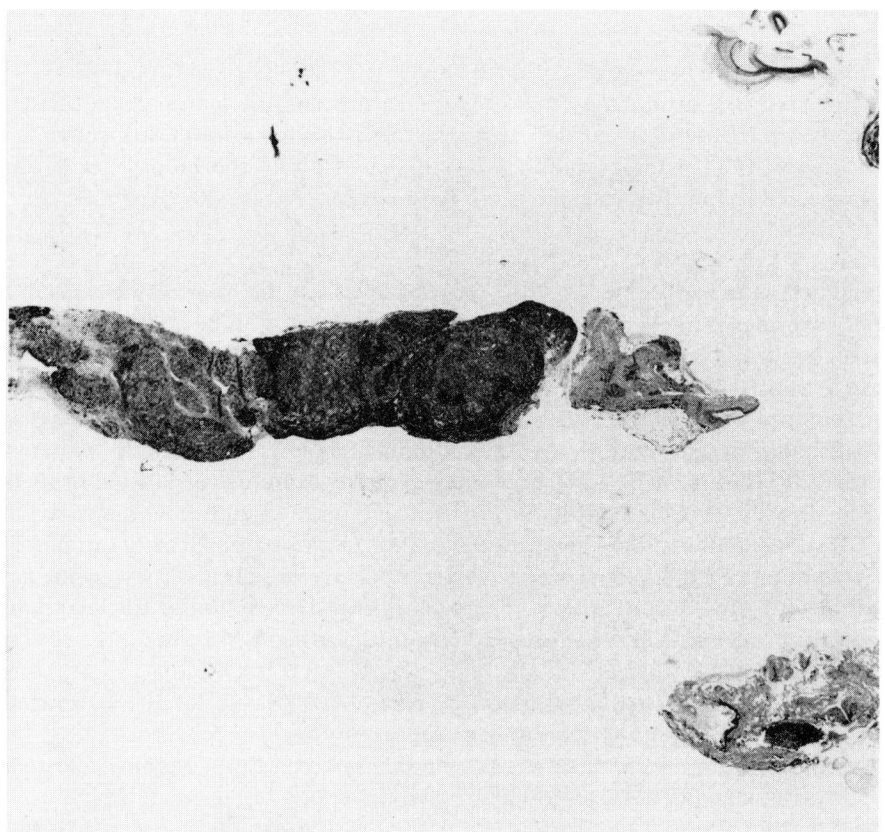

FIGURE 1.. Low power view of needle biopsy core shows dark area which proved to be heavily infiltrated by lymphocytes. (Magnification × 2.)

ogy in the U.S. until recently, and (c) fear of tumor cell dissemination along the needle tract.[21-23] Despite these problems, a few studies in America advocated the value of aspiration cytology.[1,3-5,29-32] In experienced hands, a high degree of accuracy is achieved.[1,22,29-32]

A. Techniques

The procedure for obtaining the sample, resembling that for needle biopsy, is as follows:

1. After positioning the patient, the skin is cleansed.
2. A local anesthetic may be used but is not always needed.
3. Some authors recommend a small skin incision to reduce contamination with epidermal cells.[22,31]
4. A 20 cc. syringe attached to a 22-gauge (or smaller) needle is utilized.
5. The needle is inserted into the thyroid, suction is applied and negative pressure is maintained by keeping the plunger retracted. When aspiration is completed, the pressure in the syringe is allowed to equalize by releasing the plunger; then the needle is withdrawn.
6. Two or more punctures into different areas may be required to obtain adequate material.

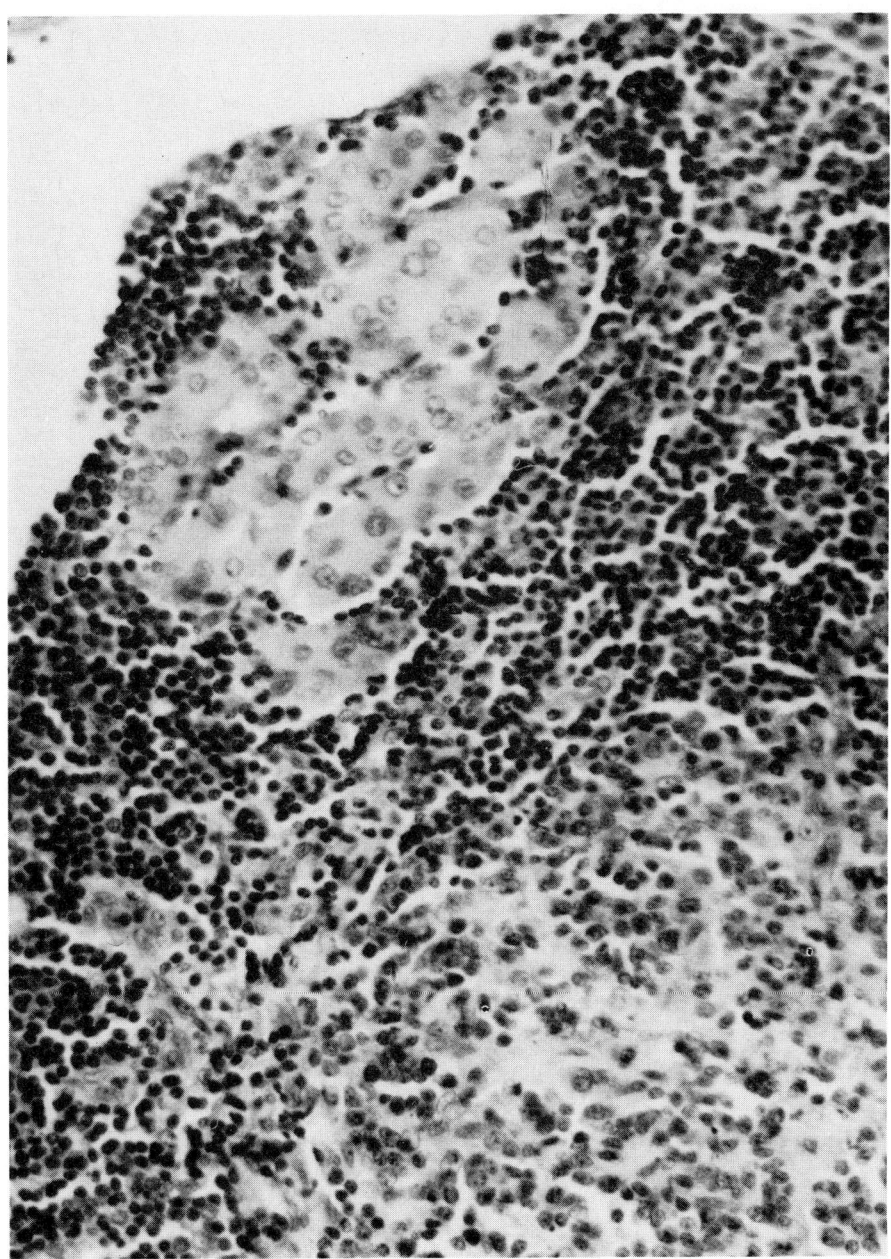

FIGURE 2.. Same case as Figure 1, showing dark area. Lymphocytes, plasma cells and Hurthle cells lining small follicles are seen. A germinal center is represented by the light area at the lower right. Case of Hashimoto's thyroiditis. (Magnification × 300.)

7. After withdrawal, the aspirated material retained in the needle is expressed as droplets onto a clean glass slide and smears are made.
8. Fixation in alcohol or air drying is followed by staining with any of a variety of techniques (Papanicolaou stain, hematoxylin-eosin, May-Grunwald-Giemsa).[22,28,31,33-48]

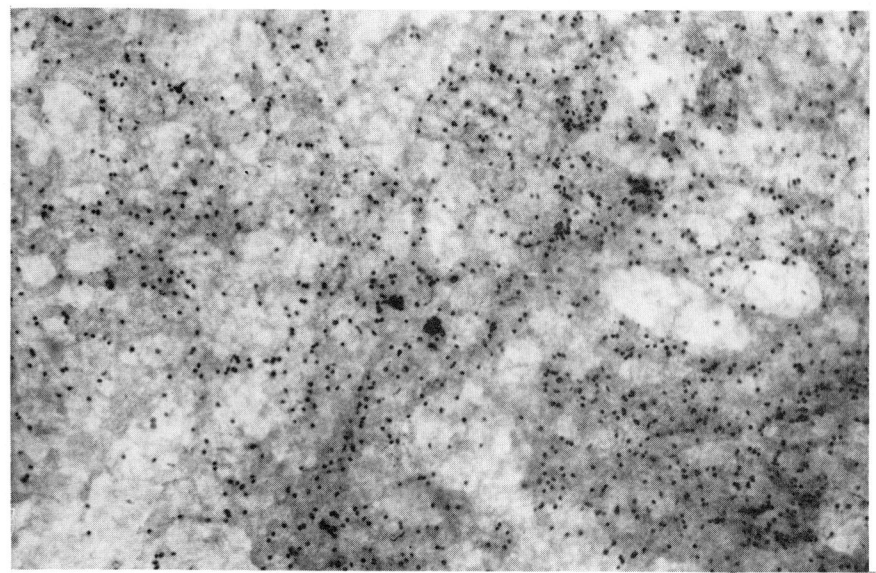

FIGURE 3.. Aspiration cytology smear of goiter shows moderate inflammatory background and a few larger darker cells in the center. (Magnification × 100.)

B. Results

When rapid fixation is effected, preservation of cellular detail is excellent. Accuracy in the range of 90 to 95% has been claimed for thyroid lesions.[33-48] These include inflammatory disorders of the thyroid, although it must be recognized that thyroid cytology has found most use in tumor diagnosis.[43]

Complications are rare; a small hematoma may occur. Because of the rich vascular supply of the gland, bleeding may be a problem.[31] This is noted most often in Graves' disease.[18,31] In tumor work, dissemination of cancer cells has not been found with aspiration cytology.[22]

In thyroiditis, the cellular sample will show (a) granulocytes and debris in acute thyroiditis,[41,43] (b) many macrophages, giant cells, and degenerative changes in follicular epithelium in subacute disease,[41,43] and (c) a lymphoplasmatic infiltrate and Hurthle cells in Hashimoto's disease[16,17,41,43,46] (Figures 3 and 4). Riedel's struma, because of its fibrotic nature, does not lend itself to diagnosis by this technique.[27]

IV. SUMMARY

In conclusion, the role of needle biopsy in thyroiditis is to prove and confirm a diagnosis suspected by symptoms or laboratory data, and to decrease the need for formal surgery with its attendant risks. The diagnostic accuracy appears excellent (90%) in experienced hands, especially if a team approach is used (clinician-surgeon-pathologist). Complications are few and minor. The role of aspiration cytology seems small in the thyroiditides, although this technique has proven extremely useful in tumor diagnosis.

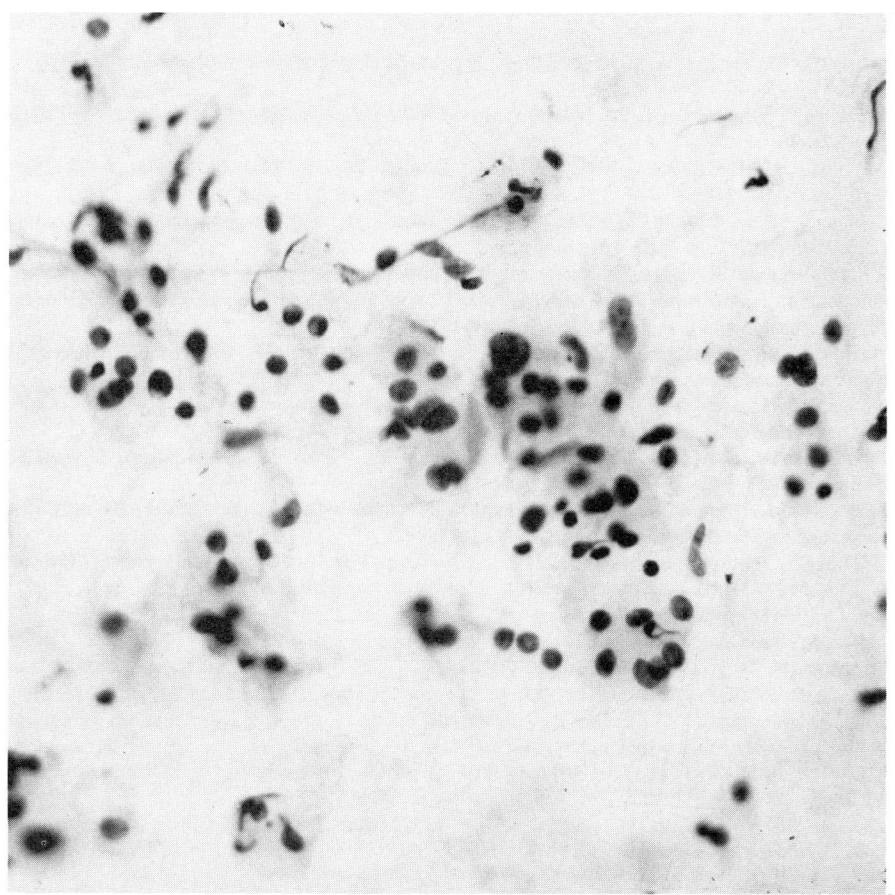

FIGURE 4.. At higher power, group of epithelial cells demonstrate oxyphilia of the cytoplasm and focal nuclear enlargement, consistent with Hashimoto's disease. (Magnification × 250.)

REFERENCES

1. **Frable, W. J.**, Thin-needle aspiration biopsy. A personal experience with 460 cases, *Am. J. Clin. Pathol.*, 65, 168, 1976.
2. **Evered, D.**, Diseases of the thyroid gland, *Clin. Endocrinol. Metab.*, 3, 425, 1974.
3. **Guthrie, C. G.**, Gland puncture as a diagnostic measure, *Johns Hopkins Med. J.*, 366, 269, 1921.
4. **Martin, H. E. and Ellis, F. G.**, Aspiration biopsy, *Surg. Gynecol. Obstet.*, 59, 579, 1934.
5. **Stewart F. W.**, The diagnosis of tumors by aspiration, Am. J. Pathol., 9 (Suppl.), 801, 1933.
6. **Crile, G. and Hazard, J. B.**, Classification of thyroiditis with special reference to the use of needle biopsy, *J. Clin. Endocrinol. Metab.*, 11, 1123, 1951.

7. Crile, G. and Hawk, W. A., Aspiration biopsy of thyroid nodules, *Surg. Gynecol. Obstet.*, 136, 241, 1973.
8. Wang, C. A., Vickery, A. L., and Maloof, F., Needle biopsy of the thyroid, *Surg. Gynecol. Obstet.*, 143, 365, 1976.
9. Esselstyn, C. B. and Crile, G., Needle aspiration and needle biopsy of the thyroid, *World J. Surg.*, 3, 321, 1978.
10. Maloof, F., Wang, C. A., and Vickery, A. L., Nontoxic goiter-diffuse or nodular, *Med. Clin. North Am.*, 59, 1221, 1975.
11. Sachdeva, H. S., Wig, J. D., Kanta, C., and Dutta, B. N., High speed pneumatic drill for biopsy of thyroid lesions, *Arch. Surg.*, 108, 744, 1974.
12. Hamlin, E. and Vickery, A. L. Needle biopsy of the thyroid gland, *N. Engl. J. Med.*, 254, 742, 1956.
13. Boehme, K. J., Winship, T., Lindsay, S., and Kypridakis, G., An evaluation of needle biopsy of the thyroid gland, *Surg. Gynecol. Obstet.*, 119, 831, 1964.
14. Beahrs, O. H., Woolner, L. B., Einhorn, S., and McConahey, W. M., Needle biopsy of thyroid gland and management of lymphocytic thyroiditis, *Surg. Gynecol. Obstet.*, 114, 636, 1962.
15. Vickery, A. L. and Hamlin, E., Struma lymphomatosa (Hashimoto's thyroiditis). Observations on repeated biopsies in sixteen patients, *N. Engl. J. Med.*, 264, 226, 1961.
16. Hamburger, J. I., Miller, J. M., and Kini, S. R., *Clinicopathologic Evaluation of Thyroid Nodules Handbook and Atlas*, J. Hamburger, Detroit, 1979.
17. Miller, J. M., Hamburger, J. I., and Kini, S., Diagnosis of thyroid nodules. Use of fine-needle aspiration and needle biopsy, *JAMA*, 241, 481, 1979.
18. Refetoff, S., Thyroid function tests, in *Endocrinology*, Vol. 1, deGroot, L. J., Cahill, G. F., Martin, L., Nelson, D. H., Odell, W. D., Potts, J. T., Steinberger, E., and Winegrad, A. I., Eds., Grune and Stratton, New York, 1979, 387.
19. Volpe, R., Subacute (de Quervain's) thyroiditis, *Clin. Endocrinol. Metab.*, 8, 81, 1979.
20. Gluck, F. B., Nusynowitz, M. L., and Plymate, S., Chronic lymphocytic thyroiditis, thyrotoxicosis and low radioactive iodine uptake, *N. Engl. J. Med.*, 293, 624, 1975.
21. Enzgell, U., Esposti, P. L., Rubio, C., Sigurdson, A., and Zajicek, J., Investigation on tumor spread in connection with aspiration biopsy, *Acta Radiol.*, 10, 385, 1971.
22. Zajicek, J., *Aspiration Biopsy Cytology, Part I. Cytology of Supradiaphragmatic Organs*, S. Karger, Basel, 1974.
23. Gibbons, R. P., Bush, W. H., and Burnett, L. L., Needle tract seeding following aspiration of renal cell carcinoma, *J. Urol.*, 118, 865, 1977.
24. Hurley, J. R., Thyroiditis, *Disease-a-Month*, December, 1977.
25. Kohler, P. O., Floyd, W. L., and Wynn, J., Indications for thyroid needle biopsy: Suppurative thyroiditis, *South. Med. J.*, 59, 182, 1966.
26. Adler, M. E., Jordan, G., and Walter, R. M., Acute suppurative thyroiditis, *West. J. Med.*, 128, 165, 1978.
27. Katsikas, D., Shorthouse, A. J., and Taylor, S., Riedel's thyroiditis, *Br. J. Surg.*, 63, 929, 1976.
28. Soderstrom, N., *Fine Needle Aspiration Biopsy*, Almquist and Wiksells, Stockholm, 1966.
29. Godwin, J. T., Cytologic diagnosis of aspiration biopsies of solid or cystic tumors, *Acta Cytol.*, 8, 206, 1964.
30. Hajdu, S. E. and Melamed, H. R., The diagnostic value of aspiration smears, *Am. J. Clin. Pathol.*, 59, 350, 1973.
31. Koss, L. G., *Diagnostic Cytology and Its Histopathologic Basis*, J. B. Lippincott, Philadelphia, 1979.
32. Kline, T. S. and Neal, H. S., Needle aspiration biopsy: A critical appraisal, *JAMA*, 239, 36, 1978.
33. Soderstrom, N., Aspiration biopsy puncture of goiters for aspiration biopsy, *Acta Med. Scand.*, 144, 237, 1952.
34. Einhorn, J. and Franzen, S., Fine needle biopsy in the diagnosis of thyroid disease, *Acta Radiol.*, 58, 321, 1962.
35. Nilsson, L. R. and Persson, P. S., Cytological aspiration biopsy in adolescent goitre, *Acta Paediatr. Scand.*, 53, 333, 1964.
36. Ofstad, E., Baardsen, A., and Refsum, S. B., Cylinder-biopsies in thyroid disorders, *Acta Chir. Scand.*, 139, 148, 1973.
37. Jensen, F. and Rasmussen, S. N., The treatment of thyroid cysts by ultrasonically guided fine needle aspiration, *Acta Chir. Scand.*, 142, 209, 1976.
38. Crockford, P. M. and Bain, G. O., Fine needle aspiration biopsy of the thyroid, *Can. Med. Assoc. J.*, 110, 1029, 1974.
39. Kolendorf, K., Hansen J. B., Engberg, L., Friis, T., and Lindenberg, J., Fine needle and open biopsy in thyroid disorders, *Acta Chir. Scand.*, 141, 20, 1975.

40. **Walfish, P. G., Hazani, E., Strawbridge, H. T. G., Miskin, M., and Rosen, I. B.**, A prospective study of combined ultrasonography and needle aspiration biopsy in the assessment of the hypofunctioning thyroid nodule, *Surgery,* 82, 474, 1977.
41. **Lowhagen, T., Granberg, P. O., Lundell, G., Skinnari, P., Sundblad, R., and Willems, J. S.**, Aspiration biopsy cytology (ABC) in nodules of the thyroid gland suspected to be malignant, *Surg. Clin. North Am.,* 59, 3, 1979.
42. **Lowhagen, T. and Sprenger, E.**, Cytologic presentation of thyroid tumors in aspiration biopsy smears, *Acta Cytol.,* 18, 192, 1974.
43. **Persson, P. S.**, Cytodiagnosis of thyroiditis, *Acta Med. Scand. Suppl.,* 483, 7, 1967.
44. **Schnurer, L. B. and Widstrom, A.**, Fine needle biopsy of the thyroid gland: A cytohistological comparison in cases of goiter, *Ann. Otol. Rhinol. Laryngol.,* 87, 224, 1978.
45. **Bonneau, H.**, Thyroid cytological diagnosis, *Int. Coll. Tumor Thyroid Gland,* Marseilles, 1964, S. Karger, Basel, 1966, 126.
46. **Friedman, M., Shimaoka, K., and Getaz, P.**, Needle aspiration of 310 thyroid lesions, *Acta Cytol.,* 23, 194, 1979.
47. **Gershengorn, M. C., McClung, M. R., Chu, E. W., Hanson, T. A. S., Weintraub, B. D., and Robbins, J.**, Fine needle aspiration cytology in the preoperative diagnosis of thyroid nodules, *Ann. Intern. Med.,* 87, 265, 1977.
48. **Walfish, P. G., Hazani, E., Strawbridge, H. T. G., Miskin, M., and Rosen, I. B.**, Combined ultrasound and needle aspiration cytology in the assessment and management of hypofunctioning thyroid nodules, *Ann. Intern., Med.,* 87, 270, 1977.

Chapter 14

SURGICAL MANAGEMENT OF THYROIDITIS

Carey Dolgin and Paul LoGerfo

TABLE OF CONTENTS

I.	Introduction	174
II.	Surgery in Acute Thyroiditis	174
III.	Surgery in Subacute Thyroiditis	174
VI.	Surgery in Hashimoto's Thyroiditis	175
	A. Pressure Symptoms	175
	B. Neck Pain	175
	C. Cosmetic Deformity	175
	D. Thyroid Mass	175
	E. Surgical Management	176
V.	Surgery in Riedel's Struma	176
VI.	Summary	177
References		177

I. INTRODUCTION

The place of surgery in patients with thyroiditis is limited. Clinical features, laboratory results, aspiration cytology, and needle biopsy will usually render a diagnosis. Therapeutic management centers on pharmacologic means (antibiotics, analgesics, steroids, and hormone replacement for acute, subacute, and chronic thyroiditis, respectively). However, some cases of thyroiditis require surgical intervention. Reasons for this are twofold: diagnostic and therapeutic.[1-4] These include:

1. Diagnostic
    (a) Mass lesions suspicious for carcinoma
2. Therapeutic
    (a) Tracheal compression
    (b) The presence of suppuration
    (c) Toxicity not controlled by medications
    (d) Cosmetic deformity

This chapter will briefly summarize the role of surgery in the four major types of thyroiditis. (The reader is referred to other works for the techniques of thyroid surgery.[5,6])

II. SURGERY IN ACUTE THYROIDITIS

This disorder represents a bacterial infection of the thyroid which may be superimposed upon a previously normal gland or on a nodular goiter. The latter tends to suppurate more often.[7-10]

As discussed in Chapter 2, the organisms cultured most often in acute thyroiditis include *Staphylococcus, Streptococcus* and *Pneumococcus*.[11,12] Needle biopsy can obtain diagnostic material. Following appropriate cultures and identification of the offending organism, antibiotic therapy will produce a cure in the overwhelming majority of patients.[1,7,8,11,12]

Surgical therapy for acute thyroiditis is limited to those patients who do not respond to antibiotics. Although Colcock[4] recommended waiting for fluctuation to occur, Volpe[7] and Thomas[1] agreed that prompt intervention is necessary if the infection is not controlled by antimicrobial drugs.

If the infection has remained confined to the thyroid (intracapsular), lobectomy is curative.[1,7] It is advisable to remove the abscess cavity intact. Acute suppurative thyroiditis with periglandular involvement requires drainage of pus.[1,7] In each instance, appropriate systemic antibiotic therapy must be maintained. Recovery is more rapid in the confined infections, but in general, all patients so treated fare well.[1,7]

III. SURGERY IN SUBACUTE THYROIDITIS

Subacute thyroiditis (granulomatous thyroiditis, giant cell thyroiditis) is a self-limiting inflammation of the thyroid gland, possibly of viral origin.[13,14] The disease responds to symptomatic treatment for pain with aspirin and/or corticosteroids. The characteristic history and course make surgical intervention unnecessary and unwarranted (see Chapter 4). However, in those cases wherein pain is minimal or absent, or in which a dominant mass is recognized raising the suspicion of a neoplasm, surgery may be undertaken.[1,3,14-16] Needle biopsy may suffice to obtain a diagnosis.[4]

Rarely, a rapidly growing, undifferentiated thyroid carcinoma presents as a painful mass simulating clinically and chemically subacute thyroiditis.[17] Surgery may be required to obtain a correct diagnosis in such a case.[1]

IV. SURGERY IN HASHIMOTO'S THYROIDITIS

Hashimoto's thyroiditis is the most common form of chronic thyroiditis, seen primarily in women and thought to be of autoimmune origin. The thyroid gland is diffusely enlarged, usually lobulated.

In addition to symptoms of hypothyroidism, the presence of a goiter may produce pressure symptoms, neck discomfort, or dysphagia.[8,14,18] Occasionally, localized nodules of thyroiditis may simulate tumors[4,18] (see also Chapters 6 and 7).

Over the past 20 yr, the frequency of diagnostic neck exploration for thyroiditis has decreased as our ability to diagnose the disease with less invasive measures, such as thyroid autoantibodies and needle biopsy, has improved. As thyroid hormone and analgesic therapy alleviate the symptoms in the majority of the patients, surgery for Hashimoto's thyroiditis has been performed on patients with intractable symptoms unresponsive to medical therapy. Presently, the indications for neck exploration and thyroidectomy in chronic thyroiditis include: pressure symptoms, neck pain, cosmetic deformity, and nonresolving thyroid mass.

A. Pressure Symptoms

Symptoms secondary to the effects of pressure from an enlarged thyroid and inflammation include hoarseness, dyspnea, stridor, dysphagia, and persistent cough. (We recently treated a patient who required surgery because of a superior vena caval syndrome, secondary to Hashimoto's disease in a substernal thyroid.)

Hashimoto's thyroiditis progresses with chronic inflammatory changes, leading to the replacement of epithelium with thickened scar. The incidence of pressure symptoms in patients with thyroiditis undergoing neck exploration has been noted between 46 to 49%.[11]

B. Neck Pain[15]

Neck pain includes pain over the area of the thyroid gland as well as symptoms referred to the jaw and chest. These complaints are caused by both active inflammatory changes and scar formation with pulling on the thyroid and surrounding structures. Involvement of the recurrent laryngeal nerves is rare.

C. Cosmetic Deformity[14]

Although the thyroid gland usually shrinks in size after institution of thyroid hormone therapy, intraparenchymal and capsular fibrosis limits the extent to which involution can take place. Persistent unsightly thyroid masses should be excised.

D. Thyroid Mass[14,15,18]

Hashimoto's thyroiditis involves the whole gland, but the extent of inflammation and reaction may vary in different parts of the gland. Thus, a nodule may be appreciated on examination. Neck exploration can be avoided in most cases since needle biopsy will often demonstrate characteristic histologic changes. In cases where fibrosis precludes adequate interpretation of the specimen, or the mass persists or enlarges despite thyroid suppression, neck exploration and thyroidectomy are indicated.

An association of Hashimoto's thyroiditis with thyroid carcinoma has been documented in the literature. In groups of patients undergoing thyroidectomy for either a diagnosis of thyroiditis or evaluation of a thyroid mass, the incidence of thyroid carcinoma associated with thyroiditis ranges between 3 and 22.4%.[19-29]

Most thyroidectomies in the above series were performed on patients with thyroiditis and an associated neck mass or local symptoms in the neck. This population does not exemplify the larger group of patients without masses or localized findings; thus the incidences of associated carcinoma quoted above may not represent the true incidence in the total population of patients with Hashimoto's thyroiditis. Surgical intervention should be limited to patients with findings on examination or thyroid scan consistent with an unresolving thyroid mass.

E. Surgical Management

The surgical procedure indicated in the patient with Hashimoto's thyroiditis depends on the appearance of the thyroid gland at the time of surgery. Patients with local symptoms and exaggerated lobulation of the thyroid without a discrete mass require bilateral partial thyroidectomies and removal of the isthmus, releasing the thyroid gland from the trachea and alleviating pressure symptoms.

Patients with Hashimoto's thyroiditis undergoing operation for clinical nodules should receive the appropriate operation based on the character of the nodule present, irrespective of the presence of thyroiditis. Unilateral nodules are treated with ipsilateral total lobectomy and isthmusectomy. When a nodule of the isthmus is noted, isthmusectomy and bilateral partial thyroidectomy should be performed. Bilateral thyroid nodules are treated by bilateral subtotal thyroidectomies and isthmusectomy. If carcinoma is found, total thyroidectomy is indicated.

Postoperative management includes thyroid hormone replacement to prevent recurrence of thyroid enlargement and nodule formation in the remaining gland. Block et al.[29] has reported a 21% incidence (20 of 99) of recurrent thyroid enlargement or masses after thyroidectomy for Hashimoto's thyroiditis. All 20 patients either failed to continue hormone treatment or were never started on a therapeutic regimen of thyroid hormone. Three of the 20 patients underwent reoperation and were noted to have recurrent chronic lymphocytic thyroiditis.

Hashimoto's thyroiditis has been associated with malignant lymphoma of the thyroid gland[30,31] (see Chapters 7 and 10). Hence, any enlarging mass in a patient with this form of thyroiditis represents an indication for surgery, since needle biopsy may provide difficulties in distinguishing the lymphocytic infiltrate of the underlying disease from the lymphoid neoplasm.

V. SURGERY IN RIEDEL'S STRUMA

Riedel's struma is a chronic inflammatory disease of unknown etiology, involving one or both lobes of the thyroid, trachea, surrounding fascia, nerves, and blood vessels[32] (see Chapter 11). No association between this disease and either acute thyroiditis or Hashimoto's struma has been identified; indeed it may represent a disorder of connective tissue and not a thyroiditis. The intense, chronic inflammation produced eventually causes fibrosis and tracheal constriction, and symptoms of neck pain, hoarseness, stridor, and dysphagia. Surgery is undertaken primarily to relieve tracheal compression.

When the disease is unilateral, lobectomy, isthmusectomy, and partial contralateral thyroidectomy are indicated. Bilateral disease is usually associated with thick scarring of the overlying fascia and strap muscles. Lahey[33] has described a technique for thyroidectomy for Riedel's struma. First, isthmusectomy and partial bilateral thyroidectomy are performed. Next, the strap muscles are sutured to the lateral wall of the trachea. Finally, the inferior aspect of the sternocleidomastoid muscles are apposed in the area of the thyroid to prevent the thyroid gland from becoming adherent to skin.

This maneuver prevents a new bridge of fibrosis from developing across the thin strap muscles, and prevents recurrence.

VI. SUMMARY

This chapter has reviewed the indications for surgery in the major forms of thyroiditis. Surgery is not primary therapy in any, although it may be life saving when suppuration occurs in acute thyroiditis, or for relief of tracheal compression in Riedel's disease.

The role of surgery in subacute and chronic lymphocytic thyroiditis (Hashimoto's) remains confined to those cases in which mass effect is a problem or in which there is strong clinical suspicion of a neoplasm.

REFERENCES

1. **Thomas, C. G.**, Surgery of the thyroid, *Med. Clin. North Am.,* 59, 1247, 1975.
2. **Linden, M. C. and Clark, J. H.,** Indications for surgery in thyroiditis, *Am. J. Surg.,* 118, 829, 1969.
3. **Colcock, B. P. and Pena, O.**, Diagnosis and treatment of thyroiditis, *Postgrad. Med.,* 44, 83, 1968.
4. **Colcock, B. P.**, Thyroiditis, in *Surgery of the Thyroid Gland,* Sedgwick, C. E., Ed., W. B. Saunders, Philadelphia, 1974, 126.
5. **Perzik, S. L.**, *Surgery in Thyroid Disease,* Stratton Book Co., New York, 1976.
6. **Sedgwick, C. E.**, Surgical techniques, in *Surgery of the Thyroid Gland,* Sedgwick, C. E., Ed., W. B. Saunders, Philadelphia, 1974, 170.
7. **Volpe, R.,** Acute suppurative thyroiditis, in *The Thyroid,* Werner, S. C. and Ingbar, S. H., Eds., Harper and Row, New York, 1971, 849.
8. **Volpe, R.,** Etiology, pathology and clinical aspects of thyroiditis, Part 2, *Pathol. Annu.,* 13, 399, 1978.
9. **Mann, C. H.**, Thyroid abscess in a 3½ year old child, *Arch. Otolaryngol.,* 103, 299, 1977.
10. **Montgomery, G. H.**, Acute thyroiditis progressing to suppuration, *J. Med. Assoc. Ala.,* 30, 497, 1961.
11. **Hendrick, J. W.**, Diagnosis and treatment of thyroiditis, *Ann. Surg.,* 144, 176, 1956.
12. **Altermeir, W. A.**, Acute pyogenic thyroiditis, *Arch. Surg.,* 61, 76, 1950.
13. **Volpe, R.,** Subacute (de Quervain's) thyroiditis, *Clin. Endocrinol. Metab.,* 8, 81, 1979.
14. **Bastenie, P. A., Bonnyms, M., and Neve, P.**, Subacute and chronic granulomatous thyroiditis, in *Thyroiditis and Thyroid Function, Clinical, Morphological and Physiopathological Studies,* Bastenie, P. A. and Ermans, A. M., Eds., Pergamon Press, Oxford, 1972, 69.
15. **Crile, G.**, Thyroiditis, *Ann. Surg.,* 127, 640, 1948.
16. **Harland, W. A. and Frantz, V. K.**, Clinicopathologic study of 261 surgical cases of so-called thyroiditis, *J. Clin. Endocrinol.,* 16, 1433, 1956.
17. **Rosen, F., Row, V. V., Volpe, R., and Erzin, C.**, Anaplastic carcinoma of the thyroid with abnormal circulating iodoproteins: A case simulating subacute thyroiditis, *Can. Med. Assoc. J.,* 95, 1039, 1966.
18. **Katz, S. M. and Vickery, A. L.**, The fibrosing variant of Hashimoto's thyroiditis, *Hum. Pathol.,* 5, 161, 1974.
19. **Dailey, M., Lindsay, S., and Skahen, R.**, The relation of thyroid neoplasm to Hashimoto's disease of the thyroid gland, *Arch. Surg.,* 70, 291, 1955.
20. **Lindsay, S., Dailey, M. E., Friedlander, J., Yee, G., and Soley, M. H.**, Chronic thyroiditis: Clinical and pathologic study of 354 patients, *J. Clin. Endocrinol.,* 12, 1578, 1952.
21. **Hirabayashi, R. N. and Lindsay, S.**, The relation of thyroid carcinoma and chronic thyroiditis, *Surg. Gynecol. Obstet.,* 121, 243, 1965.
22. **Blackburn, G. and O'Gorman, P.**, Hashimoto's disease, *Guy's Hosp. Rep. London,* 110, 379, 1961.

23. O'Hara, G. L., MacDonald, I., and Weber, R. A., Carcinoma of the thyroid gland: A review of 106 cases, *Calif. Med.,* 86, 16, 1957.
24. Pollock, W. F. and Sprorz, D. H., Jr., Surgical aspects of thyroiditis, *Arch. Surg.,* 80, 720, 1960.
25. Peterson, C. A. and Shilder, F. P., Lymphocyte thyroiditis in 757 thyroid operations, *Am. J. Surg.,* 94, 223, 1957.
26. Schlicke, C. P., Hill, J. E., and Schultz, G. F., Carcinoma in chronic thyroiditis, *Surg. Gynecol. Obstet.,* 111, 552, 1960.
27. Woolner, L. B. McConahey, W. M., and Beahrs, D. H., Struma lymphomatosa (Hashimoto's thyroiditis) and related thyroid disorders, *J. Clin. Endocrinol.,* 19, 53, 1959.
28. Crile, G. J. and Hazard, J. B., Incidence of cancer in struma lymphomatosa, *Surg. Gynecol. Obstet.,* 115, 101, 1962.
29. Block, M. A., Horn, R. C., and Miller, J. M., Unilateral thyroid nodules with lymphocytic thyroiditis, *Arch. Surg.,* 87, 280, 1963.
30. Woolner, L. B., McConahey, W. M., Beahrs, O. H., and Black, B. M., Primary malignant lymphoma of the thyroid, *Am. J. Surg.,* 111, 502, 1966.
31. Lindsay, S. and Dailey, M. E., Malignant lymphoma of the thyroid gland and its relationship to Hashimoto's disease: A clinical and pathological study of 8 cases, *J. Clin. Endocrinol.,* 15, 1332, 1955.
32. Woolner, L. B., McConahey, W. M., and Beahrs, O. H., Invasive fibrous thyroiditis (Riedel's struma), *J. Clin. Endocrinol.,* 17, 201, 1957.
33. Lahey, F. H., Thyroiditis, *Surg. Gynecol. Obstet.,* 60, 969, 1934.

Chapter 15

EXPERIMENTAL THYROIDITIS: A REVIEW

Thomas A. Colacchio

TABLE OF CONTENTS

I. Introduction 180

II. Experimental Models 181
    A. Spontaneous Autoimmune Thyroiditis (SAT) 181
        1. Chickens 181
        2. Rats 182
        3. Mice 183
        4. Beagles 183
        5. Monkeys 184
    B. Experimental Autoimmune Thyroiditis (EAT) 184
        1. Rabbits 184
        2. Guinea Pigs 185
        3. Mice 185
        4. Rats 186
        5. Monkeys 186

III. Summary: Correlation with Human Disease 187

References 187

I. INTRODUCTION

The study of human disease is often hampered because true experimental investigation in human subjects is often unjustified and may be dangerous. Consequently, we are limited to the observation of disease processes as they present and progress in our patients. Certain immunologic disorders (the primary deficiency diseases) provide "experiments of nature" and allow insight into pathogenetic mechanisms,[1] but these occur rarely.

"Experimental models", in which a particular disease has been induced, do simulate the human counterpart. Although much can be learned from these studies, their artificial (induced) nature imparts a certain unreliability and lack of true correlation. Occasionally, there occur spontaneously in animals, diseases which closely mimic human disorders; these may provide greater insight into pathogenetic mechanisms.

In this review, I will describe some of the current investigations with animal models of thyroiditis, both spontaneous and induced, and compare and contrast these with human autoimmune thyroiditis (Hashimoto's disease).

Hashimoto's thyroiditis, an autoimmune disease of uncertain etiology, has been discussed in Chapters 6 and 7. It represents a specific clinicopathologic spectrum. Histologically, it is characterized by a diffuse lymphocytic infiltration of the thyroid, fibrosis, follicular atrophy, and an eosinophilic change of the follicular epithelium. However, the range and intensity of clinical and pathologic changes are so broad as to raise the question: is it one disease or many grouped under one inclusive term? Thus, some patients with Hashimoto's disease manifest symptoms of hyperthyroidism; some are euthyroid, and a considerable number are hypothyroid.[2] The pathologic alterations also vary widely, from moderate lymphoplasmacytic infiltrate to an exaggerated form that simulates malignant lymphoma. A spectrum of atrophy and fibrosis also exists: thus, fibrosing Hashimoto's thyroiditis produces a large goiter, whereas the gland in idiopathic myxedema is so small as to barely recognizable. The role of host response in these conditions must also be taken into account in explaining the final result.

Yet, the degree of overlap and similarity have led to the inclusion of these disorders as a spectrum of autoimmune thyroiditis. Over the past few years, attempts to define the mechanism of injury, i.e., the loss of self-tolerance, have led to several different theories of pathogenesis. Evidence for cell-mediated immunity in this disorder has been suggested since, using various techniques, activity of sensitized T-lymphocytes in affected patients can be detected.[3] In addition, a variety of circulating autoantibodies against thyroglobulin, a colloid component other than thyroglobulin, and an antinuclear antibody are found in high titer in patients with autoimmune thyroiditis.[4] Indeed, both humoral and cell-mediated immunity derangements may be needed to produce the parenchymal thyroid damage.[3]

Debate continues, however, over the mechanism of production of autoimmunity. Some suggest viral infection may lead to antigenic change or thyroid injury with consequent antigen release. Genetic predilection, sex ratio, and the coexistence of other autoimmune disease require explanation and are, as yet, poorly understood. Volpe[2] suggests that an inherited defect in the suppression of a specific T-cell clone directed against normal self-constituents may be present. If this clone appeared by random mutation, it could not be controlled; when stimulated by contact with its complementary antigen, it could lead to its own replication and then sensitization of B-lymphocytes.

Because autoimmune thyroiditis represents a spectrum of disease in man, and because of the many unanswered (and as yet unasked) questions concerning this disorder, no satisfactory model which simulates this condition entirely has been identified. I shall review the common, currently available animal models of autoimmune thyroiditis and compare them with the human disease.

II. EXPERIMENTAL MODELS

Two major types of animal models for thyroiditis have been described: spontaneous and experimental (or induced).

A. Spontaneous Autoimmune Thyroiditis (SAT)

Two varieties of spontaneous thyroiditis have been described: that occurring in certain species without immunologic or other manipulation, and thyroiditis arising in hosts whose immune systems have been altered in general, but not specifically directed at the thyroid. Five animal species manifesting "spontaneous" thyroiditis have been described; these are summarized below.

1. Chickens

vanTienhoven and Cole[5] noted that about 1% of chickens of the white leghorn strain were clinically hypothyroid. These birds demonstrated large fat deposits, small dry combs, brittle bones, and small abnormal thyroids. These abnormalities resembled those seen in thyroidectomized chicks and were reversed by thyroxine.[5,6] Since this initial description in 1962,[5] inbreeding has produced the Obese Strain (OS) of white leghorn; about 90% of these birds are hypothyroid (both male and female) and exhibit an hereditary spontaneous autoimmune thyroiditis which resembles Hashimoto's disease in man.[6,7]

Numerous studies of these animals have disclosed several significant findings. These birds are truly hypothyroid, exhibit slow maturation, infertility, marked lipemia, elevated thyroid-stimulating hormone, and nearly absent thyroid hormones.[5,6,8,9] Abnormalities in thyroid function are identified as early as 2 weeks of age.[10,11]

Pathologically, the thyroids in these birds show extensive lymphocytic infiltration associated with plasma cells and the formation of germinal centers. At 1 to 5 weeks of age, the lymphoid infiltrate is found perivascularly.[6,9,12] The follicles are small and deformed. The lesion becomes more severe with more intense cellular infiltration, follicular atrophy, and the development of fibrosis. Almost 100% of the animals show the thyroiditis by 7 to 15 weeks.[6,9,12]

Ultrastructurally, the thyroids of 1-week-old chicks show epithelial cell degeneration without the participation of lymphocytes.[13] When lymphocytes and plasma cells invade, they closely adhere to degenerating follicles and infiltrate between epithelial elements. The basement membrane disintegrates and, following follicular necrosis, colloid leaks out into surrounding tissue. An increase in cellular infiltration and the development of germinal centers ensues.[8,13] Viral particles have been identified in affected animals by some[13] but not all investigators.[14]

After 7 weeks of age, ultrastructural studies disclose the presence of electron-dense deposits in the follicular basement membrane.[15] These presumed antigen-antibody complexes are not identified in very young chicks nor in normal white leghorn birds.[15] Hurthle cells have not been identified by light or electron microscopy in these thyroids.[8] The bursal basement membrane is thickened also in affected animals; no differences in lymphoid cell morphology have been identified.[9]

Circulating antibodies to thyroglobulin and thyroid extract can be demonstrated in 65% of OS chickens.[7,12,16,17] In vivo binding of antibodies to OS colloid can be identified by direct immunofluorescence, a characteristic shared by human disease but not by other animal models.[18,19]

In an attempt to define the pathogenesis of this disease, Wick et al.[6] have manipulated these animals in varied ways. Neonatal bursectomy (equivalent to B-cell ablation) produced a marked decrease in severity and incidence of the thyroiditis, whereas, neonatal thymectomy (T-cell ablation) resulted in more severe SAT. Further studies have shown that reconstitution of B-cell function led to total restoration of the severity of SAT. These experiments indicate that the OS form of SAT represents a B-cell dependent entity (induced thyroiditis, in contrast, is T-cell dependent).[7,9,20-25] Recently Luster et al.[26,27] have noted a selective IgA deficiency in affected animals; the significance of this finding remains unclear.

Normal leghorn chicks, if injected with thyroglobulin, develop an autoimmune thyroiditis, i.e., an experimental (induced) type of lesion.[9,28] In addition, in both normal and OS chickens, injection of thyroglobulin into foot-web or mattle disclosed a delayed-type hypersensitivity reaction which developed only after the thyroid pathology was established.[28]

Based upon these data and the study of experimental autoimmune encephalitis (EAE) in normal and OS chickens (in normal, bursectomized, and thymectomized states), Wick et al.[6] proposed a new classification of autoimmune disease: (a) those due to B-cell action primarily (as SAT in OS chickens), (b) those due mainly to T-cells (as experimental autoimmune thyroiditis and EAE in normal chickens), and (c) a group involving both B- and T-dependent portions of the immune system (as EAE in OS chickens).

Wick et al.[6,16] have concluded that SAT in OS chickens must be caused by both a genetic defect in the immune system *and* some alteration of the thyroid gland itself. Studies by Rose et al.[29] have helped to define the genetic determinants of OS thyroiditis. By genotypic inbreeding experiments and T- and B-cell manipulations, these authors identified three genetically determined defects in the OS strain. These include: (a) an influence (possibly an immune-response gene) determined by the major histocompatibility complex which predisposes to a more vigorous reaction of these animals to thyroglobulin,[30] (b) a thymus-dependent suppressor function which either decreases early or develops abnormally in OS chicks, and (c) an intrinsic, functional defect in the thyroid gland itself.[29,30]

2. Rats

Penhale et al.[31] developed a model using various strains of adult rats prepared by a combination of thymectomy and sublethal X-radiation. These investigators found marked variability among the different strains in their susceptibility to thyroiditis after T-cell depletion; thus, 80 to 100% of members of highly responsive strains developed thyroiditis, whereas only 9% of poorly responsive strains did. This illustrates the significance of genetic background in the development of the autoimmune disorder.

Penhale et al. felt that the "spontaneous" onset, chronic nature, and presence of high titers of autoantibodies in their rat model closely resembled human thyroiditis.[31] These studies supported the role of T-cells in the regulation of autoimmunity. Further, they suggested that thymectomy plus irradiation leads to selective depletion of those T-cells specifically involved in the suppression of autoimmune activity to thyroid components, while leaving the autoreactive "helper" T-cells unimpaired and able to trigger autoreactive B-cells.[31]

Irvine[32] expanded these studies and demonstrated that the infusion of normal thymocytes into the affected rats had no effect, while normal spleen and lymph node cells were effective in preventing autoimmune thyroiditis in these animals. From these results, this author concluded that normal T-cells need to mature or be processed through the peripheral lymphoid organs before they develop suppressor cell function.[32]

The development of thyroiditis in these animals can be prevented by injections of rat thyroid extract before the onset of the lesion. Whitmore and Irvine[33] postulate that the specific antigen induces the production of blocking antibodies which inhibit the subsequent cellular responses.[33]

The strain of rat most extensively studied has been the Buffalo strain (BUF) in which 25% of a nonmanipulated population develop autoimmune thyroiditis with males more commonly affected.[9,34,35] Neonatal thymectomy in these rats results in an earlier onset of thyroiditis (26% at 4 months) and an increased overall occurrence (87%).[9,34]

The affected rats showed high levels of antithyroid antibodies; the titer correlated directly with the severity of the thyroid lesion.[36] Immunofluorescence studies of diseased thyroids showed the presence of rat immunoglobulins.[36,37] Attempted reconstitution by intravenous injection of BUF thymus cells did not alter the incidence or severity of thyroiditis.[9,37] Skin testing for delayed hypersensitivity with thyroid antigens was negative in these animals.[36,37] These findings suggested that autoantibodies to thyroid antigens play a role in the pathogenesis of SAT in the BUF rat either by antibody-mediated, lymphocyte-dependent cytotoxicity, or by immune complex formation in the thyroid, or both.[9,36,37]

3. Mice

Kojima et al.[38,39] have investigated a highly susceptible strain of hybrid mice (C3H/HeMS × 129/J)F_1, in which neonatal thymectomy leads to the development of thyroiditis in 25% of female and 6% of male animals. This form of thyroiditis occurs spontaneously a few months after thymectomy, lasts for about a year, and subsides with aging. Affected mice demonstrated circulating antithyroid antibodies.[38] Pathologically, lymphoplasmacytic infiltration, occasionally with germinal centers, was seen.[38] In addition, lymphocytic infiltrations of ovary and stomach were seen in some of the animals;[38] this resemblance to human Hashimoto's disease was noted by the authors. (In the OS chicken model, rarely similar nonthyroidal parenchymal infiltration has been noted.)[40]

The Kojima model was then manipulated to determine possible pathogenetic mechanisms and means of prevention of the thyroiditis.[38,39] Grafting of neonatal thymus, or cell injections from adult thymus, spleen, or nodes (but not bone marrow) can prevent development of the thyroid lesion.[39] However, thymic cells from 7-day-old or older animals were effective, whereas those from younger mice were not.[39] These data suggest that the cells responsible for the prevention of postthymectomy thyroiditis are T-cells and that these elements *acquire* this ability after birth while in the thymus and then migrate to the periphery, i.e., a maturation or processing is needed for their function.[39]

4. Beagles

A relatively uninvestigated model for spontaneous autoimmune thyroiditis was found in certain purebred beagle colonies.[41-45] This entity resembles the human disease more closely than does the OS chicken since most of the dogs were not severely hypothyroid.

The entity occurs in certain family lines with an incidence of 13% in females and 11% in males.[43] Pathologic examination showed scattered foci to diffuse infiltration of lymphoplasmacytic cells, well-developed germinal centers, and the presence of Hurthle cells.[43,44] Beirewaltes and Nishiyama[44] investigated these dogs and concluded that since this thyroiditis resembles the human disease in its histopathology and functional correlation, this model offers an opportunity to study the effects of heredity, virus infection, and diet on the etiology and pathogenesis of this disease. Mizejewski[45] found antibodies to thyroglobulin, colloid antigen (CA-2) and cytoplasmic microsomal antigen in these dogs; this author concluded that canine thyroiditis parallelled the human disease since the last antibody is found only in affected beagles and humans.[45] Another similarity is the finding of positive skin tests to thyroid antigens in beagles with SAT, which present early in the course of the disease, suggesting a cell-mediated component at this stage as compared to its late development in the OS chicken model.[9]

Recently, Fritz et al.[42] described the coexistence of lymphocytic orchitis and thyroiditis with consequent sterility in affected males. Hypoadrenalism has also been reported in these dogs.[9,46]

These observations suggest that the beagle model differs from SAT in OS chickens, BUF rats, and mice, so that the dog thyroiditis approximates human Hashimoto's disease most closely. Intense immunologic evaluation of this model is awaited.

5. Monkeys

Recently, Levy and co-workers[47] have reported the occurence of spontaneous thyroiditis in marmosets. The incidence ranged from 9 to 12% in the wild to up to 60% in colony-born animals. Females are affected twice as frequently as males.[47] This model, in a species more closely aligned with man than any previously reported, appears to offer exciting prospects for our understanding of autoimmune thyroiditis. Immunologic studies are awaited eagerly.

B. Experimental Autoimmune Thyroiditis (EAT)

Much data has been accumulated from studies of models of experimental (induced) autoimmune thyroiditis. Different techniques of immunization with and without adjuvants have been employed with varying degrees of success. The validity of these models in understanding human thyroiditis has been questioned because of the obvious biases involved with the inducing techniques. Nevertheless, some information about the immune system has been acquired and several comparisons with the human disease have been made. I will review some of these models, stressing their significance and proposed similarity to human thyroiditis.

1. Rabbits

Neonatal injection of bovine serum albumin (BSA) into rabbits induces immunologic tolerance to BSA.[48] Weigle[48,49] postulated that this tolerance resembled that which exists to self-constituents. This author proposed that immunization with cross-reacting antigen or an altered form of a normal self-component might lead to autoimmunity.

Thyroiditis was produced in rabbits by immunization with altered rabbit thyroglobulin with and without complete Freund's adjuvant (CFA). In addition, these animals developed antibodies to native thyroglobulin, although their levels did not correlate with the severity of the thyroiditis. LoGerfo et al. confirmed these findings and demonstrated that thyroglobulin, altered with both arsanilic and sulfanilic acids plus CFA, leads to the highest incidence of thyroiditis (75 to 90%).[50] Later studies by Weigle and Romball[51] attempted to elucidate the mechanism of development of cell-mediated hypersensitivity to native thyroglobulin in rabbits. These workers demonstrated that prolonged immunization with altered thyroglobulin led to the development of cell-mediated hypersensitivity to the native protein with no significant reduction in thyroid lesions or circulating antibody. This finding suggests that a loss in the unresponsive state of T-lymphocytes occurs when persistent levels of antithyroglobulin antibody prevent thyroglobulin from contacting new T-cells. This mechanism, they say, may be similar to that in humans with Hashimoto's thyroiditis.

A small number of rabbits also develop a kidney lesion accompanied by glomerular depostion of antigen-antibody complexes (thyroglobulin-antithyroglobulin, in this case). Whether similar complexes occur in the thyroid itself remains unknown.[49]

Another group of investigators has produced thyroiditis in rabbits by immunization with homologous thyroid microsomes in CFA; these animals develop severe thyroiditis and circulating antimicrosomal antibodies. By immunofluorescence, these antibodies are localized in thyroid epithelial cells.[52]

2. Guinea Pigs

The guinea pig thyroiditis model has been used for lymphocyte subpopulation studies by several investigators.[53-57] Paget, McMaster, and van Boxel[53] induced EAT in guinea pigs by injecting them with thyroid extract in CFA, digested the thyroid parenchyma with its dense lymphocytic infiltrates, and prepared viable single-cell suspensions. In testing these, these workers found that 75% of the lymphocytes were T-cells and only 16% were B-cells[53] suggesting the presence of cell-mediated immunity. However, they also found within these infiltrates some lymphocytes capable of mediating antibody-dependent lymphoid cell-mediated cytotoxicity. Thus, an antibody- mediated component in the pathogenesis of this form of thyroiditis was present also.

Lin and Salvin[54] took thyroid cell cultures (capable of making thyroglobulin in vitro) from normal guinea pigs and investigated their interaction with sensitized lymphocytes from guinea pigs with EAT. In vitro, these lymphocytes were able to lyse the target thyroid cells, but only when an adequate amount of antigen (thyroglobulin) was present. Thus, sensitized lymphocytes without antigen, normal lymphocytes, purified macrophages, and hyperimmune antithyroglobulin serum produced no cell lysis.

Furthermore, sensitized lymphocytes in suspension with thyroglobulin released a product (called thyroid cytotoxic factor — TCF) capable of thyroid cell lysis without cell to cell contact.[54,55] TCF was then investigated[56] and several properties were elucidated: (1) it is not tissue specific (i.e., it can lyse other cell types), (2) it inhibits the synthesis of macromolecules and DNA by thyroid cells, (3) it is thermolabile and therefore different from macrophage inhibitory factor (MIF), and (4) it developed simultaneously with delayed skin responses and thyroid lesions in vivo. These investigators noted that circulating antibodies peaked about 6 weeks after the thyroid lesions had reached a maximum, suggesting that cell-mediated immunity represents the primary causative lesion in EAT in guinea pigs.

It has been shown by Bocker and Lietz that EAT production in the guinea pig can be suppressed by injection of thyroglobulin (homologous or heterologous) in CFA.[57] These workers also noted good correlation between thyroiditis and delayed hypersensitivity in their animals, but poor correlation with antithyroid antibody titers.[57] They suggest that this supports further the primary role of cell-mediated immunity in this model of thyroiditis.

The role of genetic factors has also been noted in the guinea pig model with some strains showing a much higher incidence of thyroiditis than others under identical experimental conditions.[58]

3. Mice

Mice have been used as a model for SAT after thymectomy and irradiation (see above.) These studies have shown that the response to thyroglobulin is T-cell dependent, and that the severity of this mononuclear cell infiltration is genetically determined.[59]

Esquivel et al. studied the role of T-cells in the loss of self-tolerance to native thyroglobulin in EAT.[60] Using bacterial lipopolysaccharide (LPS — a known mitogen for B-cells) and mouse thyroglobulin, these investigators were able to induce thyroiditis equivalent to that seen with thyroglobulin in CFA injections. A variety of T-cell and B-cell manipulations disclosed that this reaction required both cell types. Differences were noted among various strains in the development of thyroid lesions;[61] some of these were attributed to thyroglobulin heterogeneity among differing species.

Tomazic and Rose[62] attempted to compare cell-mediated and antibody-mediated immunity with the development of thyroid damage during EAT. They used the macrophage dependence reaction (MDR) as a test for cell-mediated immunity and found essentially no difference between the good and poor responder strains of mice. Thus it appears unlikely that cell-mediated immunity alone is responsible for the genetically determined differences in the thyroid lesion. Although good responder mice generally have higher antibody titers, this correlated poorly with the extent of infiltration within the strains, and therefore was unlikely to be responsible for interstrain differences.

Based upon these and previous experiments, two alternate models for the development of EAT were proposed.[61,62] The first suggests that antibody capable of fixing complement establishes a local Arthus reaction in the thyroid, leading to the accumulation of polymorphonuclear cells. This is then followed by lymphocyte and macrophage infiltration, either by reaction to local inflammation or a specific cell-mediated immunity. The alternative model proposes that antibodies react with normal sensitized lymphocytes locally in the thyroid. From this, a process of antibody-dependent, cell-mediated tissue damage develops. If either of these mechanisms is correct, it appears that cell-mediated immunity does not play a primary pathogenic role in the development of tissue damage in EAT.

However, Wick et al.[63] examined the development of thyroiditis in nude mice and found that no thyroid lesions occurred in homozygous animals immunized with murine thyroid extract in CFA. Similar experiments in heterozygous nude mice demonstrated the development of autoimmune thyroiditis.[63] These findings suggest strongly that EAT in mice depends upon the presence of T-cells, differs from spontaneous thyroiditis (a B-effector cell lesion), and that thyroglobulin is a T-dependent antigen.[63] Understanding the basic mechanisms involved in the mouse models awaits further experimentation.

4. Rats

The rat model of spontaneous autoimmune thyroiditis has been reviewed above. Several workers have described an induced thyroiditis in rats produced by injection of rat thyroid extract in CFA.[64-66] In this model, the incidence of thyroiditis peaks at 3 months. At this time, thyroid antibodies are identified and thyroid function parameters were abnormal (high PBI and BEI); goiters were also noted. Histologically, follicular hyperplasia, focal atrophy, and lymphoplasmacytic infiltration (both focal and diffuse) were seen.[66] Various strains of rat react to induction of thyroiditis according to genotype, with the most susceptible strains showing an AG-B5 major histocompatibility genotype and the least susceptible having an AB-B2 genotype.[67] In all cases, females developed more severe lesions than males. Although variable, autoantibodies were present in all affected animals, but their presence did not correlate well with severity of the thyroiditis.[67]

Evaluation of immunologic parameters in the rat model remains an area of investigation.[68] However, Paterson and Drobish[69] have found that cyclophosphamide immunosuppression can totally reverse induced thyroiditis in Wistar rats.

5. Monkeys

Pudifin et al.[70] studied the development of EAT in monkeys immunized with *human* thyroid extract. These animals not only developed thyroiditis as expected, but also developed cytotoxic antibodies to cultures of human thyroid and other cells. Preheating decreased this activity, suggesting its association with complement fixation. A second factor was identitied which was not affected by preheating, and which sensitized human target cells and rendered them susceptible to lysis by normal (nonsensitized) human lymphocytes. These results strongly point to an antibody-dependent, cell-mediated cytotoxicity in the pathogenesis of autoimmune thyroiditis in this model.[70]

III. SUMMARY: CORRELATION WITH HUMAN DISEASE

Several animal models of autoimmune thyroiditis, both spontaneous and induced, have been defined and partially characterized. However, it is clear from this review that no single model approximates, in pathogenesis or clinicopathologic features, human Hashimoto's disease. Similarly, no clearcut advantage of spontaneous over-induced models is recognized, since both share similarities and differences with human thyroiditis. Despite these shortcomings, the models afford us the opportunity to examine and separate components of the immune system and their function. Mechanisms of autoimmune reactions can also be studied in these animals.

Both circulating antibody and cell-mediated hypersensitivity reactions have been implicated in experimental autoimmune thyroiditis.[49] The role of these two arms of the immune system varies among species and it appears likely that both T- and B-cells are involved in most animals. Differences among the models reflect a predominance of one of these subsystems. Thus B-cells seem more important in spontaneous thyroiditis in the chicken, whereas cell-mediated immunity seems to be the primary effector in the guinea pig.[49,54,55] Recent work suggests the importance of genetic susceptibility. Thus, in mice, mutation at the H-2K locus altered the susceptibility of the animals to develop EAT.[71] This area of research may yield essential clues to our understanding of human "autoimmune" thyroiditis.

Incomplete evidence suggests that human thyroiditis is effected via both cell-mediated immune mechanism and a humoral response. Certain genetic groups appear more susceptible (see Chapter 6).

In man and animals, thyroglobulin is present in the circulation in very small amounts, but this concentration appears adequate to maintain tolerance at the T-cell level. A genetic mutation, a virus, an altered autoantigen, or the addition of an adjuvant can bypass the T-cell tolerance mechanism (either by inducing helper T-cells or inhibiting suppressor cells) and allow normally responsive B-cells to manufacture antibody to thyroglobulin, i.e., autoimmunity occurs.[72]

Results from animal studies have disclosed that an intact immune system is required for normal self-tolerance; and that some genetically determined defect of either the target organ, the immune system, or both allows a situation of autoimmune reactivity (either antibody-mediated, cell-mediated, or both) to develop, resulting in the development of "autoimmune" disorders. Further investigative efforts of these and other models may define the pathogenetic mechanisms involved in these diseases.

REFERENCES

1. Good, R. A., Finstad, J., Cain, W. A., Fish, A., Perey, D. Y., and Gatti, R. A., Models of immunologic diseases and disorders, *Fed. Proc.*, 28, 191, 1969.
2. Volpe, R., Thyroiditis: Current views on pathogenesis, *Med. Clin. North Am.*, 59, 1166, 1975.
3. Volpe, R., Farid, N. R., and von Westarp, C., The pathogenesis of Graves' disease and Hashimoto's thyroiditis, *Clin. Endocrinol.*, 3, 239, 1974.

4. Hall, R., Immunological aspects of thyroid function, *N. Engl. J. Med.*, 266, 1204, 1962.
5. van Tienhoven, A. and Cole, R. K., Endocrine disturbances in obese chickens, *Anat. Rec.*, 141, 111, 1962.
6. Wick, G., Sundick, R. S., and Albine, B. A., A review: The obese strain (OS) of chickens: An animal model with spontaneous autoimmune thyroiditis, *Clin. Immunol. Immunopathol.*, 3, 272, 1974.
7. Cole, R. K., Kite, J. H., and Witebsky, E., Hereditary autoimmune thyroiditis in the fowl, *Science*, 160, 1357, 1968.
8. Witebsky, E., The clinical pathology of autoimmunization, *Am. J. Clin. Pathol.*, 49, 301, 1968.
9. Bigazzi, P. E. and Rose, N. R., Spontaneous autoimmune thyroiditis in animals as a model of human disease, *Prog. Allergy*, 19, 245, 1975.
10. Newcomer, W. S., Accumulation of radioiodine in thyroids of chicks of the obese strain with hereditary thyroiditis and of their parental strain, *Gen. Comp. Endocrinol.*, 21, 322, 1973.
11. Sundick, R. S., Bagchi, N., Livezey, M. D., Brown, T. R., and Mack, R. E., Abnormal thyroid regulation in chickens with autoimmune thyroiditis, *Endocrinology*, 105, 493, 1979.
12. Kite, J. H., Wick, G., Twarog, B., and Witebsky, E., Spontaneous thyroiditis in an obese strain of chickens. II. Investigations on the development of the disease, *J. Immunol.*, 103, 1331, 1969.
13. Wick, G. and Graf, J., Electron microscopic studies in chickens of the obese strain with spontaneous hereditary autoimmune thyroiditis, *Lab. Invest.*, 27, 400, 1072.
14. Ziegel, R. F., Barron, A. L., Kite, J. H., and Witebsky, E., Virological investigations of chickens with spontaneous autoimmune thyroiditis. II. Examination of tissues by electron microscopy, *Avian Dis.*, 14, 617, 1970.
15. Kalderon, A. E., Bogaars, H. A., Jolly, G., and Diamond, I., Electron-dense deposits in the follicular basal lamina of obese strain chickens with spontaneous hereditary autoimmune thyroiditis, *Lab. Invest.*, 37, 487, 1977.
16. Wick, G., Witebsky, E., Kite, J. H., and Beutner, E. H., Immunofluorescent studies of thyroid autoantibodies in chickens of the obese strain (OS), *Clin. Exp. Immunol.*, 7, 173, 1970.
17. Witebsky, E., Kite, J. H., Wick, G., and Cole, R. K., Spontaneous thyroiditis in the obese strain of chickens. Demonstration of circulating autoantibodies, *J. Immunol.*, 103, 708, 1969.
18. Mellors, R. C., Brzosko, W. J., and Sonkin, L. S., Immunopathology of chronic nonspecific thyroiditis (autoimmune thyroiditis), *Am. J. Pathol.*, 41, 425, 1962.
19. Schauenstein, K. and Wick, G., Local production of immunoglobulin in the thyroid gland of obese strain (OS) chickens, *Clin. Exp. Immunol.*, 17, 637, 1974.
20. Nilsson, L. A. and Rose, N. R., Restoration of autoimmune thyroiditis in bursectomized-irradiated OS chickens by bursa cells, *Immunology*, 22, 13, 1972.
21. Welch, P., Rose, N. R., and Kite, J. H., Neonatal thymectomy increases spontaneous autoimmune thyroiditis, *J. Immunol.*, 110, 575, 1973.
22. Wick, G., Kite, J. H., Cole, R. K., and Witebsky, E., Spontaneous thyroiditis in the obese strain of chickens. III. The effect of bursectomy on the development of the disease, *J. Immunol.*, 104, 45, 1970.
23. Wick, G., Kite, J. H., and Witebsky, E., Spontaneous thyroiditis in the obese strain of chickens. IV. The effect of thymectomy and thymo-bursectomy on the development of the disease, *J. Immunol.*, 104, 54, 1970.
24. Wick, G. Kite, J. H., and Witebsky, E., Spontaneous thyroiditis in the obese strain of chickens. V. The effect of sublethal total body x-irradiation on the development of the disease, *J. Immunol.*, 104, 344, 1970.
25. Bacon, L. D., Sundick, R. S., and Rose, N. R., Genetic and cellular control of spontaneous autoimmune thyroiditis in OS chickens, *Adv. Exp. Med. Biol.*, 88, 309, 1977.
26. Luster, M. I., Leslie, G. A., and Cole, R. K., Selective IgA deficiency in chickens with spontaneous autoimmune thyroiditis, *Nature*, 263, 331, 1976.
27. Luster, M. I., Bacon, L. D., Rose, N. R., and Leslie, G. A., Immunogenetic and ontogenetic studies of chickens with selective IgA deficiency and autoimmune thyroiditis, *Cell. Immunol.*, 32, 417, 1977.
28. Welch, P. C. and Kite, J. H., Delayed hypersensitivity in spontaneous and experimentally induced autoimmune thyroiditis in chickens, *Fed. Proc.*, 30, 306, 1971.
29. Rose, N. R., Bacon, L. D., and Sundick, R. S., Genetic determinants of thyroiditis in the OS chicken, *Transplant. Rev.*, 31, 264, 1976.
30. Rose, N. R., Kite, J. H., Vladutiu, A. O., Tomazic, V., and Bacon, L. D., Genetic aspects of autoimmune thyroiditis, *Int. Arch. Allergy*, 45, 138, 1973.
31. Penhale, W. J., Farmer, A., and Irvine, W. J., Thyroiditis in T-cell depleted rats, *Clin. Exp. Immunol.*, 21, 362, 1975.
32. Irvine, W. J., Autoimmune thyroiditis in T-cell depleted rats, *Proc. R. Soc. Med.*, 69, 873, 1976.
33. Whitmore, D. B. and Irvine, W. J., Prevention of autoimmune thyroiditis in T-cell depleted rats by injection of crude thyroid extract, *Clin. Exp. Immunol.*, 29, 474, 1977.

34. Noble, B., Yoshida, T., Rose, N. R., and Bigazzi, P. E., Thyroid antibodies in spontaneous autoimmune thyroiditis in the Buffalo rat, *J. Immunol.*, 117, 1447, 1976.
35. Silverman, D. A. and Rose, N. R., Neonatal thymectomy increases the incidence of spontaneous and methylcholanthrene-enhanced thyroiditis in rats, *Science*, 184, 162, 1974.
36. Rose, N. R., Bigazzi, P. E., and Noble, B., Spontaneous autoimmune thyroiditis in the BUF rat, *Adv. Exp. Med. Biol.*, 73, 209, 1976.
37. Penhale, W. J., Irvine, W. J., Inglis, J. R., and Farmer, A., Thyroiditis in T-cell depleted rats: Suppression of the autoallergic response by reconstitution with normal lymphoid cells, *Clin. Exp. Immunol.*, 25, 6, 1976.
38. Kojima, A., Tanaka-Kojima, U., Sakakura, T., and Nishizuka, Y., Spontaneous development of autoimmune thyroiditis in neonatally thymectomized mice, *Lab. Invest.*, 34, 550, 1976.
39. Kojima, A., Tanaka-Kojima, Y., Sakakura, T., and Nishizuka, Y., Prevention of postthymectomy autoimmune thyroiditis in mice, *Lab. Invest.*, 34, 601, 1976.
40. Wick, G., The effect of bursectomy, thymectomy and x-irradiation on the incidence of precipitating liver and kidney autoantibodies in chickens of the obese strain (OS), *Clin. Exp. Immunol.*, 7, 187, 1970.
41. Fritz, T. E., Zeman, R. C., and Zelle, M. R., Pathology and familial incidence of thyroiditis in a closed beagle colony, *Exp. Molecul. Pathol.*, 12, 14, 1970.
42. Fritz, T. E., Lombard, L. S., Tyler, S. A., and Norris, W. P., Pathology and familial incidence of orchitis and its relation to thyroiditis in a closed beagle colony, *Exp. Molecul. Pathol.*, 24, 142, 1976.
43. Musser, E. and Graham, W. R., Familial occurrence of thyroiditis in purebred beagles, *Lab. Anim. Care*, 18, 58, 1968.
44. Beierwaltes, W. H. and Nishiyama, R. H., Dog thyroiditis: Occurrence and similarity to Hashimoto's struma, *Endocrinology*, 83, 501, 1968.
45. Mizejewski, G. J., Baron, J., and Poissant, G., Immunologic investigations of naturally occurring canine thyroiditis, *J. Immunol.*, 107, 1152, 1971.
46. Freudiger, U., Die Nebennierenrinden-Insuffizienzen beim Hund, *Dtsch. Tieraerztl Wochenschr.*, 72, 60, 1966.
47. Levy, B. M., Hampton, S. Dreizen, S., and Hampton. J. K., Thyroiditis in the marmoset, *J. Comp. Pathol.* 82, 99, 1972.
48. Wiegle, W. O., The induction of autoimmunity in rabbits following injection of heterologous or altered homologous thyroglobulin, *J. Exp. Med.*, 121, 289, 1965.
49. Weigle, W. O., Experimental autoimmune thyroiditis, *Pathol. Annu.*, 8, 329, 1973.
50. LoGerfo, P. and Colacchio, D., Unpublished data.
51. Weigle, W. O. and Romball, C. G., Humoral and cell-mediated immunity in experimental and progressive thyroiditis in rabbits, *Clin. Exp. Immunol.*, 21, 351, 1975.
52. Mangkornkanok, M. M., Markowitz, A. S., and Battifora, H. A., Chronic thyroiditis in the rabbit induced with homologous thyroid microsomes, *Science*, 178, 316, 1972.
53. Paget, S. A. McMaster, P. R., and van Boxel, J. A., Experimental autoimmune thyroiditis in the guinea pig. Characterization of infiltrating lymphocyte populations, *J. Immunol.*, 117, 2267, 1976.
54. Lin, M. S. and Salvin, S. B., In vitro and in vivo studies on the mechanism of experimental thyroiditis in guinea pigs, *Cell. Immunol.*, 27, 117, 1976.
55. Lin, M. S. and Salvin, S. B., Further studies on the mechanism of autoimmune thyroiditis in the guinea pig, *Cell. Immunol.*, 27, 188, 1976.
56. Kosunen, T. U. and Flax, M. H., Experimental allergic thyroiditis in the guinea pig, *Lab. Invest.*, 15, 606, 1966.
57. Bocker, W. and Leitz, H., Suppression of experimental allergic thyroiditis in guinea pigs by homologous and heterologous thyroglobulin, *Virchows Arch. A*, 361, 307, 1973.
58. McMaster, P. R. B., Owens, J. D., and Kyriakos, M., A comparison of autoimmunity and experimental allergic thyroiditis in Strain 2 and Hartley strain guinea pigs, *Cell. Immunol.*, 14, 39, 1974.
59. Vladitiu, A. O. and Rose, N. R., Autoimmune murine thyroiditis: Relation to histocompatibility, *Science*, 174, 1137, 1971.
60. Esquivel, P. S., Rose, N. R., and Kong, Y. M., Induction of autoimmunity in good and poor responder mice with mouse thyroglobulin and lipopolysaccharide, *J. Exp. Med.*, 145, 1250, 1977.
61. Tomazic, V. and Rose, N. R., Autoimmune murine thyroiditis. VIII. Role of different thyroid antigens in the induction of experimental autoimmune thyroiditis, *Immunology*, 30, 63, 1976.
62. Tomazic, V. and Rose, N. R., Autoimmune murine thyroiditis: Relationship of humoral and cellular immunity in high and low responder mice, *Eur. J. Immunol.*, 7, 40, 1977.
63. Wick, G., Schwarz, S., and Miller, P. U., No development of experimental autoimmune thyroiditis in nude mice, *Z. Immunitaetsforsch. Immunobiol.*, 154, 162, 1978.
64. Biorklund, A., Testing *in vitro* of lymphoid cells from rats with experimental autoimmune thyroiditis, *Lab. Invest.*, 13, 120, 1964.

65. **Willoughby, D. A. and Coote, E.**, The lymph node permeability factor: A possible mediator of experimental allergic thyroiditis in the rat, *J. Pathol. Bacteriol.*, 92, 281, 1966.
66. **Anderson, J. W., Wakim, K. G., and McConahey, W. M.**, The influence of experimental thyroiditis on thyroid function, *Mayo Clin. Proc.*, 44, 711, 1969.
67. **Penhale, W. J., Farmer, A., Urbaniak, S. J., and Irvine, W. J.**, Susceptibility of inbred rat strains to experimental thyroiditis, *Clin. Exp. Immunol.*, 19, 179, 1975.
68. **Tonooka, N., Leslie, G. A., Greer, M. A., and Olson, J. C.**, Lymphoid thyroiditis following immunization with group A streptococcal vaccine, *Am. J. Pathol.*, 92, 681, 1978.
69. **Paterson, P. Y. and Drobish, D. G.**, Reversal of experimental allergic thyroiditis in cyclophosphamide treated rats, *Clin. Exp. Immunol.*, 20, 125, 1975.
70. **Pudifin, D. J., Duursma, J., and Brain, P.**, Experimental autoimmune thyroiditis in the vervet monkey, *Clin. Exp. Immunol.*, 29, 256, 1970.
71. **Maron, R. and Cohen, I. R.**, Mutation of H-2K locus influence susceptibility to autoimmune thyroiditis, *Nature*, 279, 715, 1979.
72. **Nakamura, R. M.**, *Mechanisms of Autoimmune Disease*, American Society of Clinical Pathologists, Chicago, 1979.

INDEX

A

Abscess, 8—10, 15, 18
Acid-butanol extraction, see Butanol-extractable iodine
Acid-fast organisms, 14
Actinomyces sp., 14
Activator activity, lymphocyte, 54—55
Acute bacterial thyroiditis, 6—10, 18, 27
Acute strumitis, 6
Acute suppurative thyroiditis, 6, 8, 10, 17, 172
Acute thyroiditis
 antibiotic therapy, 172
 aspiration cytology, 166
 clinical features, 6—7
 defined, 6
 diagnosis, course, prognosis, and treatment, 9—10
 etiology, 8
 fibrosis, 10, 83
 general discussion, 2—3, 6
 incidence, 6
 laboratory findings, 7—8, 148, 150, 152—153, 163, 166
 needle biopsy, 9, 163, 172
 occurrence, 6
 pathology and pathogenesis, 8—9
 pus, 9, 172
 Riedel's struma and, 174
 scanning in, 152
 subacute thyroiditis and, 6, 9, 22, 27, 34
 suppurative, 6, 8, 10, 17, 172
 surgery in, 172
 thyroid function tests, 7—8, 148
 treatment, 10, 172
Acute viral thyroiditis, 8
Adenocarcinoma, 27
Adenoma, 18, 34, 79, 121—122, 136, 138, 140
 Riedel's struma characterized by, 136, 138, 140
Adenomatous goiter, 75, 79
Adherent tissue, Riedel's struma, 75, 136
Adolescent lymphocytic goiter, see also Hashimoto's thyroiditis, 52
Adrenal failure, Hashimoto's thyroiditis and, 82
Age, effect of, see Occurrence (age, sex)
 thyroid antibodies in, 150
 thyroid function tests, 148, 153
 thyroid-stimulating hormones in, 148, 153
Albumin, thyroxine-binding, 146
Allergic reaction, lithium, 99
Amenorrhea-galactorrhea syndrome, 82
^{241}Americum, 151
Amyloid, 79, 84
 goiter, 84
Anabolic steroid, 98
Analgesic, 172—173
Anamnestic response to inflammation, 25, 150
Anaplastic carcinoma and other tumors, 75, 84, 86, 110, 122, 137—139, 163

 occurrence, 75, 139
 pathology, 138—139
 Riedel's struma and, 137—139, 163
Angiography, neoplasm differentiation, 154
Animal models, see also specific animals by name
 experimental autoimmune, thyroiditis, 54—55, 182—185
 experimental thyroiditis, review, 178—185
  general discussion, 178—179, 185
 Hashimoto's thyroiditis, 54—55
 human correlations, 178—179, 185
 palpation thyroiditis, 44
 radiation effects on thyroid, 112—113
 spontaneous autoimmune thyroiditis, 54—55, 179—182
Antibiotics, see also specific types by name, 10, 17—19, 24, 34—35, 102, 172
Antiadrenal antibody, 82
Antibody
 antiadrenal, 82
 antimicrosomal, 149—151, 183
 antinuclear, 149, 178
 antiovarian, 82
 antithyroglobulin, 149—151, 178—179, 181—183
 antiviral, 150
 auto-, see Autoantibody
 chronic nonspecific thyroiditis, 79
 colloid antigen, 150—151
 diagnostic methods using, 149—151
 drug-associated thyroiditis, 101—102
 experimental autoimmune thyroiditis, 182—185
 fibrosing Hashimoto's thyroiditis, 137, 150
 Graves' disease, 150
 Hashimoto's thyroiditis, 53—58, 66, 70, 74, 137, 149—151
 microsomal, 56—57, 66
 Riedel's struma, 136—137, 151
 spontaneous autoimmune thyroiditis, 179—182
 subacute thyroiditis, 25—26, 31, 36, 137, 150
 thyroid carcinoma, 150
 thyroxine, 150
 triiodothyronine, 150
 tumor-associated thyroiditis, 123—125
 types, 149
Antibody-mediated immunity, 184—185
Antifungals, 19
Antigen
 colloid, see Colloid, antigen
 histocompatability, see also HLA antigen, 53
 microsomal, 182
 nuclear, 53
Antigen-antibody complex, 102, 179, 183
Antiinflammatory agents, 35—36
Antimicrosomal antibody, 149—151, 183
Antinuclear antibody, 149, 178
Antiovarian antibody, 82
Antithyroglobulin antibody, 149—151, 178—179, 181—183

Antiviral antibody, 150
APUD-amyloid, 84
Arteritis, 136
Askanazy cell, see also Hurthle cell, 66—67, 78
Aspergillus sp., 14—16, 140
Asphyxia, tracheal compression and, 141
Aspiration cytology
  acute thyroiditis, 9, 166
  complications, 166
  general discussion, 162—164, 166
  Graves' disease, 166
  Hashimoto's thyroiditis, 166
  results, 166—167
  Riedel's struma, 166
  subacute thyroiditis, 166
  team approach, 166—167
  techniques, 164—165
  tumor cell dissemination, 162, 164, 166
Aspirin, 35, 172
Associations, see Differential diagnosis
Asymptomatic thyroiditis, see also Hashimoto's thyroiditis, 52
Atherosclerosis, 82
Atrophy
  fibrous, 75
  follicular, see Follicular atrophy
Atypical mycobacteria, see also Mycobacteria, 14
Autoantibody, 8, 33, 52—55, 101—102, 150, 173, 178, 180—181, 184
Autoimmune reaction
  cancer-associated thyroiditis, 125—126
  Dilantin® and, 101
  Hashimoto's thyroiditis, 52—58, 68—69, 75, 82—83, 149
  Riedel's struma, 139
  subacute thyroiditis, 25—26, 34—35
  theory and mechanism, 25—26, 178, 182, 185
Autoimmune thyroiditis, see Experimental autoimmune thyroiditis; Hashimoto's thyroiditis; Spontaneous autoimmune thyroiditis
Aw30, HLA, Hashimoto's thyroiditis, 53

B

B8, HLA, Hashimoto's thyroiditis, 53
Bacterial thyroiditis, acute, 6—10, 18, 27
Bacteroides sp., 8
Basaloid cell, 75, 77
Batten's disease, 50, 84
Beagle models, spontaneous autoimmune thyroiditis, 54, 181—182
BEI, see Butanol-extractable iodine
Biopsy
  closed, see Needle biopsy
  open, 162
Black thyroid, minocycline-induced, 102
Brucella sp., 14
BUF, see Buffalo strain, rats
Buffalo strain, rat, studies of, spontaneous autoimmune thyroiditis, 181
Butanol-extractable iodine, test
  experimental autoimmune thyroiditis, 184
  Hashimoto's thyroiditis, 148
  methodology, 147
  subacute thyroiditis, 29, 148
  thyroid hormone measurement, 147
BW35, HLA haplotype, subacute thyroiditis and, 25, 36

C

CA-2, see Colloid, antigen, second
Cancer, 15—17, 57, 65, 71, 75—76, 79, 83—85
  Hashimoto's thyroiditis and, 57, 65, 71, 75—76, 83, 85
  Hurthle cells and, 79
  occurrence, thyroid cancer, 108, 110
  radiation exposure and, 15—17, 78, 108, 110, 112
  thyroiditis associated with, see Tumor-associated thyroiditis
Candida sp., 14—15
Capsule, thyroid
  fibrosing Hashimoto's thyroiditis, 75, 139
  Hashimoto's thyroiditis, 71—72, 75
  Riedel's struma, 75, 136
Carcinoma, see also specific types by name, 9, 15—16, 27, 34—35, 44—46, 50, 55, 57, 66, 71, 75—77, 83—85, 108—110, 118—126, 136—140, 150—151, 172—174
  antibody, 150
  Hashimoto's thyroiditis and, 55, 57, 66, 71, 75—77, 83, 125—126, 163, 173—174
  radiation caposure and, 108—110, 151
  Riedel's struma and, 136—140
  subacute thyroiditis and, 172—173
  thyroiditis and, see Tumor-associated thyroiditis
Cardiovascular system, hypothyroidism and, 82
Caseation, 14, 18
Case histories
  Dilantin®-associated thyroiditis, 99—101
  fungal thyroiditis, 15—17
  fibrosing Hashimoto's thyroiditis, 71—74
  hypothyroidism, 80—81
  nodular goiter, lithium-induced, 98—100
  Riedel's struma, 132—135
  subacute thyroiditis, 26—29
  tumor-associated thyroiditis, 121
Cell
  aspiration cytology, 163—164, 166
  basaloid, 75, 77
  clear, 75
  clear cytoplasm-containing, 78
  epidermoid, 75, 77
  epithelial, see Epithelial cell; Giant cell
  follicular, desquamation of, 48
  giant, see Giant cell
  Hurthle, see Hurthle cell

immunity, impaired, 17
parafollicular, 75, 77
pleomorphism, 75—76, 138—139
radiation effects on, 108—109
squamous, in thyroid, 75—77
tumor, dissemination, aspiration cytology, 162, 164, 166
vacuolization, 109, 113
B-Cell, see also B-Lymphocyte
    activity, 54—55, 180, 183—185
    immunoblastic sarcoma of, 86—88, 101
C-Cell, 47—48, 75
    hyperplasia of, 47—48
T-Cell, see also T-Lymphocyte
    abnormality, 32
    activity, 54—55, 180—185
    clone, autoimmunity and, 178
Cell-mediated hypersensitivity, 182, 185
Cell-mediated immunity, 54, 58, 68, 139, 178, 182—184
Cell-surface components, 53
Cell-undifferentiated carcinoma, 85
^{131}Cesium, 151
Chemotherapy, immune system and, 15—17
Chicken models
    experimental autoimmune thyroiditis, 54—55
    spontaneous autoimmune thyroiditis, 54—55, 179—180
Cholangitis, sclerosing, 141
Chromosomal aberrations, radiation, and, 109
Chronic lymphocytic thyroiditis, see Hashimoto's thyroiditis, Lymphocytic thyroiditis
Chronic nonspecific thyroiditis, 64, 79, 118
Chronic thyroiditis
    fibrosis in thyroid, 70—77, 83
    general discussion, 2—3, 64—65, 86—87
    Hashimoto's, see Hashimoto's thyroiditis
    Hurthle cell, see also Hurthle cell, 78—79
    hypothyroidism, pathology see also Hypothyroidism, 80—82, 84
    infectious, 14
    lymphocytic, see Hashimoto's thyroiditis
    lymphocytes in thyroid, 69—70, 76, 84—88
    nonspecific, 64, 79, 118
    pathologic aspects, 64—88
    Riedel's struma, see Riedel's struma
    tumor-associated, see Tumor-associated thyroiditis
Circumferential collection, histiocytes, palpation thyroiditis, 44—46
Classification, thyroiditis, 3
Clear cell, 75
Clear cytoplasm, cells with, 78
Clinical features, see also Diagnosis; Differential diagnosis
    acute thyroiditis, 6—7
    fibrosing Hashimoto's thyroiditis, 74, 178
    Hashimoto's thyroiditis, 55, 74, 125—126, 173—174, 178
    infectious thyroiditides, 15—18
    palpation thyroiditis, 44
    radiation-associated thyroiditis, 111
    Riedel's struma, 132, 135—137, 174
    subacute thyroiditis, 23, 27—29, 34
    thyroid-associated thyroiditis, 125—126
Clinicopathologic correlation, Hashimoto's thyroiditis, see also Clinical features; Pathology and pathogenesis, 74
Closed biopsy, see Needle biopsy
Coccidioidomycosis sp., 14
Collagen disease, 139—140
Colloid
    anaplastic carcinoma, 138
    antigen
        antibody to, 150—151
        second, 53, 149, 182
    cretinism, 82
    fibrosarcoma, 138
    fibrosing Hashimoto's thyroiditis, 138
    Hashimoto's thyroiditis, 53, 64, 66—68, 83, 178
    palpation thyroiditis, 47—48, 50
Radiation-associated thyroiditis, 112
    Riedel's struma, 138
    shrinkage, Hashimoto's thyroiditis, 64
    spontaneous autoimmune thyroiditis, 179, 182
    subacute thyroiditis, 24, 26, 30—32, 138
Colloidophagy, 48
Competitive protein binding, thyroid hormone measurement, 147
Congenital immunodeficiencies, 17
Congestive heart failure, 82
Constipation, hypothyroidism symptom, 82
Coronary heart disease, chronic thyroiditis and, 57
Corticosteroid hormone, see also Steroid hormone, 35, 58, 172
Contraceptive pills, 98
Cosmetic deformity, Hashimoto's thyroiditis, 173
Coumadin, 98
Course, see also Prognosis
    acute thyroiditis, 10
    Hashimoto's thyroiditis, 57—58, 137
    infectious thyroiditides, 18
    Riedel's struma, 137, 141
    subacute thyroiditis, 23, 26, 30, 35, 137
Creeping thyroiditis, see also Subacute thyroiditis, 22
Culture, tissue, infectious thyroiditis, 17
Cyclophosphamide, 78
Cyst, 9—10, 18
Cytology
    aspiration, see Aspiration cytology
    Riedel's struma, 137
    subacute thyroiditis, 31—32
Cytoplasm
    clear cells with, 78
    vacuolization of, 109

D

Damage, follicular, see Follicular destruction
Decreased immunoglobulin concentration, 17

Deformity, cosmetic, Hashimoto's thyroiditis, 173
Delayed hypersensitivity, 181, 183
de Quervain's thyroiditis, see also Subacute thyroiditis
   general discussion, 2, 22
   Riedel's struma and, 132
Desmoid-like fibrosarcoma, see also Fibrosarcoma, 139
Desmoplasia, 83, 140
Desquamation, follicular cells, 48
Destruction
   follicular, see Follicular destruction
   thyroid tissue, complete, Riedel's struma characterized by, 136
Diagnosis, see also Clinical features; Differential diagnosis; Laboratory findings
   acute thyroiditis, 9
      differential, 9—10
   fibrosing Hashimoto's thyroiditis, differential, 75—77, 83
   Hashimoto's thyroiditis, 55
      differential, 75—77, 82—86, 163, 173—174
   infectious thyroiditides, 17
      differential, 18
   methods, 146—154, 162—167
      aspiration cytology, see Aspiration cytology
      needle biopsy, see Needle biopsy
      palpation thyroiditis, differential, 44—50
   Riedel's struma, 137
      differential, 132, 136—140, 174
   subacute thyroiditis, 34
      differential, 34—35
   tumor, 162, 166—167
   tumor-associated thyroiditis, 125
Differential diagnosis, see also Clinical features; Diagnosis; Laboratory findings
   acute thyroiditis, 9—10
   fibrosing Hashimoto's thyroiditis, 75—77, 83
   fibrosis, in thyroid, 83
   Hashimoto's thyroiditis, 75—77, 82—86, 163, 173—174
   infectious thyroiditides, 18
   palpation thyroiditis, 44—50
   Riedel's struma, 132, 136—140, 174
   subacute thyroiditis, 34—35
   surgical, see Surgical management
Dilantin®, 99—101
Diphenylhydantoin, 99—101
Division delay, cell, 109
Dog models, see Beagle models
Down's syndrome, 53, 57
Drainage, 10, 18
Drug-associated thyroiditis, 79, 98—103, 139—140
   general discussion, 79, 98, 103
   lymphocytic infiltration, 99—100, 102
   Riedel's struma and, 139—140
   types of drug implicated, 98—102
DRw3, HLA, Hashimoto's thyroiditis, 53
Dyshormonogenesis, 56
Dysphagia, 7, 16, 34, 55, 173—174
Dyspnea, 7, 26, 55, 136, 173

E

EAE, see Experimental autoimmune encephalitis
EAT, see Experimental autoimmune thyroiditis
Echinococcus sp., 14
Echography, see Ultrasound techniques
Endothelial cell damage, 109
Enzyme
   Hurthle cell content, 78
   makeup, abnormal, lithium-induced thyroiditis and, 99
Eosinophilia, 99
Eosinophilic change, follicular epithelium, 64, 178
Epidemiologic studies, subacute thyroiditis, 24—25
Epidermoid cell, 75, 77
Epilepsy, Dilantin® treatment, 99
Epithelial cell, see also Giant cell, 32, 47, 66—68, 75—77, 179, 183
   lymphocyte penetrating, 67
Epithelial medullary carcinoma, 79
Epithelial tumor, 86, 121—122
Epithelioid histiocyte, see also Giant cell, 32
Epithelium, follicular, see Follicular epithelium
Ergot-like drugs, 139—140
Escherichia coli, 8
Etiology
   acute thyroiditis, 8
   infectious thyroiditides, 14—16
   iodide and thyroiditis, 101—102
   palpation thyroiditis, 44
   Riedel's struma, 139—140
   subacute thyroiditis, 23—26
Euthyroid phase, subacute thyroiditis, 26, 30
Exophthalmos, 55
Experimental autoimmune encephalitis, 180
Experimental autoimmune thyroiditis, models, see also Autoimmune thyroiditis, 54—55, 180, 182—185
Experimental models, see Animal models
External radiation, thyroid and, see also Radiation-associated thyroiditis, 110
Extraabdominal desmoid tumor, see also Fibrosarcoma, 139
Extrathyroid conditions, see Nonthyroid conditions

F

Fever, subacute thyroiditis, 28—29
Fibromatosis, see also Fibrosarcoma, 139
Fibrosarcoma
   pathology, 138—139
   Riedel's struma and, 137—139
Fibrosclerosis, invasive, see also Riedel's struma, 135

Fibrosing Hashimoto's thyroiditis, see also Hashimoto's thyroiditis
  antibody, 137, 150
  clinical features, 74, 178
  diagnosis, differential, 75—77, 83
  general discussion, 52, 70—71
  Hurthle cell, 78, 139
  hypothyroidism and, 148
  laboratory findings, 148
  lymphocytic infiltration, 138
  pathology, 66, 71—74, 138—139
  pressure symptoms, goiter size and, 74
  primary myxedema and, 81
  Riedel's struma and, 132, 137—139, 163
  squamous cells, 75—77
  surgery, 74
  thyroid capsule, nonviolation, 75, 139
Fibrosis
  acute thyroiditis, 10, 83
  cretinism, 82
  Grave's disease, 84
  Hashimoto's thyroiditis, see also Fibrosing Hashimoto's thyroiditis, 56, 64, 66, 71, 75—76, 83, 139, 173, 178
    differential diagnosis, 83
  hypothyroidism, 81
  mediastinal, 140—141
  myxedema, 81
  nodular goiter, 83
  palpation thyroiditis, 83
  radiation-associated thyroiditis, 83, 110, 112—113
  radioiodine and, 83
  retriperitoneal, 139—141
  Riedel's struma, 83, 133—136, 140—141, 152, 174
    genetic basis, 140
  spontaneous autoimmune thyroiditis, 179
  subacute thyroiditis, 23, 27—28, 31, 34, 47, 83, 163
  thyroid site of, differential diagnosis, 83
  traumatic thyroiditis, 83
Fibrosis-associated malignancies, 140
Fibrotic zone, central, of healing, subacute thyroiditis, 31
Fibrous atrophy, see also Atrophy, 75
Fibrous proliferation, 75
Fibrous replacement, extensive, myxedema, 81
Fibrous thyroiditis, invasive, see also Riedel's struma, 135
Firmness, lesion, Hashimoto's thyroiditis, 65—66, 71—72
Fluid excretion, cardiovascular, impaired, 82
Fluorescent scanning, see also Scanning, 56, 151—152
Focal lymphoid thyroiditis, 79
Follicles, isolated, palpation thyroiditis, 44—45
Follicular atrophy
  chronic nonspecific thyroiditis, 79
  experimental autoimmune thyroiditis, 184
  Hashimoto's thyroiditis, 64, 66, 68—69, 71, 74—75, 118, 178
  hypothyroidism, 81
  myxedema, 81
  spontaneous autoimmune thyroiditis, 179
Follicular basement membrane deposits, 67, 179
Follicular carcinoma and adenoma, 79, 110, 118—122, 140
  follicular adenoma and carcinoma differentiated, 121—122
  Riedel's struma and, 140
Follicular cell, desquamation of, 48
Follicular destruction
  Hashimoto's thyroiditis, 71, 75—76
  palpation thyroiditis, 44—45
  spontaneous autoimmune thyroiditis, 179
  subacute thyroiditis, 31—32, 166
Follicular epithelium
  eosinophilic change in, 64, 178
  Hashimoto's thyroiditis, 64, 66, 69, 71, 74—77, 85, 178
  Hurthle cell and, 78—79
  hyperplasia of
    cretinism, 82
    experimental autoimmune thyroiditis, 184
    Hashimoto's thyroiditis, 66, 69, 85
  metaplasia of, 71, 74—77
  tangential sectioning of, 48
Follicular-papillary carcinoma, mixed, thyroiditis and, see also Tumor-associated thyroiditis, 118—121
Free radical, 108
Fuchsinophilic material, 67
Function, thyroid, tests of, see also specific tests by name
  acute thyroiditis, 7—8, 148
  Hashimoto thyroiditis, 55—56, 148—149, 153
  methodology, 146—151, 153
  Riedel's struma, 136, 148, 153
  subacute thyroiditis, 29—30, 33, 47, 148, 153
Fungal infection, Riedel's struma, 140
Fungal thyroiditis, 6, 14—18, 32, 34, 46

G

^{67}Gallium, 151
Gammopathy, polyclonal, 139
Gas-forming organisms, 8
Gastrointestinal tract, hypothyroidism and, 82
Gaucher's disease, 50
Genetic basis, fibrosis in Riedel's struma, 140
Genetic damage, radiation, 109
Genetics, subacute thyroiditis, 25
Geographical incidence, see Incidence (geographical)
Germinal center
  Hashimoto's thyroiditis, 64, 68—69, 71, 84—85, 118, 165
  spontaneous autoimmune thyroiditis, 179, 181
  thyroiditides, various, 84
  tumor-thyroiditis, 118—120
Giant cell

anaplastic carcinoma, 138
fibrosarcoma, 138
fibrosing Hashimoto's thyroiditis, 138
Hashimoto's thyroiditis, 66
palpation thyroiditis, 44—45, 47—49
Riedel's struma, 138
subacute thyroiditis, 22—23, 27—29, 31—33, 47, 85, 138, 166
Giant cell thyroiditis, see also Subacute thyroiditis, 22, 172
Globulin, thyroxine-binding, 146—147
Glossitis, 9—10
Goiter, see also specific thyroiditides by name
adenomatous, 75, 79
adolescent lymphocytic, see also Hashimoto's thyroiditis, 52
amyloid, 84
fibrosing Hashimoto's thyroiditis, large, 74
Hashimoto's, 55—58
nodular, see Nodular goiter
painless thyroiditis and, 33
Goiterogen, 113
Gram-negative bacteria, 8
Gram-positive bacteria, 8
Granuloma, in thyroid, 46
Granulomatous reactions, 8, 14, 18, 23, 26—27, 31, 33—34, 66, 136, 163
lack of, Riedel's struma characterized by, 136
subacute thyroiditis, 23, 26—27, 31, 33—34, 132, 137, 163
Granulomatous thyroiditis, see also Infectious thyroiditides, Palpation thyroiditis; subacute thyroiditis, 22, 28, 44—46, 56, 132, 137, 172
Granulomatous vasculitis, necrotizing, 46—47
Graves' disease
antibody, 150
aspiration cytology, 166
fibrosis, 84
general discussion, 2—3
Hashimoto's thryoiditis and, 53—54, 56—57, 68—70, 78, 82, 84—85
iodine and, 101—102
lymphocytic infiltration, 84—85
palpation thyroiditis and, 47
radiation effects on, 112
subacute thyroiditis and, 23, 32—34
thyroid-stimulating globulins, 150
tumor-associated thyroiditis and, 125
Gross pathology, see also Pathology and pathogenesis
anaplastic carcinoma, 138—139
fibrosarcoma, 138—139
fibrosing Hashimoto's thyroiditis, 71—72, 138—139
Hashimoto's thyroiditis, 65—66, 71—72
myxedema, 81
Riedel's struma, 136, 138
subacute thyroiditis, 31, 138
Guinea pig models, experimental autoimmune thyroiditis, 55, 183

H

Hapten, iodide as, 79, 102
Hardness, lesion
Hashimoto's thyroiditis, 65—66
Riedel's struma, 75, 132, 136—137
Hashimoto's thyroiditis, see also Chronic lymphocytic thyroiditis
animal models, 54—55
antibody, 53—58, 66, 70, 74, 137, 149—151
aspiration cytology, 166—167
autoimmune character, 52—58, 68—69, 75, 82—83, 149
cancer and, 57, 65, 71, 75—76, 83, 85
carcinoma and, 55, 57, 66, 71, 75—77, 83, 125—126, 163, 173—174
chronic nonspecific thyroiditis and, 79
classic, 52—58, 66, 70, 74, 77—78, 82—83, 150
clinical features, 55, 74, 125—126, 173—174, 178
course, 57—58, 137
diagnosis, course, prognosis, and treatment, 55, 57—58, 66, 75—77, 82—86, 137
differential diagnosis, 75—77, 82—86, 163, 173—174
experimental autoimmune thyroiditis and, 178—185
fibrosing variant, see Fibrosing Hashimoto's thyroiditis
fibrosis, 56, 64, 66, 71, 75—76, 83, 139, 173, 178
differential diagnosis, 83
firmness, lesion, 65—66, 71—72
follicular involvement, 64, 66, 68—69, 71, 77, 85, 118, 178
form, 65—69
general discussion, 2—3, 52, 58, 64, 178
germinal centers, 64, 68—69, 71, 84—85, 165
Graves' disease and, 53—54, 56—57, 68—70, 78, 82, 84—85
hardness, lesion, 65—66
histology, 58, 64, 178
HLA frequencies, 53
Hurthle cell in, 64, 66—70, 78—79, 85, 118, 165—166
hyperthyroidism and, see also Hashitoxicosis, 55—58, 69—70, 148, 178
hypothyroidism and, 55—58, 74—75, 137, 148—149, 152, 173, 178
incidence, 52—53, 66, 101, 137
iodine and, 101—102
juvenile, 66, 69—70, 78, 150
antibody, 150
laboratory findings, 55—57, 148—153, 163—167
lobular appearance, 65—66, 71—73, 75
pyramidal shape, 65
lymphocytic infiltration, 52, 56, 58, 64, 66, 68—72, 74—76, 84, 163—166, 174, 178
lymphoma and, 57, 76, 86, 122—123, 126, 174, 178

myxedema and, 55—56, 69—70, 75—76, 81, 178
needle biopsy, 163—165, 173—174
nodule, 77, 121
occurrence, 52, 66, 69, 137
painless thyroiditis and, 33—34, 163
pathology and pathogenesis, 53—54, 65—77, 82—84, 178
  classic form, 65—69
patient groups, thyroid function determining, 149
premalignant potential, 85, 125—126
prognosis, 66
Riedel's struma and, 64, 70—71, 75, 132, 135, 137—140, 174
scanning in, 152
subacute thyroiditis and, 23, 32—35, 55—56, 66, 70, 85, 163
surgery in, 58, 173—174
symmetrical enlargement, thyroid, 65
thyroid function tests, 55—56, 148—149, 153
thyroid hormone and, 53, 56—57, 173—174
thyroid-stimulating hormones in, 56—57, 149, 153
treatment, 58, 173—174
tumor-associated thyroiditis and, 77, 83, 85, 118—126, 163
types, table, 66
woodiness, lesion, 65
Hashitoxicosis, 56, 69—70, 85, 148
Heart failure, congestive, 82
Helper activity, lymphocyte, 54—55
Hemochromatosis, 50, 84
Hemorrhage, into thyroid, 9—10, 18, 48—49
Hemosiderin, 48—49
Hereditary spontaneous autoimmune thyroiditis, 179
Heterogeneous lesion groups, chronic nonspecific thyroiditis, 79
Histiocyte, see also Giant cell
  circumferential collection of, palpation thyroiditis, 44—46
  palpation thyroiditis, 44—50
  subacute thyroiditis, 32—34, 47
Histiocytic lymphoma of Rappaport, 86
Histiocytic reaction, hemorrhage in thyroid, 48—49
Histochemistry, Hurthle cell, 78
Histocompatability antigen, see also HLA, antigen, 53, 180, 184
Histology, see also Laboratory findings; Pathology and pathogenesis
  experimental autoimmune thyroiditis, 184
  fibrosarcoma, 139
  Hashimoto's thyroiditis, 58, 64, 178
  infectious thyroiditis, 17
  lithium-induced thyroiditis, 99
  myxedema, 81
  palpation thyroiditis, 44—46
  Riedel's struma, 136—137
  subacute thyroiditis, 31
  tuberculous thyroiditis, 14

Histopathology, see also Laboratory findings; Pathology and pathogenesis
  acute thyroiditis, 8
  Riedel' struma, 136
Histoplasmosis, 140
Historical aspects
  acute thyroiditis, 6
  case histories, see Case histories
  Hashimoto's thyroiditis, 52, 64
  Riedel's struma, 2, 132
  subacute thyroidites, 22
  thyroiditis (general), 2
HLA, antigen
  Aw30, Hashimoto's thyroiditis, 53
  B8, Hashimoto's thyroiditis, 53
  BW35, subacute thyroiditis, 25, 36
  drug-associated thyroiditis, 99, 102
  DRw3, Hashimoto's thyroiditis, 53
Hoarseness, 7, 26, 55, 136, 173—174
Hodgkin's disease, 86, 101
Hormone
  corticosteroid, see Corticosteroid hormone
  steroid, see Steroid hormone
  thyroid, see Thyroid hormone; specific thyroid hormones by name
  thyroid-stimulating, see Thyroid-stimulating hormone
  thyrotropin-releasing, 56
Host-immune reaction, secondary, cancer-associated thyroiditis, 125
Human thyroiditis, correlation with animal experimental models, see also Animal models, 178—179, 185
Humoral immunity, 54, 68, 139, 178, 185
Hurthle cell
  cancer and, 79
  chronic nonspecific thyroiditis, 79
  follicular epithelium and, 78—79
  fibrosing Hashimoto's thyroiditis, 78, 136
  Graves' disease, 84
  Hashimoto's thyroiditis, 64, 66—70, 78—79, 85, 118, 165—166
  hypothyroidism, 81
  mitochondria, numerous, 67, 78
  myxedema, 81
  pathology, 78—79
  radiation-associated thyroiditis, 112
  Riedel's struma, 136
  spontaneous autoimmune thyroiditis, 179, 181
  subacute thyroiditis, 33, 85
  tumor, 79
  tumor-associated thyroiditis, 118, 121
Hypercholesterolemia, 82
Hyperplasia
  C-cell, 47—48
  follicular epithelium, see Follicular epithelium, hyperplasia of
Hypersensitivity
  cell-mediated, 182, 185
  delayed, 181, 183
Hyperthyroidism
  Hashimoto's thyroiditis and, see also

Hashitoxicosis, 55—58, 69—70, 148, 178
iodine-induced, 101—102
laboratory findings, 146—147
palpation thyroiditis and, 47—48
radiation-associated thyroiditis and, 110—111
subacute thyroiditis and, 25—26, 29, 31, 33, 35, 47, 153
transient, 57
Hypertrophied thymus, 65
Hypofunctioning nodule, Hashimoto's thyroiditis, 77
Hypoparathyroidism, 82, 136, 141
Hypothyroidism
acute thyroiditis and, 10
case history, 80—81
clinical grades of, 87
drug-associated thyroiditis and, 98, 101—102
fibrosing Hashimoto's thyroiditis and, 148
fibrosis, 81
Hashimoto's thyroiditis and, 55—58, 74—75, 137, 148—149, 152, 173, 178
infiltrative disorders causing, 84
iodine-induced, 101—102
laboratory findings, 146—148
pathology, 80—82, 84
extrathyroid, 82
palpation thyroiditis and, 47—48
permanent, 74
primary, 82
radiation-associated thyroiditis and, 110—113
radioiodide uptake, 151
radioiodine and, 110—112
mechanism, 111
Riedel's struma and, 136—137, 141, 148—149, 152
Schmidt's syndrome, 82
spontaneous autoimmune thyroiditis and, 179
subacute thyroiditis and, 26, 29—31, 35, 47, 152—153
subclinical, 55—56, 58
Hypothyroiditis, 70, 85

I

Idiopathic myxedema, see Myxedema, primary
Idiosyncratic reactions, to drugs, thyroiditis and, 99—101
Immune complex, 54, 67, 181
Immune system and immune response
autoimmune response, see Autoimmune response
Dilantin® and, 101
experimental autoimmune thyroiditis, 182—185
Hashimoto's thyroiditis and, 52—54, 57—58, 67
iodide and, 79
Riedel's struma and, 139
spontaneous autoimmune thyroiditis, 179—182, 185
suppression of, see Immunosuppression
thyroid cancer and, 125—126

Immunity
antibody-mediated, 184—185
cell-mediated, 54, 58, 68, 139, 178, 182—184
humoral, 54, 68, 139, 178, 185
Immunoamyloid, 84
Immunoblastic lymphadenopathy, 101
Immunoblastic sarcoma, B-cell, 86—88, 101
Immunocompromised patients, 17—18
Immunodeficiencies, congenital, 17
Immunofluorescence
experimental autoimmune thyroiditis, 183
spontaneous autoimmune thyroiditis, 179, 181
thyroid antibody detection, 149—150
Immunoglobulin
concentration, decreased, 17
thyroid-stimulating, 53, 124, 149—150
Immunological aspects, tumor-associated thyroiditis, 123—125
Immunologically mediated vasculitis, see also Vasculitis, 140
Immunologic status, impaired, 14
Immunosuppression, 14—18, 184
Impairment
cellular immunity, 17
immunologic system, 14
interferon production, 17
Incidence (geographical), see also Occurrence (age, sex)
acute thyroiditis, 6
Hashimoto's thyroiditis, 52—53, 66, 101, 137
lymphocytic thyroiditis, increase in, 101
Riedel's struma, 135, 137
subacute thyroiditis, 22—23, 137
tumor-associated thyroiditis, 121
Indomethacin, 35
Infection
cancer patients and, 15
granulomatous, see Granulomatous infection
routes to thyroid, 8
Infectious granulomatous thyroiditis, see also Granulomatous thyroiditis, 46
Infectious thyroiditides, see also specific types by name, 6, 14—19
clinical features
diagnosis, course, prognosis, and treatment
etiology, 14—16
general discussion, 14
laboratory findings
Infiltrates
lymphocytic
anaplastic carcinoma, 138
chronic infiltration, see Chronic lymphocytic thyroiditis; Hashimoto's thyroiditis; Lymphocytic thyroiditis
chronic nonspecific thyroiditis, 79
drug-associated thyroiditis, 99—100, 102
experimental autoimmune thyroiditis, 184
fibrosarcoma, 138
fibrosing Hashimoto's thyroiditis, 138
Graves' disease, 84—85
Hashimoto's thyroiditis, 52, 56, 58, 64, 66, 68—72, 74—76, 84, 163—166, 174, 178

hypothyroidism, 81
iodine and, 102
lymphoma of thyroid, 85—88
myxedema, 81, 85
nodular goiter, 85
radiation-associated thyroiditis, 112
Riedel's struma, 136, 138—139
Schmidt's syndrome, 82
spontaneous autoimmune thyroiditis, 179, 181
subacute thyroiditis, 138
thyroiditides, various, 85
tumor-associated thyroiditis, 118—122
lymphocytic-plasmacytic, thyroid neoplasm, 118
nonlymphocytic, hypothyroidism and, 84
Infiltration, lymphocytic, see Infiltrates, lymphocytic
Interferon production, cancer therapy and, 17
Internal radiation, effects of, 110—113
Invasive fibrosclerosis, see also Riedel's struma, 135
Invasive fibrous thyroiditis, see also Riedel's struma, 135
Involvement, thyroid, Riedel's struma, 75, 140—141
Iodate, 101
Iodide
   dietary, effect of, 101—102, 118
   drug-associated thyroiditis and, 85, 101—102
   lymphocytic infiltration and, 85
   organification defects, 151
   radioiodide, 151—152
   thyroid hormone synthesis and, 146
   water supply (U.S.) containing, effect of, 79
Iodine
   accumulation, lithium interference, 99
   acute thyroiditis and, 8
   butanol-extractable, see Butanol-extractable iodine
   compounds containing, 98, 147
   cretinism and, 102
   dietary, effect of, 101—102, 118
   hapten, role as, 79, 102
   Hashimoto's thyroiditis and, 52—53
   hyperthyroidism induced by, 101—102
   hypothyroidism induced by, 101—102
   protein-bound, see Protein-bound iodine
   radioiodine, see Radioiodine
   thyroid hormone and, 101, 146
   thyroiditis unmasked by, 101—102
^{123}Iodine, 151
^{125}Iodine, 110, 151
^{131}Iodine, 110, 112—113, 151, 153
Iodized salt, 101
Iodoprotein, 146—149
Isolated follicles, palpation thyroiditis, 44—45
Isthmusectomy, 174

J

Juvenile lymphocytic thyroiditis, see Hashimoto's thyroiditis, juvenile

K

Keratinizing squamous cell, 75
Killer lymphocyte, see K-Lymphocyte
Klebsiella sp., 8

L

Laboratory findings, see also Diagnosis; Differential diagnosis; Histology; Histopathology; Pathology and pathogenesis
   acute thyroiditis, 7—8, 148, 150, 152—153, 163, 166
   fibrosing Hashimoto's thyroiditis, 148
   Hashimoto's thyroiditis, 55—57, 148—153, 163—167
   hyperthyroidism, 146—147
   hypothyroidism, 146—148
   infectious thyroiditides, 17
   methods, 146—154, 162—167
      aspiration cytology, see Aspiration cytology
      general discussion, 146
      needle biopsy, see Needle biopsy
      nuclear medicine, 151—152
      other techniques, 154
      thyroid function tests, 146—151, 153
      ultrasound, 152—154
   palpation thyroiditis, 44—46
   Riedel's struma, 136—137, 148—149, 151—153, 163, 166
   subacute thyroiditis, 29—31, 148—150, 152—153, 163, 166
Lactotroph, 82
Laryngospasm, 140—141
LATS, see Long-acting thyroid stimulator
Levothyroxine, 57—58
Lipofuscin, 50, 102
Lipoprotein, microsomal, 53
Lithium, 85, 98—100
Lobectomy, 10, 18, 27, 137, 172, 174
Lobular appearance, Hashimoto's thyroiditis, 65—66, 71—73, 75
   pyramidal shape, 65
Long-acting thyroid stimulator, 123—124, 149—150
Lymphadenopathy, immunoblastic 101
Lymphocyte
   epithelial cell penetrated by, 67
   helper activity, 54—55
   immunity, impaired, 17
   infiltration, see Infiltrates, lymphocytic
   killer activity, 54—55
   stimulation by tumor extract, 125
   suppressor activity, 54—55, 101
   thyroid, activity, 84—88, 118
   thyroiditis and, see Lymphocytic thyroiditis

B-Lymphocyte, activity, see also B-Cell, 54—55, 178
K-Lymphocyte, activity, 54—55
T-Lymphocyte, activity, see also T-Cell, 54—55, 178
Lymphocytic infiltration, see Infiltrate, lymphocytic
Lymphocytic thyroiditis
　chronic, see Hashimoto's thyroiditis
　drug-related, see also Drug-associated thyroiditis, 79, 99—102
　Hashimoto's see Hashimoto's thyroiditis
　incidence, increase in, 101
　juvenile, see Hashimoto's thyroiditis, juvenile
　lymphocytic infiltration, 84—88
　nonspecific, 85
　tumor-associated, see Tumor-associated thyroiditis
Lymphocytosis, 99
Lymphography, neoplasm differentiation, 154
Lymphoid thyroiditis, focal, 79
Lymphoma, 15, 17, 34, 57, 76, 85—88, 122—124, 163, 174
　Hashimoto's thyroiditis and, 57, 76, 86, 122—123, 126, 163, 174, 178
　malignant, 76, 85—86, 122—124, 140, 163, 174, 178
　occurrence, 85—86, 122
　primary, 85—88, 122
　systemic, 85
　varieties recorded, 86

M

Macrophage, see also Giant cell, 32, 48, 76, 166, 183—184
Macrophage dependence reaction test, cell-mediated immunity, 184
Macrophage inhibitory factor, 183
Malignancies, see also specific malignancies by name, 78—79, 110, 113, 122—124, 136, 139—140
Malignant lymphoma, see Lymphoma, malignant
Malignant pseudothyroiditis, 83
Mass, thyroid
　acute thyroiditis, 10
　dominant, painless thyroiditis and, 33
　Hashimoto's thyroiditis, 173—174
　tuberculous thyroiditis, 18
MDR, see Macrophage dependence reaction
Mediastinal fibrosis, 140—141
Medullary carcinoma, 79, 84, 121
Metaplasia
　follicular epithelium, 71, 74—77
　oxyphil, 66
　squamous, 71, 74—75, 81, 138—139
Metastases, to thyroid, 84
Metastatic carcinoma, 86
MGI virus, 25
Mice, see Mouse models
Microabscess, 8—9, 15, 31

Microscopic features
　anaplastic carcinoma, 138—139
　fibrosarcoma, 138
　fibrosin Hashimoto's thyroiditis, 71—74, 138—139
　Hashimoto's thyroiditis, 66—69, 71—74
　Hurthle cell, 78
　myxedema, 81
　Riedel's struma, 133—135, 138
　subacute thyroiditis, 31, 138
　tuberculous thyroiditis, 18
Microsomal antibody, 56—57, 66
Microsomal antigen, 182
Microsomal lipoprotein, 53
MIF, see Macrophage inhibitory factor
Migrating thyroiditis, see also Subacute thyroiditis, 22
Minocycline, 102
Mitochondria, Hurthle cell, 67, 78
Mitosis, 138—139
Mixed papillary-follicular carcinoma, 118—121
Monkey models
　experimental autoimmune thyroiditis, 184—185
　spontaneous autoimmune thyroiditis, 182
Mouse models
　experimental autoimmune thyroiditis, 183—184
　spontaneous autoimmune thyroiditis, 181
Mucopolysaccharide, 82
Multifocal granulomatous folliculitis, see Palpation thyroiditis
Multinucleate, follicular epithelial cell, see also Giant cell, 32
Multinucleation, cell, 109
Mycobacteria, 8, 14, 18, 23
Myocardial infarct, premature, 82
Myxedema
　fibrosis, 81
　Hashimoto's thyroiditis and, 55—56, 69—70, 75—76, 81, 178
　lymphocytic infiltration, 81, 85
　primary, 75—76, 81, 83, 112, 178
　radiation-associated thyroiditis and, 112
　Riedel's struma and, 136
　secondary, 75, 81
　subacute thyroiditis and, 34
　thyrotropes in, 82

N

Neck pain, see also Pain
　acute thyroiditis, 6—7, 10
　Hashimoto's thyroiditis, 55, 173
　infectious thyroiditis, 17
　Riedel's struma, 174
　subacute thyroiditis, 22, 26—27, 34, 47
Necrotizing granulomatous vasculitis, see also Vasculitis, 46—47
Needle biopsy
　acute thyroiditis, 9, 163, 172
　general discussion, 162, 166
　Hashimoto's thyroiditis, 56, 77, 163—165,

173—174
  infectious thyroiditis, 17—18
  results, 163—165
  Riedel's struma, 137, 163
  subacute thyroiditis, 23, 33—34, 163, 172
  team approach, 166—167
  techniques, 162—163
  ultrasound techniques and, 154
Neonatal thymectomy, 181
Neoplasm, 17, 77, 79, 83, 109—110, 113, 118—121, 132, 154, 172, 174
  differentiation techniques, 154
  periphery, lymphocytic-plasmacytic infiltrates, 118
  radiation-induced, 109—110, 113
  thyroiditis associated with, see also Tumor-associated thyroiditis, 118—121
Neutropenia, 99
Nodular goiter, 6, 8, 33—34, 46, 49, 77—79, 83, 85, 98—100, 121, 172
  fibrosis, 83
  Hashimoto's thyroiditis and, 77, 121
  lithium-induced, case history, 98—100
  lymphocytic infiltration, 85
Nonspecific thyroiditis
  chronic, 64, 79, 118
  lymphocytic, 85
Nonsuppurative thyroiditis, see also Subacute thyroiditis, 22
Nonthyroid conditions
  hypothyroidism, pathology of, 82
  Riedel's struma and, 141
  subacute thyroiditis, 35
Nontoxic disease, painless, 33
Nonviolation, thyroid capsule, by fibrosing Hashimoto's thyroiditis, 75
Noxious stimuli thyroid response to, see also Palpation thyroiditis, 50
Nuclear antigen, 53
Nuclear medicine, thyroiditis diagnosis by, 151—152
Nucleomegaly, 112

O

Obese strain, white leghorn chicken, studies of, autoimmune thyroiditis 54—55, 179—180
Occlusive phlebitis, see also Phlebitis, 140
Occult thyroiditis, 102
Occurence (age, sex), see also Incidence (geographical)
  acute thyroiditis, 6
  anaplastic carcinoma, 75, 139
  focal lymphoid thyroiditis, 79
  Hashimoto's thyroiditis, 52, 66, 69, 137
  Hashitoxicosis, 69
  lymphoma, 85—86, 122
  Riedel's struma, 135, 137
  subacute thyroiditis, 23, 137
  thyroid cancer, 108, 110
  thyroid function abnormalities, 79

tumor-associated thyroiditis, 118, 122
Oncocyte, see also Hurthle cell, 67, 75, 78, 139
Open biopsy, 162
Organisms, thyroiditis-producing
  acute thyroiditis, 8, 10
  Riedel's struma, 139
  subacute thyroiditis 23
  unusual, see Unusual organisms
OS, see Obese strain, white leghorn chicken
Outcome, see Course; Prognosis
Ovarian failure, Hashimoto's thyroiditis and, 82
Oxyphil, see also Hurthle cell, 66—71, 138, 167
  Hashimoto's thyroiditis, see Hashimoto's thyroiditis classic
  metaplasia of, 66

P

Pain, see also neck pain, 10, 27, 173
Painless nontoxic disease, 33
Painless thyroiditis, 22—23, 27, 33—34, 56—57, 69—70, 163
  Hashimoto's thyroiditis and, 33—34, 163
  subacute variety, 33—34, 56, 70
Painless thyrotoxic thyroiditis, 33
Palpation thyroiditis
  description, 44
  differential diagnosis and prognosis, 44—50
  fibrosis, 83
  general discussion, 2—3, 44, 50
  histology, 44—46
  pathogenesis, 50
  significance, 50
  subacute thyroiditis and, 24, 32—34, 44, 46—48, 50
  tuberculous thyroiditis and, 18
Papillary carcinoma and other papillary tumors, 44, 46, 76, 79, 85, 110, 113, 118—121, 125—126, 163
  thyroiditis and, see Tumor-associated thyroiditis
Parafollicular cell, 75, 77
Pathogenesis, see Pathology and pathogenesis
Pathology and pathogenesis, see also Histology; Histopathology; Laboratory findings
  acute thyroiditis, 8—9
  anaplastic carcinoma, 138—139
  chronic thyroiditis, 64—88
  cretinism, 82
  experimental autoimmune thyroiditis, 183
  extrathyroid, hypothyroidism, 82
  fibrosarcoma, 138—139
  fibrosing Hashimoto's thyroiditis, 66, 71—74, 138—139
  gross, see Gross pathology
  Hashimoto's thyroiditis, 53—54, 65—77, 82—84, 178
    classic form, 65—69
  hypothyroidism, 80—82, 84
    extrathyroid, 82
  infectious thyroiditides, 18

microscopic, see Microscopic features
myxedema, 81
palpation thyroiditis, 50
radiation-associated thyroiditis, 111—112
retroperitoneal fibrosis, 139—141
Riedel's struma, 136—140
spontaneous autoimmune thyroiditis, 179—181
subacute thyroiditis, 24, 26, 31—34, 138
tumor-associated thyroiditis, 118—120, 123—125
Pathophysiology
subacute thyroiditis, 26
tumor-associated thyroiditis, 123—125
PBI, see Protein-bound iodine
Penicillin, 10
Perchlorate discharge test, 56, 151—152
Perithyroidal vessel wall, degeneration of, 134
Peritumor thyroiditis, see Tumor-associated thyroiditis
Permanent hypothyroidism, see also Hypothyroidism
Phagocytosis, 16, 32, 48—49
Phenylbutazone, 35
Phlebitis, 136, 140
occlusive, 140
Physical findings, see also Clinical features
acute thyroiditis, 7
Riedel's struma, 136
subacute thyroiditis, 29
Pituitary changes, myxedema, 82
Plasmacytoid tumor cell characteristics, 86
Pleomorphism, cellular, 75—76, 138—139
Pneumococcus sp., 8, 172
Polyclonal gammopathy, 139
Postpartum period, Hashimoto's thyroiditis in, 57
Prealbumin, thyroxine-binding, 146
Premalignant potential, Hashimoto's thyroiditis, 85, 125—126
Prednisone, 98
Pressure symptoms, 136, 173
Primary hypothyroidism, see also Hypothyroidism, 82
Primary lymphoma, see also Lymphoma, 85—88, 122
Primary myxedema, see Myxedema, primary
Prognosis, see also Course
acute thyroiditis, 10
Hashimoto's thyroiditis, 66
infectious thyroiditides, 18
lymphoma, thyroid, 86
palpation thyroiditis, 50
Riedel's struma, 141
subacute thyroitidis, 35
Prohormone, 84
Prolactin, 82
Protein binding, competitive, thyroid hormone measurement, 147
Protein-bound iodine, test
acute thyroiditis, 7—8, 148
experimental autoimmune thyothyroiditis, 184
fibrosing Hashimoto's thyroiditis, 148
Hashimoto's thyroiditis, 56, 85, 148
hyperthyroidism, 146
hypothyroidism, 146
infectious thyroiditis, 17
methodology, 146—147, 153
subacute thyroiditis, 27, 29—30, 34, 85
thyroid hormone measurement, 147
Pseudolymphoma, 101
Pseudothyroiditis, malignant, 83
Pseudotuberculosis thyroiditis, see also Subacute thyroiditis, 22
Pus, acute thyroiditis, 9, 172
Pyramida shape, lobe, Hashimoto's thyroiditis, 65

R

Rabbit models, experimental autoimmune thyroiditis, 182—183
Radiation
effects of, 108—110, 112—113
carcinoma and, 108—110, 151
external, 110, 112—113
general aspects, 108—109
internal, 110—113
therapy
cancer, 15—17, 78, 108, 110, 112
radiation-associated thyroiditis and, 108—113
subacute thyroiditis, 35
Radiation-associated thyroiditis, 108—113
clinical features, 111
fibrosis, 83
general discussion, 108, 113
pathology, 111—112
radiation, effects of, 108—110
radioiodine, thyroid and, 110
thyroid, radiation and, 110, 112—113
animal models, 112—113
Radical, free, 108
Radioimmunoassay
Hashimoto's thyroiditis, 56—57
thyroid hormone measurement, 147, 151
thyroid-stimulating hormone measurement, 148
Radioiodide, 151—152
Radioiodine techniques
acute thyroiditis, 8
fibrosis and, 83
Hashimoto's thyroiditis, 56, 58, 70, 85
infectious thyroiditis, 17
radiation-associated thyroiditis, 110
subacute thyroiditis, 23, 26—27, 29—31, 33—34, 85
therapy, hypothyroidism and, 110—113
Radionuclide scanning, see also Scanning, 151, 153
Radiosensitivity, cell, 109
Rappaport's lymphoma, 86
Rat models
experimental autoimmune thyroiditis, 184

spontaneous autoimmune thyroiditis, 54, 180—181
Recovery, see Course; Prognosis
Renal tubular defects, 82
Replacement, tumoral, 84
Resin triiodothyronine uptake, test
   acute thyroiditis, 153
   fibrosing Hashimoto's thyroiditis, 153
   Hashimoto's thyroiditis, 56, 153
   Riedel's struma, 153
   subacute thyroiditis, 153
   thyroxine measurement, 147
Resolution phase, subacute thyroiditis, 26, 30
Reticulum cell sarcoma, see also Immunoblastic sarcoma, 86, 101
Retriperitoneal fibrosis, 139—141
Riedel's struma
   acute thyroiditis and, 174
   adenoma characterizing, 136, 138, 140
   adherent tissue, 75, 136
   antibodies in, 136—137, 151
   aspiration cytology, 166
   carcinoma and, 136—140, 163
   case history, 132—135
   clinical features, 132, 135—137, 174
   diagnosis, course, prognosis, and treatment, 132, 136—141, 174
     differential diagnosis, 132, 136—140, 174
   etiology, 139—140
   fibrosarcoma and, 137—139
   fibrosing Hashimoto's thyroiditis and, 132, 137—139, 163
   fibrosis, 83, 133—136, 140—141, 152, 174
     genetic basis, 140
   general discussion, 2—3, 132, 141
   giant cell in, 138
   hardness, lesion, 75, 132, 136—137
   Hashimoto's thyroiditis and, 64, 70—71, 75, 132, 135, 137—140, 174
   Hurthle cell, 136
   hypothyroidism and, 136—137, 141, 148—149, 152
   incidence, 135, 137
   laboratory findings, 136—137, 148—149, 151—153, 163, 166
   lymphocytic infiltration, 136, 138—139
   myxedema and, 136
   needle biopsy, 137, 163
   occurrence, 135, 137
   pathology and pathogenesis, 136—140
   physical findings, 136
   recurrence rate, 141
   scanning in, 152
   subacute thyroiditis and, 23, 35, 137—138, 140—141
   surgery in, 141, 174—175
   thyroid function tests, 136, 148, 153
   thyroid involvement, 75, 140—141
   thyroid-stimulating hormones in, 149, 153
   treatment, 141, 174—175
   woodiness, lesion, 75, 136
RTU, see Resin triiodothyronine uptake

S

Salicylates, 36, 98
Salmonella sp., 8
Salt, iodized, 101
Sarcoidosis, 18, 34, 46, 48—50
Sarcoma, see also specific types by name, 86—88, 101, 109
SAT, see Spontaneous autoimmune thyroiditis
Scanning, 56, 151—153
   acute thyroiditis, 152
   fluorescent, 56, 151—152
   Hashimoto's thyroiditis, 152
   radionuclide, 151, 153
   Riedel's struma, 152
   subacute thyroiditis, 152
Schmidt's syndrome, 82
Sclerosing cholangitis, 141
Secondary host-immune reaction, cancer-associated thyroiditis, 125
Secondary myxedema, see also Myxedema, 75, 81
Second colloid antigen, 53, 149, 182
^{75}Selenomethionine, 151
Self-limited nature, subacute thyroiditis, 22, 36
Sepsis, 6—7, 14
Septicemia, 10
Serratia sp., 15
Sex, effect of, see Occurrence (age, sex)
Signs, see Clinical features
Silent subacute thyroiditis, see also Painless thyroiditis, 27
Skin testing, spontaneous autoimmune thyroiditis, 181—182
Smear test, infectious thyroiditis, 17
Sore throat, subacute thyroiditis, 27—28, 34
Spontaneous autoimmune thyroiditis, models, see also Autoimmune thyroiditis, 54—55, 179—182
Squamous carcinoma, 75, 77
Squamous cell, in thyroid, 75—77
Squamous metoplasia, 71, 74—75, 81, 138—139
Stages, see Course
Staphylococcus sp., 8, 172
Steroid hormone, see also Corticosteroid hormone, 15, 36, 98, 111, 147
Storage disease, 46, 50, 84
Streptococcus sp., 8, 172
Stridor, 136, 173—174
Stroma, 138
Structure, see Microscopic features; Ultrastructure
Struma granulomatosa, see also Subacute thyroiditis, 22
Struma lymphomatosa see also Hashimoto's thyroiditis, 2, 52
Strumatitis, see Thyroiditis
Strumitis, acute, 6
Subacute thyroiditis
   acute thyroiditis and, 6, 9, 22, 27, 34
   anamnestic response to inflammation, 25, 150
   antibody, 150

aspiration cytology, 166
carcinoma and, 172—173
case history, 26—29
clinical features, 23, 27—29, 34
diagnosis, course, prognosis, and treatment, 23, 26, 34—35, 137
   euthyroid or transition phase, 26, 30
   hypothyroid phase, 26, 30
   resolution phase, 26, 30
   thyrotoxic phase, 26, 29—30
diseases associated with, 35
etiology, 23—26
fibrosis, 23, 27—28, 31, 34, 47, 83, 163
follicular involvement, 31—32, 166
general discussion, 2—3, 22—23, 36
giant cell in, 22—23, 27—29, 31—33, 47, 85, 138, 166
granulomatous reactions, 23, 26—27, 31, 33—34, 132, 137, 163
Hashimoto's thyroiditis and, 23, 32—36, 55—56, 66, 70, 85, 163
Hurthle cell in, 33, 85
hyperthyroidism and, 25—26, 29, 31, 33, 35, 47, 153
hypothyroidism and, 26, 29—31, 35, 47, 152—153
incidence, 22—23, 137
infectious thyroiditis and, 14, 17—18
laboratory findings, 29—31, 148—150, 152—153, 163, 166
lymphocytic infiltration, 138
needle biopsy, 23, 33—34, 163
occurrence, 23, 137
painless, see also Painless thyroiditis, 33—34, 56, 70
palpation thyroiditis and, 24, 32—34, 44, 46—48, 50
pathology, 24, 26, 31—34, 138
radiation associated thyroiditis and, 111, 113
Riedel's struma and, 23, 35, 137—138, 140—141
scanning in, 152
self-limited nature, 22, 36
surgery in, 35, 172—173
thyroid antibodies in, 150
thyroid function tests, 29—30, 33, 37, 148, 153
thyroid-stimulating hormones in, 24, 29—30, 148—149, 153
treatment, 34—35, 172—173
tumor-associated thyroiditis and, 125
viral causation, 8, 24—26, 32, 36, 47, 50
Subclinical hypothyroidism, see Hypothyroidism, subclinical
Sulfonamide, 98
Sulfonylurea, 98
Suppurative thyroiditis, acute, 6, 8, 10, 17, 172
Suppression, immune system, see Immunosuppression
Suppressor activity, lymphocyte 54—55, 101
Suppurative thyroiditis, 6, 8, 10, 17
Surgical management, see also specific techniques by name

acute thyroiditis, 10, 172
biopsy, 162
fibrosing Hashimoto's thyroiditis, 74
general discussion, 172, 175
Hashimoto's thyroiditis, 58, 173—174
infectious thyroiditis, 17—18
methodology, 162, 172—175
Riedel's struma, 141, 174—175
subacute thyroiditis, 35, 172—173
Symmetrical enlargement, thyroid, Hashimoto's thyroiditis
Symptoms, see clinical features; specific symptoms by name
Synthesis, thyroid hormone, 146, 148
Systemic lymphoma, see also Lymphoma, 85

T

T_3, see Triiodothyronine
T_4, see Thyroxine
Tangential sectioning, follicular epithelium, 48
Tanned red cell agglutination test, thyroid antibody detection, 149—150
TBG, see Thyroxin-binding globulin
TBPA, see Thyroxin-binding prealbumin
TCF, see Thyroid cytotoxic factor
Team approach, asperation cytology and needle biopsy, 166—167
^{99}Technetium, 151
Teratoma, 75
Tests, see also Animal models; Laboratory findings; specific tests by name, 146—154
Tetracycline, 10
Therapy, see Treatment
Thermography, neoplasm differentiation, 154
Thiazide, 98
Thymectomy, 180—181, 183
Thymic remnants, 75, 77
Thymus, hypertrophied, 65
Thymus-dependent suppressor function, 180
Thyroglobulin, 30—31, 53—57, 66, 74, 78, 125, 146, 150—151, 178—180, 182—185
   antithyroglobulin antibody, see Antithyroglobulin antibody
   experimental autoimmune thyroiditi 182—185
   spontaneous autoimmune thyroiditis, 179—180, 182, 185
   thyroid hormone release and, 146
Thyroglossal cyst, 9—10, 18
Thyroglossal duct, epidermoid cells from, 75, 77
Thyroid antibody, see Antibody
Thyroid cytotoxic factor, 183
Thyroidectomy, 173—175
Thyroid extract, 179, 181, 183—184
Thyroid gland
   black, minocycline-induced, 102
   capsule, see Capsule, thyroid
   conditions, thyroiditis associated with
      Riedel's struma, 140
      subacute thyroiditis, 35

discovery of, 2
fibrosis in, differential diagnosis, 83
function, tests of, see Function; specific tests
    by name
granulomas in, see also Granulomatous
    reactions, 46
hemorrhage into, 9—10, 18, 48—49
Hurthle cells in, 78—79
infection, routes of, 8
infiltration of, see Infiltrates, thyroid
involvement, Riedel's struma, 75, 140—141
lymphocytes in, see also Infiltrates,
    lymphocytic, 84—88
mass, see Mass, thyroid
metastases to, 84
noxious stimuli, response to, see also Palpation
    thyroiditis. 50
pain, subacute thyroiditis identified by, see also
    Neck pain; Pain, 27
radiation in, see also Radiation-associated
    thyroiditis, 110, 112—113
    animal models, 112—113
radioiodine and, see also Radioiodine, 110
squamous cells in, 75—77
symmetrical enlargement, Hashimoto's
    thyroiditis, 65
tuberculosis, immunity, 14
tumors of, see Tumor, thyroid; Tumor-
    associated thyroiditis; specific tumors by
    name or type
Thyroid hormone, see also specific hormones by
    name
  acute thyroiditis, 8
  cretinism, 82
  Hashimoto's thyroiditis, 53, 56—57, 173—174
  iodine inhibition of, 101
  measurement of, 146—147, 151
  protein binding, 146
  radiation-associated thyroiditis, 110
  spontaneous autoimmune thyroiditis, 179
  subacute thyroiditis, 24, 26, 29—30, 34—35,
      149
  synthesis, 146, 148
Thyroiditides, see also specific types by name
  infectious, see Infectious thyroiditides
  lymphocytic infiltration, Thyroiditis, see also
      specific types and topics by name
  classification of, 3
  descriptions of, classical, 2
  history, see Historical aspects
  problems in understanding, 2
Thyroid-specific autoantibody, see Autoantibody
Thyroid-stimulating hormone
  Hashimoto's thyroiditis, 56—57, 149
  hypothyroidism, 148
  laboratory diagnostic procedures, 146,
      148—149, 153
  lithium effect on, 99
  radiation effects on, 110—111
  spontaneous autoimmune thyroiditis, 179
  subacute thyroiditis, 24, 29—30, 148—149
  synthesis, 146

Thyroid-stimulating hormone-induced thyroiditis,
    121
Thyroid-stimulating immunoglobulin, 53, 124,
    149—150
Thyroid stimulator, long-acting, 123—124,
    149—150
Thyrotoxicosis, 7, 55, 57—58
  transient, 57
Thyrotoxic phase, subacute thyroiditis, 26,
    29—30
Thyrotoxic thyroiditis, painless, see also Painless
    thyroiditis, 33
Thyrotroph, 82
Thyrotropin, 24, 29, 34—35, 111, 113
Thyrotropin-releasing hormone, 56, 148—149
Thyroxine
  acute thyroiditis 7—8, 148
  antibody to, 150
  diphenylhydantoin and, 99
  fibrosing Hashimoto's thyroiditis, 148
  Hashimoto's thyroiditis, 56, 78, 148
  hyperthyroidism, 147
  hypothyroidism, 82, 147
  infectious thyroiditis, 17
  measurement of, 146—147, 153
  protein binding, 146
  subacute thyroiditis, 29—30, 34, 48
  synthesis, 146
Thyroxine-binding albumin, 146
Thyroxine-binding globulin, 146—147
Thyroxine-binding prealbumin, 146
Tracheal compression, 141, 174
Transient hyperthyroidism, 57
Transient thyrotoxicosis, 57
Transition phase, subacute thyroiditis, 26, 30
Transplantation, organs, thyroiditis and, 15, 17
Traumatic thyroiditis, see also Palpation
    thyroiditis, 6, 32, 44, 50, 83
Treatment
  acute thyroiditis, 10, 172
  cancer, thyroiditis and, 15—17, 78
  Hashimoto's thyroiditis, 58, 173—174
  infectious thyroiditides, 18—19
  radiation therapy, see Radiation, therapy
  radioiodine, hypothyroidism and, 110—112
  Riedel's struma, 141, 174—175
  subacute thyroiditis, 34—35, 172—173
  surgical, see Surgical management
Treponema sp., 14
TRH, see Thyrotropin-releasing hormone
Triiodothyronine
  acute thyroiditis, 7—8, 148
  antibody to, 150
  fibrosing Hashimoto's thyroiditis, 148
  Hashimoto's thyroiditis 56, 148
  hyperthyroidism, 147
  infectious thyroiditis, 17
  measurement of, 146—147, 153
  protein binding, 146
  resin triiodothyronine uptake, see Resin
      triiodothyronine uptake
  subacute thyroiditis, 29—30, 33—35, 148

synthesis, 146
toxicosis, 147
TSI$_g$, see Thyroid-stimulating immunoglobulin
Tuberculosis thyroiditis, 14, 18, 32, 34, 46
Tumor, thyroid, see also specific tumors by name or type
    cell dissemination, aspiration cytology, 162, 164, 166
    diagnosis aspiration cytology, 162, 166—167
    Hurthle cell, 79
    lymphocytic infiltration, 85
    radiation-produced, 108—110, 112—113
    replacement, 84
    subacute thyroiditis and, 29, 34
    thyroiditis associated with, see Tumor-associated thyroidits
    types involved in thyroiditis, 79, 118—124
Tumor-associated thyroiditis
    autoimmune response, 125—126
    clinical correlations, 125—126
    diagnosis, 125
    general discussion, 118, 126
    Graves' disease and, 125
    Hashimoto's thyroiditis and, 77, 83, 85, 118—126, 163
    Hurthle cells, 118, 121
    immunologic aspects, 123—125
    incidence, 121
    lymphocytic infiltration, 118—122
    occurrence, 118, 122
    pathology, 118—120, 123—125
    subacute thyroiditis and, 125
    tumor types involved, see also specific tumors by name or type, 79, 118—124
Tumor extract, lymphocyte stimulation by, 125

U

Ultimobranchial body, 75, 77
Ultrasonography, see Ultrasound techniques
Ultrasound techniques, thyroiditis diagnosis
    acute thyroiditis, 9
    methodology, 152—154
Ultrastructure
    anaplastic carcinoma, 139
    Hashimoto's thyroiditis, 66—68
    Hurthle cell, 78
    myxedema, 81
    spontaneous autoimmune thyroiditis, 179
    subacute thyroiditis, 32—33
Unmasking, thyroiditis, iodine and, 101—102
Unusual organisms, thyroiditis-producing
    acute thyroiditis, 10
    infectious thyroiditides, 14

V

Vacuolization, cell, 109, 113
Vasculites, 46—47, 138—140
    immunologically mediated, 140
    necrotizing granulomatous, 46—47
Vinblastine, 78
Viral causation, subacute thyroiditis, 8, 24—26, 32, 36, 47, 50
Virus-like particles, Hashimoto's and spontaneous autoimmune thyroiditis, 68, 179
Vocal cord paralysis, 136

W

Water supply, U.S. iodide in, 79
White leghorn chicken, see Obese strain, white leghorn chicken
Woodiness, lesion
    Hashimoto's thyroiditis, 65
    Riedel's struma, 75, 136

X

X-ray, fluorescent, see Fluorescent scanning

Y

Yersinia sp., 54

NO LONGER THE PROPERTY
OF THE
UNIVERSITY OF R.I. LIBRARY